a LANGE medical book

CURRENT
Practice Guidelines
In Primary Care
2013

Joseph S. Esherick, MD, FAAFP
Medical Director of Critical Care Services
Associate Director of Medicine
Ventura County Medical Center
Associate Clinical Professor of Family Medicine
David Geffen School of Medicine
Los Angeles, California

Daniel S. Clark, MD, FACC, FAHA
Director of Medicine and Cardiology
Ventura County Medical Center
Assistant Clinical Professor of Family Medicine
David Geffen School of Medicine
Los Angeles, California

Evan D. Slater, MD
Director, Hematology and Medical Oncology
Ventura County Medical Center
Assistant Clinical Professor of Medicine
David Geffen School of Medicine
Los Angeles, California

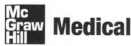 **Medical**

New York   Chicago   San Francisco   Lisbon   London
Madrid   Mexico City   Milan   New Delhi   San Juan   Seoul
Singapore   Sydney   Toronto

CURRENT Practice Guidelines in Primary Care, 2013

Copyright © 2013 by The McGraw-Hill Companies, Inc. Copyright © 2000 through 2009 by The McGraw-Hill Companies, Inc. All rights reserved. Printed in the United States of America. Except as permitted under the United States Copyright Act of 1976, no part of this publication may be reproduced or distributed in any form or by any means, or stored in a data base or retrieval system, without the prior written permission of the publisher.

1 2 3 4 5 6 7 8 9 0 DOC/DOC 17 16 15 14 13 12

ISBN 978-0-07-179750-4
MHID 0-07-179750-5
ISSN 1528-1612

Notice

Medicine is an ever-changing science. As new research and clinical experience broaden our knowledge, changes in treatment and drug therapy are required. The authors and the publisher of this work have checked with sources believed to be reliable in their efforts to provide information that is complete and generally in accord with the standards accepted at the time of publication. However, in view of the possibility of human error or changes in medical sciences, neither the authors nor the publisher nor any other party who has been involved in the preparation or publication of this work warrants that the information contained herein is in every respect accurate or complete, and they disclaim all responsibility for any errors or omissions or for the results obtained from use of the information contained in this work. Readers are encouraged to confirm the information contained herein with other sources. For example and in particular, readers are advised to check the product information sheet included in the package of each drug they plan to administer to be certain that the information contained in this work is accurate and that changes have not been made in the recommended dose or in the contraindications for administration. This recommendation is of particular importance in connection with new or infrequently used drugs.

This book was set in Times Roman by Cenveo Publisher Services.
The editor was Christine Diedrich.
The production supervisor was Jeffrey Herzich.
Project management was provided by Cenveo Publisher Services.
RR Donnelley was printer and binder.

This book is printed on acid-free paper.

McGraw-Hill books are available at special quantity discounts to use as premiums and sales promotions, or for use in corporate training programs. To contact a representative please e-mail us at bulksales@mcgraw-hill.com.

This book is dedicated to all of our current and former residents at the Ventura County Medical Center.

Contents

√ denotes major 2013 updates.
+ denotes new topic for 2013.

√ denotes major 2013 updates.
+ denotes new topic for 2013.

2. DISEASE PREVENTION

√ denotes major 2013 updates.
+ denotes new topic for 2013.

3. DISEASE MANAGEMENT

√ denotes major 2013 updates.
+ denotes new topic for 2013.

√ denotes major 2013 updates.
+ denotes new topic for 2013.

√ denotes major 2013 updates.
+ denotes new topic for 2013.

4.   APPENDICES

Preface

Current Practice Guidelines in Primary Care, 2013 is intended for all clinicians interested in updated, evidence-based guidelines for primary care topics. This pocket-sized reference consolidates information from nationally recognized medical associations and government agencies into concise recommendations and guidelines of virtually all ambulatory care topics. This book is organized into topics related to disease screening, disease prevention, and disease management for quick reference to the evaluation and treatment of the most common primary care disorders.

The 2013 edition of *Current Practice Guidelines in Primary Care* contains thirty three new chapters and updates many other primary care topics. It is a great resource for residents, medical students, midlevel providers, and practicing physicians in family medicine, internal medicine, pediatrics, and obstetrics and gynecology.

Although painstaking efforts have been made to find all errors and omissions, some errors may remain. If you find and error or wish to make a suggestion, please email us at pbg.ecommerce_custserv@mcgraw-hill.com.

Joseph Esherick, MD, FAAFP
Daniel S. Clark, MD, FACC, FAHA
Evan Slater, MD

1
Disease Screening

Disease Screening	Organization	Date	Population	Recommendations	Comments	Source
Abdominal Aortic Aneurysm (AAA)	USPSTF ACC/AHA Canadian Society for Vascular Surgery	2005 2006	Men aged 65–75 years who have ever smoked	One-time screening for AAA by ultrasonography. No recommendation for or against screening for AAA in men aged 65–75 years who have never smoked.	1. Cochrane review (2007): Significant decrease in AAA-specific mortality in men but not for women. (OR, 0.60, 95% CI 0.47–0.99) but not for women. (*Cochrane Database Syst Rev.* 2007;2:CD002945; http://www. thecochranelibrary.com) 2. Early mortality benefit of screening (men aged 65–74 years) maintained at 7-year follow-up. Cost-effectiveness of screening improves over time. (*Ann Intern Med.* 2007;146:699) 3. Surgical repair of AAA should be considered if diameter ≥5.5 cm or if AAA expands ≥0.5 cm over 6 months to reduce higher risk of rupture. Meta-analysis: endovascular repair associated with fewer postoperative adverse events and lower 30-day and aneurysm-related mortality but not all-cause mortality compared with open repair. (*Br J Surg.* 2008;95(6):677)	http://www.ahrq.gov/ clinic/uspstf/uspsaneu. htm *J Vasc Surg.* 2007; 45:1268–76. *Circulation.* 2006;113(11): e463–e654 *J Vasc Surg.* 2007;45:1268–1276
	USPSTF	2005	Women	Routine screening is not recommended.		
	CMS	2007	Men aged 65–75 years who have smoked at least 100 cigarettes in their lifetime or who have a family history of AAA	Recommend one-time ultrasound screening for AAA.	4. Asymptomatic AAA between 4.4 and 5.5 cm. should have regular ultrasound surveillance with surgical intervention when AAA expands > 1 cm per year or diameter reaches 5.5 cm. (*Cochrane Database Syst Rev.* 2008, CD001835) http://www.thecochranelibrary.com) 5. Medicare covers one-time limited screening.	http://www.medicare. gov/navigation/ manage-your-health/ preventive-services/ abdominalaortic- aneurysm.aspx

Disease Screening	Organization	Date	Population	Recommendations	Comments	Source
Alcohol Abuse & Dependence	AAFP USPSTF VA/DOD ICSI	2010 2004 2009 2010	Adults	Screen all adults in primary care settings, including pregnant women, for alcohol misuse.	1. Screen annually using validated tool. 2. AUDIT score ≥ 4 for men and ≥ 3 for women and SASQ reporting of ≥ 5 drinks in a day (men) or ≥ 4 drinks in a day (women) in the past year are valid and reliable screening instruments for identifying unhealthy alcohol use. 3. The TWEAK and the T-ACE are designed to screen pregnant women for alcohol misuse.	http://www.guidelines.gov/content.aspx?id=36873 http://www.ahrq.gov/clinic/pocketgd1011/pocketgd1011.pdf http://www.icsi.org/preventive_services_for_adults/preventive_serv ces_for_adults_4.html
	VA/DOD	2009	Adults	Provide brief intervention to those who have a positive alcohol misuse screen. Brief interventions during future visits.		http://www.guidelines.gov/content.aspx?id=15676
	AAFP USPSTF ICSI	2010 2004 2010	Adolescents Children and adolescents	Insufficient evidence to recommend for or against screening or counseling interventions to prevent or reduce alcohol misuse by adolescents.	1. AUDIT and CAGE questionnaires have not been validated in children or adolescents. 2. Reinforce not drinking and driving or riding with any driver under the influence. 3. Reinforce to women the harmful effects of alcohol on fetuses.	http://www.guidelines.gov/content.aspx?id=36873 http://www.icsi.org/preventive_services_for_children__guideline_/preventive_services_for_children_and_adolescents_2531.html

AUDIT: alcohol use disorders identification test; SASQ: single alcohol screening question.

	ANEMIA					
Disease Screening	Organization	Date	Population	Recommendations	Comments	Source
Anemia	AAFP	2006	Infants aged 6–12 months	Perform selective, single hemoglobin or hematocrit screening for high-risk infants.[a]	Reticulocyte hemoglobin content is a more sensitive and specific marker than is serum hemoglobin level for iron deficiency. One-third of patients with iron deficiency will have a hemoglobin level > 11 g/dL.	http://www.aafp.org/online/en/home/clinical/exam.html
	USPSTF	2010	Infants aged 6–12 months	Evidence is insufficient to recommend for or against routine screening, but risk assessment based on diet, socioeconomic status, prematurity, and low-birth-weight should be done.	Recommends routine iron supplementation in asymptomatic high-risk children aged 6–12 months but not in those who are of average risk for iron deficiency anemia.	

ANEMIA

Disease Screening	Organization	Date	Population	Recommendations	Comments	Source
Anemia (continued)	USPSTF	2010	Pregnant women	Screen all women with hemoglobin or hematocrit at first prenatal visit.	1. Insufficient evidence to recommend for or against routine use of iron supplements for nonanemic pregnant women (USPSTF). 2. When acute stress or inflammatory disorders are not present, a serum ferritin level is the most accurate test for evaluating iron deficiency anemia. Among women of childbearing age, a cut-off of 30 ng/mL has sensitivity of 92%, specificity of 98% (*Blood* 1997;89:1052–1057). 3. Severe anemia (hemoglobin < 6) associated with: abnormal fetal oxygenation and transfusion should be considered. In iron-deficient women intolerant of oral iron, intravenous iron sucrose or iron dextran should be given.	http://www.ahrq.gov/clinic/cpgsix.htm

[a]Includes infants living in poverty, Blacks, Native Americans and Alaska natives, immigrants from developing countries, preterm and low-birth-weight infants, and infants whose principal dietary intake is unfortified cow's milk or soy milk. Less than two servings per day of iron-rich foods (iron-fortified breakfast cereals or meats).

ATTENTION-DEFICIT/HYPERACTIVITY DISORDER

Disease Screening	Organization	Date	Population	Recommendations	Comments	Source
Attention Deficit/ Hyperactivity Disorder (ADHD)	AAFP AAP	2000	Children aged 6–12 years with inattention, hyperactivity, impulsivity, academic underachievement, or behavioral problems	Initiate an evaluation for ADHD. Diagnosis requires the child meet DSM-IV criteriaᵃ and direct supporting evidence from parents or caregivers and classroom teacher. Evaluation of a child with ADHD should include assessment for coexisting disorders.	1. The rise in stimulant prescriptions since 1990 plateaued in 2002. (*Am J Psychiatr.* 2006;163:579) 2. Current estimates are that 8.7% of U.S. children/ adolescents and 5% of adults meet criteria for ADHD. (*Arch Pediatr Adolesc Med.* 2007;161:857. *Am J Psychiatr.* 2006;163:716) Worldwide prevalence is estimated at 5.3%. (*Am J Psychiatr.* 2007;164:942) 3. The U.S. Food and Drug Administration (FDA) approved a "black box" warning regarding the potential for cardiovascular side effects of ADHD stimulant drugs. (*N Engl J Med.* 2006;354:1445)	*Pediatrics.* 2000; 105:1158

ᵃDSM-IV Criteria for ADHD:

I: Either A or B.

A: *Six or more of the following symptoms of inattention have been present for at least 6 months to a point that is disruptive and inappropriate for developmental level. Inattention:* (1) Often does not give close attention to details or makes careless mistakes in schoolwork, work, or other activities. (2) Often has trouble keeping attention on tasks or play activities. (3) Often does not seem to listen when spoken to directly. (4) Often does not follow instructions and fails to finish schoolwork, chores, or duties in the workplace (not due to oppositional behavior or failure to understand instructions). (5) Often has trouble organizing activities. (6) Often avoids, dislikes, or does not want to do things that take a lot of mental effort for a long period of time (such as schoolwork or homework). (7) Often loses things needed for tasks and activities (eg, toys, school assignments, pencils, books, or tools). (8) Is often easily distracted. (9) Is often forgetful in daily activities.

B: *Six or more of the following symptoms of hyperactivity-impulsivity have been present for at least 6 months to an extent that is disruptive and inappropriate for developmental level. Hyperactivity:* (1) Often fidgets with hands or feet or squirms in seat. (2) Often gets up from seat when remaining in seat is expected. (3) Often runs about or climbs when and where it is not appropriate (adolescents or adults may feel very restless). (4) Often has trouble playing or enjoying leisure activities quietly. (5) Is often "on the go" or often acts as if "driven by a motor." (6) Often talks excessively.

Impulsivity: (1) Often blurts out answers before questions have been finished. (2) Often has trouble waiting one's turn. (3) Often interrupts or intrudes on others (eg, butts into conversations or games).

II: Some symptoms that cause impairment were present before age 7 years.

III: Some impairment from the symptoms is present in two or more settings (eg, at school/work and at home).

IV: There must be clear evidence of significant impairment in social, school, or work functioning.

V: The symptoms do not happen only during the course of a pervasive developmental disorder, schizophrenia, or other psychotic disorder. The symptoms are not better accounted

BACTERIURIA, ASYMPTOMATIC						
Disease Screening	Organization	Date	Population	Recommendations	Comments	Source
Bacteriuria, Asymptomatic	AAFP USPSTF	2010 2008	Pregnant women	Recommend screening for bacteriuria at first prenatal visit or at 12–16 weeks gestation.	http://www.guidelines.gov/content.aspx?id=34005 http://www.uspreventiveservicestaskforce.org/uspstf08/asymptbact/asbactrs.htm	
	AAFP USPSTF	2010 2008	Men and nonpregnant women	Recommends against routine screening for bacteriuria.		

BACTERIAL VAGINOSIS

Disease Screening	Organization	Date	Population	Recommendations	Comments	Source
Bacterial Vaginosis	AAFP USPSTF	2010 2008	Pregnant women at high risk for preterm delivery	Insufficient evidence to recommend for or against routine screening.	http://www.guidelines.gov/content.aspx?id=34005 http://www.uspreventiveservicestaskforce.org/uspstf08/bv/bvrs.htm	
	AAFP USPSTF	2010 2008	Low-risk pregnant women	Recommend against routine screening.		

	BARRETT'S ESOPHAGUS				
Disease screening	Organization	Date	Population	Recommendations	Comments	Source
Barrett's Esophagus (BE)	AGA	2011	General population with GERD	Against screening general population with GERD for BE (strong recommendation).	—Despite lack of evidence of benefit of screening general population with GERD for BE, endoscopic screening is common and wide-spread.	
			High risk population with GERD (multiple risk factors including age >50, male gender, Caucasian, chronic GERD, hiatal hernia, BMI >30, intra-abdominal distribution of body fat)	Screening should be strongly considered in this population especially patients with multiple risk factors (weak recommendation).	—40% of patients with BE and esophageal cancer have not had chronic GERD symptoms. —The diagnosis of dysplasia in BE should be confirmed by at least one additional pathologist, preferably one who is an expert in esophageal pathology (*Gastroenterology* 2011;140:1084).	

Disease Screening	Organization	Date	Population	Recommendations	Comments	Source
CANCER, BLADDER						
Cancer, Bladder	AAFP	2011	Asymptomatic persons	Recommends against routine screening for bladder cancer (CA) in adults. Evidence is insufficient to assess balance of benefits and harms of screening for bladder CA in asymptomatic adults.	1. *Benefits:* There is inadequate evidence to determine whether screening for bladder CA would have any impact on mortality. *Harms:* Based on fair evidence, screening for bladder CA would result in unnecessary diagnostic procedures and overdiagnosis (70% of bladder CA is in-situ) with attendant morbidity. (NCI, 2008) 2. A high index of suspicion should be maintained in anyone with a history of smoking (4–7-fold increased risk),[a] exposure to industrial toxins (aromatic amines, benzene) or therapeutic pelvic radiation, cyclophosphamide chemotherapy, history of *Schistosoma haematobium* cystitis, hereditary nonpolyposis colon CA (Lynch syndrome), and history of transitional cell carcinoma of ureter (50% risk of subsequent bladder CA). Large screening studies in these high-risk populations have not been performed.	http://www.aafp.org/online/en/home/clinical/exam.html
	USPSTF	2011				http://www.ahrq.gov/clinic/uspstf/uspsblad.htm

Disease Screening	Organization	Date	Population	Recommendations	Comments	Source
Cancer, Bladder (continued)					3. Urine cytology with only 10% positive predictive value, urinary biomarkers (nuclear matrix protein 22, telomerase) with suboptimal sensitivity and specificity.	http://www.cancer.gov

[a]Individuals who smoke are four to seven times more likely to develop bladder CA than are individuals who have never smoked. Additional environmental risk factors: exposure to aminobiphenyls; aromatic amines; azo dyes; combustion gases and soot from coal; chlorination by-products in heated water; aldehydes used in chemical dyes and in the rubber and textile industries; organic chemicals used in dry cleaning, paper manufacturing, rope and twine making, and apparel manufacturing; contaminated Chinese herbs; arsenic in well water. Additional risk factors: prolonged exposure to urinary *Schistosoma haematobium* bladder infections, cyclophosphamide, or pelvic radiation therapy for other malignancies.

Disease Screening	Organization	Date	Population	Recommendations[a,b]	Comments	Source
					CANCER, BREAST	
Cancer, Breast	ACS	2008	Women aged 20–39 years	Inform women of benefits and limitations of breast self-exam (BSE). Educate concerning reporting a lump or breast symptoms. Clinical breast exam (CBE) every 2–3 years. Breast imaging not indicated for average-risk women.	1. *Benefits of mammography screening:* Based on fair evidence, screening mammography in women aged 40–70 years decreases breast CA mortality. The benefit is higher in older women (reduction in risk of death in women aged 40–49 years = 15%–20%, 25%–30% in women aged ≥ 50 years). *Harms:* Based on solid evidence, screening mammography may lead to potential harm by overdiagnosis (indolent tumors that are not life-threatening) and unnecessary biopsies for benign disease. (*CA Cancer J Clin.* 2012;62:5. *Ann Intern Med.* 2012;156:491)	http://www.cancer.org
	ACP	2007	Women aged 40–49 years	Perform individualized assessment of breast CA risk; base screening decision on benefits and harms of screening (see Comment 1) as well as on a woman's preferences and CA risk profile. (*Ann Intern Med.* 2012;156:635. *Ann Intern Med.* 2012;156:662)	2. BSE does not improve breast CA mortality (*Br J Cancer.* 2003;88:1047) and increases the rate of false-positive biopsies. (*J Natl Cancer Inst.* 2002;94:1445) 3. Twenty-five percent of breast CAs diagnosed before age 40 years are attributable to *BRCA1* or 2 mutations.	*Ann Intern Med.* 2007;146:511

CANCER, BREAST

Disease Screening	Organization	Date	Population	Recommendations[a,b]	Comments	Source
Cancer, Breast (continued)	UK-NHS	2006	Women aged 40–49 years	Based on current evidence, routine screening is not recommended.	4. The sensitivity of annual screening of young (aged 30–49 years) high-risk women with magnetic resonance imaging (MRI) and mammography is superior to either alone, but MRI is associated with a significant increase in false-positives. (*Lancet.* 2005;365:1769. *Lancet Oncol.* 2011;378:1804) 5. Computer-aided detection in screening mammography appears to reduce overall accuracy (by increasing false-positive rate), although it is more sensitive in women aged < 50 years with dense breasts. (*N Engl J Med* 2007;356:1399) 6. Digital mammography vs. film screen mammography equal in women 50–79 y/o but digital more accurate in women 40-49 y/o (*Ann Intern Med.* 2011;155:493).	http://www.cancerscreening.nhs.uk
	AAFP	2010	Women aged ≥ 40 years	Mammography, with or without CBE, every 1–2 years after counseling about potential risks and benefits.	Evidence is insufficient to recommend for or against routine CBE alone, or teaching or performing a routine BSE; recommend against screening women > 75 y/o.	http://www.aafp.org/online/en/home/clinical/exam.html

					CANCER, BREAST	
Disease Screening	Organization	Date	Population	Recommendations[a,b]	Comments	Source
Cancer, Breast (continued)	ACS	2008	Women aged ≥40 years	Mammography and CBE yearly; if > 20% lifetime risk of breast CA, annual mammogram + MRI. *BRCA-1* and *2* mutation-positive women should begin MRI and mammogram screening at age 30 years or younger depending on family history. Lymphoma survivors with a history of mediastinal radiation should begin mammography and MRI yearly 10 years after radiation.	1. In high-risk women, probability of breast CA when mammogram is negative = 1.4% (1.2%–1.6%) versus when mammogram plus MRI are negative = 0.3% (0.1%–0.8%) (*Ann Intern Med.* 2008;148:671). MRI two to three times as sensitive as mammogram, but 2-fold increase in false-positives—use in selected high-risk population only. (*J Clin Oncol.* 2005;23:8469. *J Clin Oncol.* 2009;27:6124) 2. If lifetime risk of breast CA is between 15% and 20%, women should discuss risks/benefits of adding annual MRI to mammography screening. Sensitivity of MRI superior to mammography, especially in higher-risk women aged < 50 years with dense breasts (increasing breast density increases risk of breast CA and lowers sensitivity of mammogram). A > 75% breast density increases risk of breast CA 5-fold. (*J Clin Oncol.* 2010; 28:3830)	http://www.cancer.org *CA Cancer J Clin.* 2007;57:75

CANCER, BREAST					

Disease Screening	Organization	Date	Population	Recommendations[a,B]	Comments	Source
Cancer, Breast (continued)	UK-NHS	2006	Women aged 50–70 years Women aged >70 years	Program-initiated mammography screening of all women every 3 years. Patient-initiated screening covered by National Health Service (NHS).	Annual versus 3-year screening interval showed no significant difference in predicted breast CA mortality, although relative risk reduction among annually screened women had nonsignificant reduction of 5%–11%. (*Eur J Cancer.* 2002;38:1458)	http://www.cancerscreening.nhs.uk
	AGS	2005	Women aged 70–85 years	If estimated life expectancy ≥ 5 years, then offer screening mammography ± CBE every 1–2 years.	Incidence of breast CA highest in th s age range but significant comorbidities and competing causes of death compared with that of younger women.	http://www.americangeriatrics.org
	AAFP	2008	Women with family history associated with increased risk (breast CA aged <50 years or ovarian CA at any age) for deleterious mutations in *BRCA1* or *BRCA2* genes[c] (Gail model: *J Natl Cancer Inst.* 1999;91:1541. BRAC PRO model: *Am J Hum Genet.* 1998;62:145)	Refer for genetic counseling and evaluation for *BRCA* testing.	1. In one study, nearly half of *BRCA*-positive women with newly diagnosed breast CA developed malignant disease detected by mammography < 1 year after a normal screening mammogram. (*Cancer.* 2004;100:2079) 2. Consider mammography plus MRI screening in high-risk women. (*CA Cancer J Clin.* 2011;61:8–30) 3. Management of an inherited predisposition to breast CA is controversial. (*NEJM.* 2007;357:154). Risk-reducing surgery versus enhanced surveillance with yearly magnetic resonance imaging (MRI) and mammography.	http://www.aafp.org/online/en/home/clinical/exam.html

Disease Screening	Organization	Date	Population	Recommendations[a,b]	Comments	Source
CANCER, BREAST						
Cancer, Breast (continued)	USPSTF	2009	Women aged 50–74 years	—Biennial screening mammography —BSE teaching not recommended —Inconclusive data for screening women aged > 75 years.	These recommendations for women aged 40–50 years have been widely criticized and largely ignored by other advisory organizations as inconsistent with available data. Subsequent trial from Norway showed significant benefit in mortality reduction (28%) in the aged 40–49 years subset. Analysis of data sets continues, but there has been no major change in practice patterns. (*Am J Roentgenol.* 2011;196:112. *Am J Coll Rad.* 2010;7:18. *Cancer.* 2011;117:7. *Eur J Cancer.* 2010;46:3137. *CA Cancer J Clin.* 2012;62:129).	http:// www. ahrq. gov/ clinic/ uspstfix. htm
			Women aged 40–50 years	—Decision to begin screening mammography before age 50 years should be individualized according to benefit versus harm for each unique patient. (*Ann Intern Med.* 2012;156:609)		
	NCCN	2011	Aged 20–40 years (average risk)	CBE every 1–3 years—breast awareness education.	A woman with mediastinal radiation at age 20–25 years will have a 75-fold increased risk of breast CA at age 35 years versus age-matched controls. Salpingo-oophorectomy will decrease risk of breast CA in *BRCA1* and 2 carriers by 50% and decrease risk of ovarian CA by 90%–95%.	www. nccn. org
			Aged > 40 years (average risk)	Annual CBE, annual mammogram. MRI not recommended in average-risk patients.		
			Acquired increased risk—prior thoracic radiation therapy	CBE q6–12 months, annual mammogram and annual MRI beginning 8–10 years after radiation therapy or age 25 years, whichever occurs last.		

CANCER, BREAST						
Disease Screening	Organization	Date	Population	Recommendations[a,b]	Comments	Source
Cancer, Breast (continued)	USPSTF	2009	Lifetime risk of breast CA > 20% based on family history, genetic predisposition (*BRCA1* or 2). (http://www.cancer.gov/bcrisktoo/)	Aged < 25 years annual CBE, breast awareness education, and referral to genetic course: or:	Tamoxifen or raloxifene not studied as de novo chemo prevention in *BRCA1* or 2 patients, but tamoxifen will decrease risk of contralateral breast CA by 50% in *BRCA*-mutated breast CA patients. (*Int J Cancer.* 2006;118:2231)	http://www.ahrqgor*clinic/uspstf
	NCCN	2011	History of lobular carcinoma in situ atypical hyperplasia or history of breast CA	Aged > 25 years, annual mammogram and MRI, CBE q6–12 months, consider risk-reducing strategies (surgery, chemo prevention).	Risk-reducing bilateral mastectomy in *BRCA1* and 2 mutation carriers results in a 90% risk reduction in incidence of breast CA and a 90% rate of satisfaction with risk-reducing surgery (*NEJM.* 2001;345:159. *JAMA.* 2010;304:967)	www.nccn.org

[a]Debate about the value of screening mammograms was triggered by a Cochrane review published on October 20, 2001 (*Lancet.* 2001;358 1340–1342). This review cited a number of methodologic and analytic flaws in the large long-term mammography trials. The USPSTF and NCI concluded that the flaws were problematic but unlikely to negate the consistent and significant mortality reductions observed in the trials.

[b]Summary of current evidence: *CA Cancer J Clin.* 2011;61:8–30.

[c]1. Women not of Ashkenazi Jewish heritage:

Two first-degree relatives with breast CA, one of whom received the diagnosis at age ≤ 50 years.

A combination of ≥ 3 first- or second-degree relatives with breast CA.

A combination of both breast and ovarian CA among first- and second-degree relatives.

A first-degree relative with bilateral breast CA.

A combination of ≥ 2 first- or second-degree relatives with ovarian CA.

A first- or second-degree relative with both breast and ovarian CA.

A history of breast CA in a male relative.

2. Women of Ashkenazi Jewish heritage: Any first-degree relative (or second-degree relatives on the same side of the family) with breast or ovarian CA.

CANCER, BREAST				
TABLE A: HARMS OF SCREENING MAMMOGRAPHY				
Harm	Internal Validity	Consistency	Magnitude of Effects	External Validity
Treatment of insignificant CAs (overdiagnosis of indolent cancer) can result in breast deformity, lymphedema, thromboembolic events, and chemotherapy-induced toxicities.	Good	Good	Approximately 20%–30% of breast CAs detected by screening mammograms represent overdiagnosis. (*BMJ.* 2009;339:2587) Oncotype DX (a predictive panel of 15 breast CA genes) can reduce the use of chemotherapy by 50% in node-negative hormone receptor-positive patients.	Good
Additional testing (false-positives)	Good	Good	Estimated to occur in 30% of women screened annually for 10 years, 7%–10% of whom will have biopsies. This creates anxiety and negative quality of life impact. (*Ann Int Med.* 2009;151:738. *Ann Intern Med.* 2011;155:481)	Good
False sense of security, delay in CA diagnosis (false-negatives)	Good	Good	About 10%–30% of women with invasive CA will have negative mammogram results, especially if young with dense breasts or with lobular or high-grade CAs. (*Radiology.* 2005;235:775)	Good
Radiation-induced mutation can cause breast CA, especially if exposed before age 30 years. Latency is more than 10 years, and the increased risk persists lifelong.	Good	Good	In women beginning screening at age 40 years, benefits far outweigh risks of radiation inducing breast CA. Women should avoid unnecessary CT scanning. (*BJC.* 2005;93:590. *Ann Intern Med.* 2012;156:662)	Good
Source: NCI. 2010—http://www.cancer.gov				

CANCER, CERVICAL

Disease Screening	Organization	Date	Population	Recommendations	Comments	Source
Cancer, Cervical	ACS	2012	Women aged <21 y/o: no screening [a] Women between age 21 and 29 y/o Average risk women 30–65 y/o	Cytology alone (PAP smear) every 3 years until age 30 years Human papillomavirus (HPV) DNA testing not recommended if aged < 30 years (majority of young patients will clear the infection). HPV and cytology "co-testing" every 5 years (preferred) or cytology alone every 3 years (acceptable). If HPV positive/cytology negative—either 12-month follow-up with co-testing or test for HPV 16 or 18 genotypes with referral to colposcopy if positive. Continue to screen more frequently if high-risk factors present. [bcd]	1. Cervical CA is causally related to infection with HPV (> 70% associated with either HPV-18 or HPV-16 genotype) (See new ACIP HPV recommendations, Appendix VIII). 2. Immunocompromised women (organ transplantation, chemotherapy, chronic steroid therapy, or human immunodeficiency women [HIV]) should be tested twice during the first year after initiating screening and annually thereafter. (*CA Cancer J Clin.* 2011;61:**;** *Ann Intern Med.* 2011;155:698) 3. Women with a history of cervical CA or in utero exposure to diethylstilbestrol (DES) should continue average-risk protocol for women aged < 30 years indefinitely. 4. HPV vaccination of young women is now recommended by ACIP, UK-NHS, and others. Cervical CA screening recommendations have not changed for women receiving the vaccine because the vaccine covers only 70% of HPV serotypes that cause cervical CA. (*MMWR.* 2007;56(RR-2):1–24)	http://www.cancer.org http://www.survivorshipguidelines.org *CA Cancer J Clin.* 2012;62:147–172.

Disease Screening	Organization	Date	Population	Recommendations	Comments	Source
Cancer, Cervical (continued)	ACS	2012	Age >65 y/o After hysterectomy	No screening following adequate prior screening. No screening in women without a cervix and no history of CIN2 or worse in past 20 years or cervical CA ever.	5. Long-term use of oral contraceptives may increase risk of cervical CA in women who test positive for cervical HPV DNA (*Lancet.* 2002;359:1085). Smoking increases risk of cervical CA 4-fold. (*Am J Epidemiol.* 1990;131:945) 6. A vaccine against HPV-16 and 18 significantly reduces the risk of acquiring transient and persistent infection. (*NEJM.* 2002;347:1645. *Obstet Gynecol.* 2006;107(1):4)	http://www.uspreventiveservicestaskforce.org/ *Ann Intern Med.* 2012;156:880.
	USPSTF	2012	Women ages 21–29 y/o Women ages 30–65 y/o Women younger than 21 y/o Women younger than age 30 y/o	Screen with cytology (PAP smear) every 3 years. Screen with cytology every 3 years or co-testing (cytology/HPV testing) every 5 years. Do not screen. Do not screen with HPV testing (alone or with cytology).	7. *Benefits:* Based on solid evidence, regular screening of appropriate women with the Pap test reduces mortality from cervical CA. Screening is effective when starting at age 21 years. *Harms:* Based on solid evidence, regular screening with the Pap test leads to additional diagnostic procedures and treatment for low-grade squamous intraepithelial lesions (LSILs), with uncertain long-term consequences on fertility and pregnancy. Harms are greatest for younger women, who have a higher prevalence of LSILs. LSILs often regress without treatment. False-positives in postmenopausal women are due to mucosal atrophy. (NCI, 2008)	

	CANCER, CERVICAL					
Disease Screening	**Organization**	**Date**	**Population**	**Recommendations**	**Comments**	**Source**
Cancer, Cervical (continued)	UK-NHS UK-NHS	2011 2011	Women aged < 25 years Women aged 25–49 years Women aged 50–64 years	Routine screening is not recommended. Routine screen every 3 years—triage to HPV testing if borderline changes or mild dyskaryosis; if HPV positive refer for colposcopy. Routinely screen every 5 years with conventional cytology—HPV triage if borderline abnormal findings.	UK-NHS initiated an HPV immunization program for girls aged 12–13 years in September 2008. UK-NHS contacts all eligible women who are registered with a primary care doctor.	http://www.cancerscreening.nhs.uk http://www.cancerscreening.nhs.uk
	UK-NHS	2011	Women aged ≥ 65 years	Screen women who have not been screened since age 50 years or who have had recent abnormal test results—if all previous cervical cancer screening has been negative, cease screening.	Stop screening after age 65 years if there are three consecutive normal test results.	http://www.cancerscreening.nhs.uk
	ACOG	2009	Begin at age 21 years independent of sexual history	Every 2 years from ages 21–29.	Women aged ≥ 30 years can extend interval to every 2–3 years if: three consecutive negative screens, no history of cervical intraepithelial neoplasia 2 or 3, not immunocompromised, no HIV, and not exposed to DES. No more often than 3 years if cervical cytology and HPV testing combined.	ACOG Practice bulletin: *Obstet Gynecol.* 2009;114:1409.

CANCER, CERVICAL

Disease Screening	Organization	Date	Population	Recommendations	Comments	Source
Cancer, Cervical (continued)	USPSTF	2011	Women aged > 65 years	Recommends against routine screening if woman has had adequate recent screening and normal Pap smear results and is not otherwise at high risk for cervical CA.[c]	Beyond age 70 years, there is little evidence for or against screening women who have been regularly screened in previous years. Individual circumstances, such as the patient's life expectancy, ability to undergo treatment if CA is detected, and ability to cooperate with and tolerate the Pap smear procedure, may obviate the need for cervical CA screening.	http://www.ahrq.gov/clinic/uspstf/uspscerv.htm
	ACS	2008	Women aged ≥ 70 years	Discontinue screening if ≥ three normal Pap smear results in a row and no abnormal Pap smear results in the last 10 years.[d]		http://www.cancer.org
	ACS ACOG USPSTF	2008 2009 2012	Women without a cervix and no history of high-grade precancer or cervical cancer	Recommends against routine Pap smear screening in women who have had a total hysterectomy or removal of the cervix for benign disease and no history of abnormal cell growth.		http://www.cancer.org http://www.ahrq.gov/clinic/uspstf/uspscerv.htm ACOG practice bulletin–109 12/09

[a]Sexual history in patients < 21 y/o not considered in beginning cytological screening, which should start at age 21.

[b]New tests to improve CA detection include liquid-based/thin-layer preparations, computer-assisted screening methods, and HPV testing (*Am Fam Phys.* 2001;64:729. *N Engl J Med.* 2007;357:1579. *JAMA.* 2009;302:1757).

[c]High-risk factors include DES exposure before birth, HIV infection, or other forms of immunosuppression, including chronic steroid use.

[d]Women with a history of cervical CA, DES exposure, HIV infection, or a weakened immune system should continue to have screenings as long as they are in more than 5-year life expectancy.

CANCER, COLORECTAL						
Disease Screening	**Organization**	**Date**	**Population**	**Recommendations**	**Comments**	**Source**
Cancer, Colorectal	ACS USMTFCC[a] ACR	2008		See Table on page 26. Tests that find polyps and CA are preferred.	Although colonoscopy is the de facto gold standard for colon CA screening, choice of screening technique depends on risk, comorbidities, insurance coverage, patient preference, and availability. Above all, do something to screen for colon CA.	*CA Cancer J Clin.* 2008;58:130 *CA Cancer J Clin.* 2012;62:124–142
	AAFP USPSTF	2008 2008	Aged ≥50 years at average risk[b]	Screen with one of the following strategies.[c,d,e] 1. Fecal occult blood test (gFOBT-guiac based or iFOBT-immunochemical based—iFOBT is preferred) annually.[f] 2. Flexible sigmoidoscopy every 5 years. 3. FOBT annually plus flexible sigmoidoscopy every 5 years. 4. Colonoscopy every 10 years.[g] 5. CT colonoscopy.	1. The USPSTF "strongly recommends" colorectal cancer (CRC) screening in this group up to age 75 y/o; screening patients >75 y/o is not recommended. 2. Flexible sigmoidoscopy and one-time FOBT mandating a colonoscopy if either yields positive results will miss 25% of significant proximal neoplasia. This strategy should include yearly FOBT. (*N Engl J Med.* 2001;345:555. *N Engl J Med.* 2012;366:2345) 3. FOBT alone decreased CRC mortality by 33% compared with those who were not screened. (*Gastroenterol* 2004;126:1674) 4. Accuracy of colonoscopy is operator dependent—rapid withdrawal time, poor prep, and lack of experience will increase false-negatives. (*N Engl J Med.* 2006;355:2533. *Ann Intern Med.* 2012;156:692)	http://www.aafp. org/online/en/ home/clinical/ exam.html http://www.cancer. org *Gastrointest Endosc.* 2006;63:546 *Ann Intern Med.* 2012;156:378 *Gastroenterology.* 2003;124:544 http://www.ahrq. gov/clinic/uspstf/ uspscolo.htm

CANCER, COLORECTAL

Disease Screening	Organization	Date	Population	Recommendations	Comments	Source
Cancer, Colorectal (continued)	ACOG	2007	Women at average risk aged ≥ 50 years	Preferred method: • Colonoscopy every 10 years Other appropriate methods: • FOBT annually • Flexible sigmoidoscopy every 5 years • FOBT annually plus flexible sigmoidoscopy every 5 years • Double-contrast barium enema every 5 years	5. Percentage of U.S. adults receiving some form of CRC screening has increased from 44% in 1999 to 63% in 2008. (*Arch Intern Med.* 2011;171:647. *Arch Intern Med.* 2012;172:575) 6. Colonoscopy vs. iFOBT testing in CRC with similar detection of cancer but more adenomas identified in colonoscopy group. (*N Engl J Med.* 2012;366:697. *N Engl J Med.* 2012;366:687)	ACOG Committee Opinion, No. 357, Nov 2007
	UK-NHS	2007	Adults aged 60–69 years Adults aged ≥ 70 years	Program screened every 2 years with FOBT[c] Patient-initiated screening covered by NHS		http://www.cancerscreening.nhs.uk/bowel/index.html
	ACS USMTFCC[a]	2008	Persons at increased risk based on family history but without a definable genetic syndrome	*Group I:* Screening colonoscopy at age 40 years, or 10 years younger than the earliest diagnosis in the immediate family, and repeated every 5 years.[h] *Group II:* Follow average-risk recommendations, but begin at age 40 years.		*CA Cancer J Clin.* 2008;58:130
			Very high-risk-hereditary nonpolyposis colorectal cancer (HNPCC–Lynch syndrome) (3% to 5% of all CRCs) proven gene carrier—evaluate if Bethesda criteria is met[h]	Colonoscopy every 2 years beginning at age 20–25 y/o then yearly at age 40 years.[h]	Increased risk of non-CRC (endometrial, ovary, upper gastrointestinal, pancreas, renal pelvis, ureter) requires systematic screening. (*J Clin Oncol.* 2000;18:11. *J Clin Oncol.* 2012;30:1058).	

CANCER, COLORECTAL						

Disease Screening	Organization	Date	Population	Recommendations	Comments	Source
Cancer, Colorectal (continued)			Classic familial adenomatous polyposis (FAP)	At-risk children should be offered genetic testing at age 10–12 years. Flexible sigmoidoscopy or colonoscopy every 12 months starting at age 10–12 years. Elective colectomy based on number and histology of polyps—usually done by early 20s; upper endoscopy every 5 years if no gastric or duodenal polyps starting in early 20s.	Extraintestinal tumors in FAP include hepatoblastoma (AFP screening recommended in families with this tumor), adrenal tumors, osteomas, brain tumors, skin CA, and thyroid CA.	*Am J Gastroenterol.* 2009;104:739 *J Clin Oncol.* 2003;21:2397 *Gut.* 2008 57:704 *JAMA.* 2006;296:1507

[a] U.S. Multisociety Task Force on Colorectal Cancer. (ACG, ACP, AGA, ASGE)

[b] Risk factors indicating need for earlier/more frequent screening: personal history of CRC or adenomatous polyps or hepatoblastoma, CRC or polyps in a first-degree relative aged < 60 years or in 2 first-degree relatives of any age, personal history of chronic inflammatory bowel disease, and family with hereditary CRC syndromes (*Ann Intern Med.* 1998;128(1):900. *Am J Gastroenterol.* 2009;104:739. *N Engl J Med.* 1994;331(25):1669. *N Engl J Med.* 1995;332(13):861). Additional high-risk group: history of ≥ 30 Gy radiation to whole abdomen; all upper abdominal fields; pelvic; thoracic, lumbar, or sacral spine. Begin monitoring 10 years after radiation or at age 35 years, whichever occurs last (http://www.survivorshipguidelines.org). Screening colonoscopy may result in only 15% of the expected gain in life expectancy seen in younger patients (*JAMA.* 2006;295:2357). ACG treats African Americans as high-risk group. See separate recommendation above.

[c] A positive result on an FOBT should be followed by colonoscopy. An alternative is flexible sigmoidoscopy and air-contrast barium enema.

[d] FOBT should be performed on 2 samples from 3 consecutive specimens obtained at home. A single stool guaiac during annual physical exam is not adequate.

[e] USPSTF did not find direct evidence that a screening colonoscopy is effective in reducing CRC mortality rates.

[f] Use the guaiac-based test with dietary restriction, or an immunochemical test without dietary restriction. Two samples from each of 3 consecutive stools should be examined without rehydration. Rehydration increases the false-positive rate.

[g] Population-based retrospective analysis: risk of developing CRC remains decreased for > 10 years following negative colonoscopy findings (*JAMA.* 2006;295:2366).

[h] *Group I:* First-degree relative with colon CA or adenomatous polyps at age < 60 years or 2 first-degree relatives with CRC or adenomatous polyps at any time. *Group II:* First-degree relative with CRC or adenomatous polyps at age ≥ 60 years or 2 second-degree relatives with CRC. Revised Bethesda criteria for testing for HNPCC (Lynch syndrome)—screen for tumor microsatellite instability if CRC diagnosed in a patient aged < 50 years, presence of synchronous, metachronous CRC or other HNPCC defining tumor at any age. CRC with microsatellite unstable-type histology (mucinous, signet ring, infiltrating lymphocytes) in patients aged < 60 years. CRC diagnosed in 1 or more first-degree relatives with HNPCC-related tumor with one of the cancers diagnosed at age < 50 years. CRC diagnosed under age 50. CRC diagnosed in 2 or more first-degree or second-degree relatives with HNPCC-related tumors regardless of age. Confirmation of HNPCC is made by genetic evaluation of the involved genes (*J Natl Cancer Inst.* 2004;96:261).

CANCER, COLORECTAL

The following options are acceptable choices for CRC screening in average-risk adults beginning at age 50 years. Since each of the following tests has inherent characteristics related to prevention potential, accuracy, costs, and potential harms, individuals should have an opportunity to make an informed decision when choosing one of the following options.

In the opinion of the guidelines development committee, *colon CA prevention* should be the primary goal of CRC screening. Tests that are designed to detect both early CA and adenomatous polyps should be encouraged if resources are available and patients are willing to undergo an invasive test.

Tests that Detect Adenomatous Polyps and Cancer

Test	Interval	Key Issues for Informed Decisions
FSIG with insertion to 40 cm or to the splenic flexure	Every 5 years	Complete or partial bowel prep is required.
		Because sedation usually is not used, there may be some discomfort during the procedure.
		The protective effect of sigmoidoscopy is primarily limited to the portion of the colon examined. NCI study of 77,000 patients showed a significant decrease in CRC incidence (both distal and proximal) and a 50% reduction in mortality (distal only) (*J Natl Cancer Inst.* 2012;104:1).
		Patients should understand that positive findings on sigmoidoscopy usually result in a referral for colonoscopy.
Colonoscopy	Every 10 years	Complete bowel prep is required.
		Procedural sedation is used in most centers; patients will miss a day of work and will need a chaperone for transportation from the facility.
		Risks include perforation and bleeding, which are rare but potentially serious; most of the risk is associated with polypectomy (*Ann Intern Med.* 2009;150:1).
DCBE	Every 5 years	Complete bowel prep is required.
		If patients have one or more polyps ≥ 6 mm, colonoscopy will still be needed for biopsy or polyp removal; follow-up colonoscopy will require complete bowel prep.
		Risks of DCBE are low; rare cases of perforation have been reported—radiation exposure is a concern. USPSTF does not recommend DCBE due to lower sensitivity than other methods (*N Engl J Med.* 2007;357;1403).
CTC	Every 5 years	Complete bowel prep usually required. (*Ann Intern Med.* 2012;156:692)
		If patients have one or more polyps ≥ 6 mm, colonoscopy will be recommended; if same-day colonoscopy is not available, a second complete bowel prep will be required before colonoscopy.
		Risks of CTC are low; rare cases of perforation have been reported.
		Extracolonic abnormalities may be identified on CTC that could require further evaluation (7%–15% of CT exams). Not as sensitive as colonoscopy for polyps < 1 cm and especially for polyps ≤ 6 mm.

TESTS THAT PRIMARILY DETECT CANCER		
Test	**Interval**	**Key Issues for Informed Decisions**
gFOBT with high sensitivity for CA	Annual	Depending on manufacturer's recommendations, two to three stool samples collected at home are needed to complete testing; a single stool gathered during a digital exam in the clinical setting is not an acceptable stool test and should not be done.
FIT (iFOBT) with high sensitivity for CA	Annual	
		Positive test results are associated with an increased risk of colon CA and advanced neoplasia; colonoscopy should be recommended if the test results are positive.
		If the test result is negative, it should be repeated annually.
		Patients should understand that one-time testing is likely to be ineffective.
sDNA with high sensitivity for CA	Interval uncertain	An adequate stool sample must be obtained and packaged with appropriate preservative agents for shipping to the laboratory. USPSTF does not recommend due to insufficient evidence.
		The unit cost of the currently available test is significantly higher than are other forms of stool testing.
		If the test result is positive, colonoscopy will be recommended.
		If the test result is negative, the appropriate interval for a repeat test is uncertain. sDNA testing is not widely used at this time. (*Ann Intern Med.* 2008;149:441)
CRC, colorectal cancer; CA, cancer; FSIG, flexible sigmoidoscopy; DCBE, double-contrast barium enema; CTC, computed tomography colonography; CT, computed tomography; gFOBT, guaiac-based fecal occult blood test; FIT, fecal immunochemical test; sDNA, stool DNA.		

CANCER, ENDOMETRIAL

Disease Screening	Organization	Date	Population	Recommendations	Comments	Source
Cancer, Endometrial	ACS	2008	All postmenopausal women	Inform women about risks and symptoms of endometrial CA and strongly encourage them to report any unexpected bleeding or spotting. This is especially important for women with an increased risk of endometrial CA (history of unopposed estrogen therapy, tamoxifen therapy, late menopause, nulliparity, infertility or failure to ovulate, obesity, diabetes, or hypertension).	1. *Benefits:* There is inadequate evidence that screening with endometrial sampling or transvaginal ultrasound (TVU) decreases mortality. *Harms:* Based on solid evidence, screening with TVU will result in unnecessary additional exams because of low specificity. Based on solid evidence, endometrial biopsy may result in discomfort, bleeding, infection, and, rarely, uterine perforation. (NCI, 2008) 2. Presence of atypical glandular cells on Pap test from postmenopausal (aged > 40 years) women not taking exogenous hormones is abnormal and requires further evaluation (TVU and endometrial biopsy). Pap test is insensitive for endometrial screening. 3. Endometrial thickness of < 4 mm on TVU is associated with low risk of endometrial CA. (*Am J Obstet Gynecol.* 2001;184:70) 4. Most cases of endometrial CA are diagnosed as a result of symptoms reported by patients (uterine bleeding), and a high proportion of these cases are diagnosed at an early stage and have high rates of cure. (NCI, 2008)	http://www.cancer.org

CANCER, ENDOMETRIAL					
Disease Screening	Organization	Date	Population	Recommendations	Comments	Source
Cancer, Endometrial (continued)					5. Tamoxifen use for 5 years raises the risk of endometrial CA 2–3-fold, but CAs are low stage, low grade, with high cure rates. (*J Natl Cancer Inst.* 1998;90:1371)	
	ACS	2008	All women at high risk for endometrial CA[a] (patients with known or high suspicion for HNPCC mutation carrier)	Annual screening beginning at age 35 years with endometrial biopsy.	1. Variable screening with ultrasound among women (aged 25–65 years; $n = 292$) at high risk for HNPCC mutation detected no CAs from ultrasound. Two endometrial cases occurred in the cohort that presented with symptoms. (*Cancer.* 2002;94:1708) 2. The Women's Health Initiative (WHI) demonstrated that combined estrogen and progestin did not increase the risk of endometrial CA but did increase the rate of endometrial biopsies and ultrasound exams prompted by abnormal uterine bleeding. (*JAMA.* 2003;290)	http://www.cancer.org

[a]High-risk women are those known to carry HNPCC-associated genetic mutations, or at high risk to carry a mutation, or who are from families with a suspected autosomal dominant predisposition to colon CA (45%–50% lifetime risk of endometrial CA).

Disease Screening	Organization	Date	Population	Recommendations	Comments	Source
Cancer, Gastric			Average-risk population	There are currently no recommendations regarding screening for gastric CA.	1. Population endoscopic screening for gastric CA in moderate- to high-risk population subgroups is cost-effective (Japan, South America). (*Clin Gastroenterol Hepatol.* 2006;4:709)	
Adenocarcinoma of gastroesophageal junction	ASGE	2006	Diagnosis— Barrett's esophagus with or without gastroesophageal reflux disease	—No dysplasia—scope every 3 years —Mild dysplasia—scope in 6 months, then yearly High-grade dysplasia— surgery or endoscopic therapy	2. Patients at increased risk for gastric CA should be educated about risk and symptoms. (*Helicobacter pylori*, pernicious anemia, HNPCC, post-partial gastrectomy). 3. *Benefits:* There is fair evidence that screening would result in no decrease in gastric CA mortality in the United States. *Harms:* There is good evidence that esophagogastroduodenoscopy screening would result in rare but serious side effects, such as perforation, cardiopulmonary events, aspiration pneumonia, and bleeding. (NCI, 2008)	*Gastrointest Endosc.* 2006;63:570

	CANCER, LIVER				

Disease Screening	Organization	Date	Population	Recommendations	Comments	Source
Cancer, Liver (Hepatocellular Carcinoma [HCC])	AASLD[b]	2010 update	Adults at high risk for HCC,[a] especially those awaiting liver transplantation, should be entered into surveillance programs.	Surveillance with ultrasound at 6-month intervals.	1. Alpha fetoprotein (AFP) alone should not be used for screening unless ultrasound is not available (low sensitivity). 2. *Benefits:* Based on fair evidence, screening would not result in a decrease in HCC-related mortality.	*Hepatology.* 2005;42:1208
	British Society of Gastroenterology[b]	2003	Adults	Surveillance with abdominal ultrasound and AFP every 6 months should be considered for high-risk groups.[a]	*Harms:* Based on fair evidence, screening would result in rare but serious side effects associated with needle biopsy, such as needle-track seeding, hemorrhage, bile peritonitis, and pneumothorax. (NCI, 2008. *Ann Intern Med.* 2012;156:387)	*Gut.* 2003;52 (suppl III:iii http://www.bsg. org.uk/

[a] *HBsAg+ persons (carriers):* Asian males aged ≥ 40 years, Asian females aged ≥ 40 years; all cirrhotics; family history of HCC; Africans aged > 20 years. *Non-hepatitis B carriers:* hepatitis C; alcoholic cirrhosis; genetic hemochromatosis; primary biliary cirrhosis, alpha-1-antitrypsin deficiency with cirrhosis, hepatitis C with cirrhosis; hemochromatosis with cirrhosis.
[b] Only 2 organizations recommending screening for HCC in high-risk populations (low level evidence).

				CANCER, LUNG		
Disease Screening	Organization	Date	Population	Recommendations	Comments	Source
Cancer, Lung	AAFP USPSTF	2008 2004	Asymptomatic persons	Evidence is insufficient to recommend for or against lung CA screening.	1. Counsel all patients against tobacco use, even when aged > 50 years. Smokers who quit gain ~10 years of increased life expectancy. (*BMJ.* 2004:328) 2. *Benefits:* Based on fair evidence, screening with sputum cytology or CXR does not reduce mortality from lung CA. Evidence is inadequate to assess mortality benefit of low-dose CT (LDCT). *Harms:* Based on solid evidence, screening would lead to false-positive test results and unnecessary invasive procedures. (NCI, 2008)	http://www.aafp.org/online/en/home/clinical/exam.html http://www.ahrq.gov/clinic/uspstf/uspslung.htm
	ACCP	2012	Asymptomatic persons	Based on good evidence, routine screening for lung CA with chest x-ray (CXR), sputum cytology is not recommended. Routine screening with LDCT is not recommended except in the context of a clinical trial.	3. Spiral CT screening can detect greater number of lung CAs in smokers with a > 10-pack/year exposure. (*N Engl J Med.* 2006;355:1763–1771) 4. Although screening increases the rate of lung CA diagnosis and treatment, it may not reduce the risk of advanced lung CA or death from lung CA. (*JAMA.* 2007;297:995)	http://www.chestnet.org/education/guidelines/index.php *Chest.* 2003;123:835–885 *CA Cancer J Clin.* 2004;54:41

CANCER, LUNG						
Disease Screening	Organization	Date	Population	Recommendations	Comments	Source
Cancer, Lung (continued)	ACS	2012	Asymptomatic persons (Interim Guidance or Lung Cancer Screening)	Guidance in shared decision making regarding screening of high-risk persons.	5. The NCI has reported initial data from the National Lung Screening Trial (NLST), a randomized controlled trial comparing LDCT and CXR yearly × 3 with 8-year follow-up. 53,500 men and women aged 50–74 years, 30-pack/year smokers were randomized. A 20.3% reduction in deaths from lung CA was reported for the LDCT group (estimated that 10,000–15,000 lives could be saved per year). Problems with false-positives and cost of workup were noted, but benefits may lead to a change in guidelines. ACS 2012 interim statement on lung cancer screening recommend adults between the ages of 55 and 74 who meet eligibility criteria of NSLT may consider LDCT screening for lung cancer. This should take place in the setting where appropriate resources and expertise are available to minimize morbidity. Patients with a 30-pack year smoking but nonsmoking for > 15 years are excluded. The NCCN and ASCO have formally recommended LDCT screening for patients who meet the criteria of the NCST study (*Ann Intern Med.* 2011;155:540. *Ann Intern Med.* 2011;155:537. *N Engl J Med.* 2011;365:395. *JAMA.* 2012:307:2418).	http://www.cancer.org http://www.cancer.gov/nlst

Disease Screening	Organization	Date	Population	Recommendations	Comments	Source
CANCER, ORAL						
Cancer, Oral	AAFP USPSTF	2008 2004	Asymptomatic persons	Evidence is insufficient to recommend for or against routinely screening adults for oral CA.	1. Risk factors: regular alcohol or tobacco use. 2. A randomized controlled trial of visual screening for oral CA (at 3-year intervals) showed decreased oral CA mortality among screened males (but not females) who were tobacco and/or alcohol users over an 8-year period. (*Lancet.* 2005;365:1927)	http://www.aafp.org/online/en/home/clinical/exam.html http://www.ahrq.gov/clinic/uspstf/uspsoral.htm
	COG	2006	History of radiation to head, oropharynx, neck, or total body Acute/chronic graft-versus-host disease	Annual oral cavity exam.	Significant increase in HPV (subtypes 16 and 18)-related squamous cell cancer of the oropharynx (base of tongue and tonsil) in nonsmokers. 20%–30% improvement in cure rate versus that for smoking-related cancers. (*N Engl J Med.* 2010;363:24) Prevalence of oral HPV infection in United States is 6.9% (*JAMA.* 2012;307:693).	http://www.survivorshipguidelines.org

CANCER, OVARIAN						

Disease Screening	Organization	Date	Population	Recommendations	Comments	Source
Cancer, Ovarian	USPSTF	2012	Asymptomatic women at average risk[a]	Recommends against routine screening. Beware of symptoms of ovarian CA that can be present in early-stage disease (abdominal, pelvic, and back pain; bloating and change in bowel habits; urinary symptoms). (*J Clin Oncol.* 2005;23:7919. *Ann Intern Med.* 2012;156:182)	1. Risk factors: age > 60 years; low parity; personal history of endometrial, colon, or breast CA; family history of ovarian CA; and hereditary breast/ovarian CA syndrome. Use of oral contraceptives for 5 years decreases the risk of ovarian CA by 50%. (*JAMA* 2004;291:2705) 2. *Benefit:* There is inadequate evidence to determine whether routine screening for ovarian CA with serum markers such as CA-125 levels, TVU, or pelvic exams would result in a decrease in mortality from ovarian CA. *Harm:* Problems have been found of specificity (positive predictive value) and need for invasive procedures to make a diagnosis. Based on solid evidence, routine screening for ovarian CA would result in many diagnostic laparoscopies and laparotomies for each ovarian CA found. (NCI, 2008) (*JAMA.* 2011;305:2295) 3. Additionally, cancers found by screening have not consistently been found to be lower stage. (*Lancet Oncol.* 2009;10:327)	http://www.aafp.org/online/en/home/clinical/exam.html http://www.ahrq.gov/clinic/uspstf/uspsovar.htm
	AAFP USPSTF	2008 2005	Women whose family history is associated with an increased risk for deleterious mutations in *BRCA1* or *BRCA2* genes[b]	Recommends referral for genetic counseling and evaluation for *BRCA* testing. Does not recommend routine screening in this group. Screening with CA-125, TVU, and pelvic exam can be considered, but there is no evidence in this population that screening reduces risk of death from ovarian CA.		http://www.aafp.org/online/en/home/clinical/exam.html http://www.ahrq.gov/clinic/uspstf/uspsbrgen.htm

CANCER, OVARIAN

Disease Screening	Organization	Date	Population	Recommendations	Comments	Source
Cancer, Ovarian (continued)	ACOG NCCN	2009 2011	High-risk patients with *BRCA1* or 2 mutations or strong family history of ovarian CA	Recommends screening with CA-125 and TVUs at age 30–35 years or 5–10 years earlier than earliest onset of ovarian CA in family members.	4. Preliminary results from the Prostate, Lung, Colorectal and Ovarian (PLCO) Cancer Screening Trial: At the time of baseline exam, positive predictive value for invasive cancer was 3.7% for abnormal CA-125 levels, 1% for an abnormal TVU results, and 23.5% if both tests showed abnormal results. (*Am J Obstet Gynecol.* 2005;193:1630)	

[a]Lifetime risk of ovarian CA in a woman with no affected relatives is 1 in 70. If 1 first-degree relative has ovarian CA, lifetime risk is 5%. If 2 or more first-degree relatives have ovarian CA, lifetime risk is 7%. Women with 2 or more family members affected by ovarian cancer have a 3% chance of having a hereditary ovarian cancer syndrome. If *BRCA1* mutation, lifetime risk of ovarian CA is 45%–50%; if *BRCA2* mutation, lifetime risk is 15%–20%. Lynch syndrome = 8%–10% lifetime risk of ovarian CA.

[b]USPSTF recommends against routine referral for genetic counseling or routine BRCA testing of women whose family history is not associated with increased risk for deleterious mutation in *BRCA1* or *BRCA2* genes.

CANCER, PANCREATIC

Disease Screening	Organization	Date	Population	Recommendations	Comments	Source
Cancer, Pancreatic	AAFP USPSTF	2008 2004	Asymptomatic persons	Recommends against routine screening.	1. Cigarette smoking has consistently been associated with increased risk of pancreatic CA. *BRCA2* mutation is associated with a 5% lifetime risk of pancreatic CA. Blood group O with lower risk and diabetes with a 2-fold higher risk of pancreatic CA. (*J Nat Cancer Inst.* 2009;101:424. *J Clin Oncol.* 2009;27:433) 2. USPSTF concluded that the harms of screening for pancreatic CA due to the very low prevalence, limited accuracy of available screening tests, invasive nature of diagnostic tests, and poor outcomes of treatment exceed any potential benefits.	http://www.aafp.org/online/en/home/clinical/exam.html http://www.ahrq.gov/clinic/uspstf/uspspanc.htm

					CANCER, PROSTATE	
Disease Screening	**Organization**	**Date**	**Population**	**Recommendations**	**Comments**	**Source**
Cancer, Prostate	ACS	2010	Men aged ≥50 years[a]	Offer annual prostate-specific antigen (PSA) and digital rectal exam (DRE) if ≥10-year life expectancy.[b] Discuss risks and benefits of screening strategy.	1. Discouraging tests or not offering tests is not appropriate. 2. Men who ask their doctors to make the decision on their behalf should be tested.	http://www.cancer.org
	USPSTF	2012	Asymptomatic men	Do not use PSA-based screening for prostate CA. There is convincing evidence that PSA-based screening results in the detection of many cases of asymptomatic prostate CA and that a substantial percentage of men will have a tumor that will remain asymptomatic for the patient's lifetime. Because of the current inability to distinguish tumors that will remain indolent from those destined to be lethal, many men are subjected to the harms of treatment for a prostate CA that will never become symptomatic. The benefits of PSA-based screening for prostate CA do not outweigh the harms (this recommendation applies to high-risk patients as well—African American/ positive family history[c]). There is ongoing significant criticism of the USPSTF prostate screening recommendations. (*JAMA.* 2011;306:2715. *JAMA.* 2011;306:2719. *JAMA.* 2011;306:2721)	1. There is good evidence that PSA can detect early-stage prostate CA (2-fold increase in organ-confined disease at presentation with PSA screening), but mixed and inconclusive evidence that early detection improves health outcomes or mortality. 2. Two long-awaited studies add to the confusion. A U.S. study of 76,000 men showed increased prostate CA found in screened group, but no reduction in risk of death from prostate CA. A European study of 80,000 men showed a decreased rate of death from prostate CA by 20% but significant overdiagnosis (there was no difference in overall death rate). 1410 men needed to be screened and 48 cases of prostate CA were found to prevent one death from prostate CA. Patients older than age 70 years had an increased death rate in the screened group. (*N Engl J Med.* 2009;360:1310, 1320. *N Engl J Med.* 2012;366:981. *N Engl J Med.* 2012;366:1047).	http://www.ahrq.gov/clinic/uspstf/uspsprca.htm *Ann Intern Med.* 2012;157:published ahead of print. *Ann Intern Med.* 2011;155:762–771

CANCER, PROSTATE					
Disease Screening	Organization	Date	Population	Recommendations	Comments	Source
Cancer, Prostate (continued)					3. *Benefit:* Insufficient evidence to establish whether a decrease in mortality from prostate CA occurs with screening by DRE or serum PSA. *Harm:* Based on solid evidence, screening with PSA and/or DRE detects some prostate CAs that would never have caused important clinical problems. Based on solid evidence, current prostate CA treatments result in permanent side effects in many men, including erectile dysfunction and urinary incontinence. (NCI, 2008) 4. Men with localized, low-grade prostate CAs (Gleason score 2–4) have a minimal risk of dying from prostate CA during 20 years of follow-up (6 deaths per 1000 person-years). (*JAMA*. 2005;293:2095) 5. Radical prostatectomy (vs. watchful waiting) reduces disease-specific and overall mortality in patients with early-stage prostate CA (*N Engl J Med*. 2011; 364:1708). This benefit was seen only in men aged < 65 years. Active surveillance for low-risk patients (*J Clin Oncol*. 2010;28:126. *Ann Intern Med*. 2012;156:582) is safe and increasingly used as an alternative to radical prostatectomy. A gene signature profile reflecting virulence and treatment responsiveness in prostate CA is needed.	

Disease Screening	Organization	Date	Population	Recommendations	Comments	Source
CANCER, PROSTATE						
Cancer, Prostate (continued)					6. PSA velocity (> 0.5–0.75 ng/year rise) is predictive for the presence of prostate CA especially with a PSA of 4–10. (*Eur Urol.* 2009;56:573)	www.uroweb.org
	EAU	2007	Asymptomatic men	There is a lack of evidence to support or disregard widely adopted, population-based screening programs for early detection of prostate CA.		
	UK-NHS	2007	Asymptomatic men	Informed decision making.	See informational leaflet at: http://www.cancerscreening.nhs.uk/prostate/prostate-patient-info-sheet.pdf	www.cancerscreening.nhs.uk

[a]Men in high-risk groups (1 or more first-degree relatives diagnosed before age 65 years, African Americans) should begin screening at age 45 years. Men at higher risk due to multiple first-degree relatives affected at an early age could begin testing at age 40 years (http://www.cancer.org/).

[b]Men who ask their doctor to make the decision should be tested. Discouraging testing or not offering testing is inappropriate.

CANCER, SKIN						

Disease Screening	Organization	Date	Population	Recommendations	Comments	Source
Cancer, Skin (melanoma)	AAFP USPSTF	2009 2012	Adult general population	Evidence is insufficient to recommend for or against routine screening using a total-body skin exam for early detection of cutaneous melanoma, basal cell carcinoma, or squamous cell skin CA.[a,b] Recommends counseling children, adolescents, and young adults age 10–24 years who have fair skin to minimize exposure to ultraviolet radiation to reduce the risk of skin cancer.	*Benefits:* Evidence is inadequate to determine whether visual exam of the skin in asymptomatic individuals would lead to a reduction in mortality from melanomatous skin CA. *Harms:* Based on fair though unqualified evidence, visual exam of the skin in asymptomatic persons may lead to unavoidable increases in harmful consequences. (NCI, 2008). 28 million people in the United States use UV indoor tanning salons, increasing risk of squamous, basal cell cancer and malignant melanoma (*J Clin Oncol* 2012;30:1588). No guidelines for patients with familial atypical mole and melanoma–FAM-M) syndrome, although systematic surveillance warranted.[c]	http://www.aafp.org/online/en/home/clinical/exam.html http://www.ahrq.gov/clinic/uspstf/uspsskca.htm

[a]Clinicians should remain alert for skin lesions with malignant features when examining patients for other reasons, particularly patients with established risk factors. Risk factors for skin CA include: evidence of melanocytic precursors (atypical moles), large numbers of common moles (> 50), immunosuppression, any history of radiation. family or personal history of skin CA, substantial cumulative lifetime sun exposure, intermittent intense sun exposure or severe sunburns in childhood, freckles, poor tanning ability, and light skin, hair, and eye color.

[b]Consider educating patients with established risk factors for skin CA (see above) concerning signs and symptoms suggesting skin CA and the possible benefits of periodic self-exam. Alert at-risk patients to significance of asymmetry, border irregularity, color variability diameter > 6 mm, and evolving change in previous stable mole. All suspicious lesions should be biopsied (excisional or punch, not a shave biopsy) (*Ann Intern Med.* 2009;150:188) (USPSTF) (ACS) (COG)

[c]Consider dermatologic risk assessment if family history of melanoma in ≥ 2 blood relatives, presence of multiple atypical moles, or presence of numerous actinic keratoses.

CANCER, TESTICULAR

Disease Screening	Organization	Date	Population	Recommendations	Comments	Source
Cancer, Testicular	AAFP USPSTF	2008 2011	Asymptomatic adolescent and adult males[a]	Recommend against routine screening. Be aware of risk factors for testicular CA—previous testis CA (2%–3% risk of 2nd cancer), cryptorchid testis, family history of testis CA, HIV (increased risk of seminoma), Klinefelter syndrome. 3–5-fold increase in testis cancer in Caucasion men vs. other ethnicity.	*Benefits:* Based on fair evidence, screening would not result in appreciable decrease in mortality, in part because therapy at each stage is so effective. *Harms:* Based on fair evidence, screening would result in unnecessary diagnostic procedures. (NCI, 2011)	http://www.aafp.org/online/en/home/clinical/exam.html http://www.ahrq.gov/clinic/uspstf/uspstest.htm
	ACS	2004	Asymptomatic men	Testicular exam by physician as part of routine cancer-related checkup.		http://www.cancer.org
	EAU	2008	High-risk males[a]	Self-physical exam is advisable.		www.uroweb.org

[a]Patients with history of cryptorchidism, orchiopexy, family history of testicular CA, or testicular atrophy should be informed of their increased risk for developing testicular CA and counseled about screening. Such patients may then elect to be screened or to perform testicular self-exam. Adolescent and young adult males should be advised to seek prompt medical attention if they notice a scrotal abnormality. (USPSTF)

CANCER, THYROID

Disease Screening	Organization	Date	Population	Recommendations	Comments	Source
Cancer, Thyroid	AAFP	2010	Asymptomatic persons	Recommends against the use of ultrasound screening in asymptomatic persons. Be aware of higher-risk patients: radiation administered in infancy and childhood for benign conditions (thymus enlargement, acne) have an increased risk beginning 5 years after radiation and may appear more than 20 years later; nuclear fallout exposure; history of goiter; family history of thyroid disease; female gender; Asian race. (*Int J Cancer.* 2001;93:745)	Neck palpation for nodules in asymptomatic individuals has sensitivity of 15%–38%, specificity of 93%–100%. Only a small proportion of nodular thyroid glands are neoplastic, resulting in a high false-positive rate. (USPSTF)	http://www.aafp.org/online/en/home/clinical/exam.html http://www.cancer.org

CAROTID ARTERY STENOSIS

Disease Screening	Organization	Date	Population	Recommendations	Comments	Source
Carotid Artery Stenosis (CAS) (asymptomatic)	ASN USPSTF AHA/ASA ACCF/ACR/AIUM/ ASE/ASN/ICAVL/ SCAI/SCCT/SIR/ SVM/SVS	2007 2010 2012	Asymptomatic adults	Screening of the general population or a selected population based on age, gender, or any other variable alone is not recommended. Inappropriate to screen asymptomatic adult.	1. The prevalence of internal CAS of ≥ 70% varies from 0.5% to 8% based on population-based cohort utilizing carotid duplex ultrasound. General population > age 65 years estimated prevalence of 1%. No risk stratification tool further distinguishes the importance of CAS. No evidence suggests that screening for asymptomatic CAS reduces fatal or nonfatal strokes. 2. Carotid duplex ultrasonography to detect CAS ≥ 60%: sensitivity, 94%; specificity, 92%. (*Ann Intern Med.* 2007;147(12):860) 3. If true prevalence of CAS is 1%, number needed to screen to prevent 1 stroke over 5 years = 4368; to prevent 1 disabling stroke over 5 years = 8696. (*Ann Intern Med.* 2007;147(12):860)	*J Neuroimaging.* 2007;17:19–47 http://www.ahrq.gov/ clinic/uspstf/uspsacas. htm USPFT 2007 (AHRQ #08-05102-EF-1) *Stroke.* 2010:42 Appropriate Use Criteria for PVD part 1. *J Am Coll Cardiol.* 2012:60(3):242–276.

CELIAC DISEASE

Disease Screening	Organization	Date	Population	Recommendations	Comments	Source
Celiac Disease	NICE	2009	Children and adults	Serologic testing to screen for celiac disease should be performed for any of the following signs, symptoms, or associated conditions: chronic diarrhea, failure to thrive, persistent or unexplained gastrointestinal symptoms, prolonged fatigue, recurrent abdominal pain, cramping or distension, unexpected weight loss, unexplained anemia, autoimmune thyroid disease, dermatitis herpetiformis, irritable bowel syndrome, type 1 diabetes, or first-degree relatives with celiac disease.	1. Patients must continue a gluten-containing diet during diagnostic testing. 2. IgA tissue transglutaminase (TTG) is the test of choice. 3. IgA endomysial antibody test is indicated if the TTG test is equivocal. 4. Avoid anti–gliadin antibody testing. 5. Consider serologic testing for any of the following: Addison disease, amenorrhea, autoimmune hepatitis, autoimmune myocarditis, chronic immune thrombocytopenic purpura (ITP), dental enamel defects, depression, bipolar disorder, Down syndrome, Turner syndrome, epilepsy, lymphoma, metabolic bone disease, chronic constipation, polyneuropathy, sarcoidosis, Sjögren syndrome, or unexplained alopecia.	http://www.nice.org.uk/nicemedia/pdf/CG86FullGuideline.pdf

CHLAMYDIA

Disease Screening	Organization	Date	Population	Recommendations	Comments	Source
Chlamydia	CDC ICSI	2010 2010	Women aged ≤ 25 years who are sexually active	Annual screening.	1. Chlamydia is a reportable infection to the Public Health Department in every state.	http://www.cdc.gov/mmwr/pdf/rr/rr5912.pdf http://www.icsi.org/preventive_services_for_adults/preventive_services_for_adults_4.html
	CDC	2010	Women aged ≤ 35 years who are sexually active and in juvenile detention or jail	At intake and then annual screening.		http://www.cdc.gov/mmwr/pdf/rr/rr5912.pdf
	CDC	2010	Young heterosexual men	Insufficient evidence for or against routine screening.		http://www.cdc.gov/mmwr/pdf/rr/rr5912.pdf
	CDC	2010	Homosexual men	Annual testing for men who have had insertive or receptive intercourse in the past year.	1. Urine nucleic amplification acid test (NAAT) for chlamydia for men who have had insertive intercourse. 2. NAAT of rectal swab for men who have had receptive anal intercourse.	http://www.cdc.gov/mmwr/pdf/rr/rr5912.pdf

CHOLESTEROL & LIPID DISORDERS

Disease Screening	Organization	Date	Population	Recommendations	Comments	Source
Cholesterol & Lipid Disorders	USPSTF	2007	Infants, children, adolescents, or young adults (aged < 20 years)	Insufficient evidence to recommend for or against routine population lab screening.[a]	1. Childhood drug treatment of dyslipidemia lowers lipid levels but effect on childhood or adult outcomes pending. 2. Lifestyle approach is recommended starting after age 2 years.	http://www.ahrq.gov/clinic/uspstf/uspschlip.htm *Pediatrics.* 2007;120:e189–e214 *Circulation.* 2007;115:1948–1967. *Pediatrics.* 2008;122:198–208
	AHA	2007		Selective screening aged > 2 years with a parent aged < 55 years with coronary artery disease, peripheral artery disease, cerebrovascular disease, or hyperlipidemia should be screened with fasting panel.		
	Pediatrics Integrated Guidelines for CV Health and Risk Reduction in Children and Adolescents	2008 2011		Selective screening aged > 2 years if positive family history (FH) of dyslipidemia, presence of dyslipidemia, or the presence of overweight, obesity, hypertension, diabetes, or a smoking history. Universal screening in adolescents regardless of family history between 9 and 11 years and again between 18 and 21 years.	Fasting lipid profile is recommended. If within normal limits repeat testing in 3–5 years is recommended. Fasting lipid profile or nonfasting non-HDL cholesterol level.	www.nhlbi.nih.gov/guidelines/cvd_ped/index.htm. Accessed 12/9/2011

CHOLESTEROL & LIPID DISORDERS

Disease Screening	Organization	Date	Population	Recommendations	Comments	Source
Cholesterol & Lipid Disorders (continued)	NCEP III	2004	Adult men and women aged > 20 years	Check fasting lipoprotein panel (if testing opportunity is nonfasting, use nonfasting total cholesterol [TC] and high-density lipoprotein [HDL]) every 5 years if in desirable range; otherwise see management algorithm.[b]	3. There are no recommendation at which age screening should be discontinued. Screening should continue beyond age 65 years if the individual patient would benefit from long-term lipid management. (*Geriatrics*. 2000;55(8):48) 4. Treatment decisions should be based on at least two cholesterol levels. 5. Screen with fasting lipid panel to include TC, low-density-lipoprotein cholesterol (LDL-C), high-density-lipoprotein cholesterol (HDL-C), and triglycerides.	*Circulation.* 2002;106:3143–3421 *Circulation.* 2004;110: 227–239 http://www.nhlbi.nih.gov/guidelines/cholesterol/atp3upd04.htm
	USPSTF	2008	Men aged > 35 years	Grade A recommendation. Optimal screening interval uncertain.		http://www.ahrq.gov/clinic/uspstf/uspschol.htm
			Men aged 20–35 years	Only if at increased risk for coronary heart disease (CHD). Grade B recommendation.		
			Women aged > 45 years	Screen if at increased risk of CHD. Grade A recommendation.		
			Women aged 20–45 years	Screen if at increased risk of CHD. Grade B recommendation. No recommendation for or against routine screening in men aged 20–35 years or in women aged ≥ 20 years who are not at increased risk of CHD.		

CHOLESTEROL & LIPID DISORDERS

Disease Screening	Organization	Date	Population	Recommendations	Comments	Source
Cholesterol & Lipid Disorders (continued)	AAFP	2008	Men aged ≥ 35 years	Strongly recommends routine screening for lipid disorders.		http://www.acfp.org/exam/
	European Society of Cardiology/European Atherosclerosis Society	2011	Women aged ≥ 45 years	Strongly recommends screening only if at increased risk of CHD.[c]		http://www.ahrq.gov/clinic/uspstf/uspschol.htm
	Canadian Society of Cardiology	2009	Men aged > 40 years; women > 50 years	Random total cholesterol and HDL–C or fasting lipid profile, periodicity based on risk factors for all patients.		*Eur Heart J.* 2011:324(7); 1769–1818
			Men aged > 40 years: women > 50 years	May be considered based on age, if postmenopausal particularly in the presence of other risk factors. Universally based on age, presence of diabetes, hypertension, smoking, obesity, FH of CAD, chronic kidney disease, evidence of atherosclerosis, HIV infection. Erectile dysfunction, inflammatory disease.		*Can Soc Cardiol.* 2009:25(10) 567–579

[a]AHA: Low efficacy of targeted screening of children based on family history. Sensitivity and specificity of screening complicated by variability in TC and HDL based on race, gender, and sexual maturation (*Circulation*. 2007;115:1948–1967).

[b]Classify fasting TC < 200 mg/dL as desirable, 200–239 mg/dL as borderline, or ≥ 240 mg/dL as high. Classify HDL < 40 as low, and ≥ 60 as high. Classify LDL < 100 as optimal, 100–129 as near or above optimal, 130–159 as borderline high, 160–189 as high, and ≥ 190 as very high. If TC < 200 mg/dL and HDL ≥ 40 mg/dL, then repeat in 5 years; if nonfasting TC ≥ 200 mg/dL or HDL < 40 mg/dL, then check fasting lipids and risk-stratify based on LDL (see Management Algorithm). Advanced lipoprotein testing does not predict carotid intima-media thickness better than traditionally measured lipid values. (2005;142:742–750).

[c]Hypertension, smoking, diabetes, family history of CHD before age 50 years (male relatives), or age 60 years (female relatives), family history suggestive of familial hyperlipidemia.

CORONARY ARTERY DISEASE

Disease Screening	Organization	Date	Population	Recommendations	Comments	Source
Coronary Artery Disease	AAFP USPSTF	2008 2004	Adults at low risk of CHD events[a]	Recommends *against* routine screening in men and women with resting electrocardiogram (ECG), exercise treadmill test (ETT), or electron-beam CT for coronary calcium at low risk for CHD risk.[b]	USPSTF recommends against screening asymptomatic individuals due to the high false-positive results, the low mortality with asymptomatic disease, and the iatrogenic diagnostic and treatment risks.	http://www.aafp.org/online/en/home/clinical/exam.html *Circulation.* 2005;111:682–696 http://www.ahrq.gov/clinic/uspstf/uspsacad.htm 2004 *Ann Intern Med.* 2004;140:569 *Circulation.* 2005;112:771–776
	AHA ESC	2010 2003 2007	All asymptomatic adults aged ≥20 years	Framingham Risk Score, including blood pressure (BP) and cholesterol level, should be obtained. SCORE Risk System is an alternate choice. No benefit in genetic testing, advanced lipid testing, natriuretic peptide testing, high-sensitivity C-reactive protein (CRP), ankle-brachial index, carotid intimamedial thickness, coronary artery score on electron-beam CT, homocysteine level, lipoprotein (a) level, CT angiogram, MRI, or stress echocardiography regardless of CHD risk.		*Circulation.* 2007;115:402–426 *J Am Coll Cardiol.* 2010;56(25):2182–2199 http://www.uspreventiveservicestaskforce.org/uspstf/uspscoronaryhd.htm. 2009 *Eur Heart J.* 2007:28(19); 2375–2414. *J Am Coll Cardiol.* 2007:49; 378–402.

CORONARY ARTERY DISEASE

Disease Screening	Organization	Date	Population	Recommendations	Comments	Source
Coronary Artery Disease (continued)			Adults at intermediate risk of CHD events	May be reasonable to consider use of coronary artery calcium and high-sensitivity CRP (hsCRP) measurements in patients at intermediate risk according to Framingham Score.[b] hsCRP is not recommended in low- or high-risk individuals.		
	AAFP	2008	Adults at high risk of CHD events[a]	Insufficient evidence to recommend for or against routine screening with ECG, ETT, or electron-beam CT for coronary calcium, ankle-brachial index, carotid intima-media thickness.[b]		*Arch intern Med.* 2011;171(11):977–982
	AHA	2007				http://www.aafp.org/online/en/home/clinical/exam.html
	USPSTF	2009				http://www.ahrq.gov/clinic/uspstf/uspsacad.htm *Annals Intern Med.* 2009;151: 474–482

CORONARY ARTERY DISEASE

Disease Screening	Organization	Date	Population	Recommendations	Comments	Source
Coronary Artery Disease (continued)	ACCF/AHA	2010	Women	Cardiac risk stratification by the Framingham Risk Score should be used. High risk in women should be considered when the risk is ≥ 10% rather than ≥ 20%. An alternative 10-year risk score to consider is the Reynolds Risk Score, although it requires measurement of hsCRP.		AHA Guidelines. *J Am Coll Cardiol.* 2011;57(12): 1404–1423

[a]Increased risk for CHD events: older age, male gender, high BP, smoking, elevated lipid levels, diabetes, obesity, sedentary lifestyle. Risk assessment tool for estimating 10-year risk of developing CHD events available online, or *see Appendix VI* and *VII.* http://hp2010.nhlbihin.net/atpiii/calculator.asp?usertype=prof

[b]AHA scientific statement (2006): Asymptomatic persons should be assessed for CHD risk. Individuals found to be at low risk (< 10% 10-year risk) or at high risk (> 20% 10-year risk) do not benefit from coronary calcium assessment. High-risk individuals are already candidates for intensive risk-reducing therapies. In clinically selected, intermediate-risk patients, it may be reasonable to use electron-beam CT or multidetector computed tomography (MDCT) to refine clinical risk prediction and select patients for more aggressive target values for lipid-lowering therapies (*Circulation.* 2006;114:1761–1791).

DEMENTIA

Disease Screening	Organization	Date	Population	Recommendations	Comments	Source
Dementia	ICSI	2010	Adults	Insufficient evidence to recommend for or against routine dementia screening.		http://www.icsi.org/preventive_services_for_adults/preventive_services_for_adults_4.html

Disease Screening	Organization	Date	Population	Recommendations	Comments	Source
DEPRESSION						
Depression	USPSTF	2009	Children aged 7–11 years	Insufficient evidence to recommend for or against routine screening.		http://www.uspreventiveservicestaskforce.org/uspstf09/depression/chdeprart.pdf
	USPSTF	2009	Adolescents	Screen all adolescents aged 12–18 years for major depressive disorder (MDD) when systems are in place to ensure accurate diagnosis, appropriate psychotherapy, and adequate follow-up.	1. Screen in primary care clinics with the Patient Health Questionnaire for Adolescents (PHQ-A) (73% sensitivity; 94% specificity) or the Beck Depression Inventory-Primary Care (BDI-PC) (91% sensitivity; 91% specificity). See *Appendix 1.* 2. Treatment of adolescents with selective serotonin reuptake inhibitors (SSRIs), psychotherapy, or combined therapy decreases MDD symptoms. 3. SSRI may increase suicidality in some adolescents, emphasizing the need for close follow-up.	
	USPSTF ICSI	2009 2010	Adults	Recommend screening adults for depression when staff-assisted support systems are in place for accurate diagnosis, effective treatment, and follow-up.	1. Asking two simple questions may be as accurate as formal screening tools: a. "Over the past 2 weeks, have you felt down, depressed, or hopeless?" b. "Over the past 2 weeks, have you felt little or no interest or pleasure in doing things?" 2. Optimal screening interval is unknown.	http://www.uspreventiveservicestaskforce.org/uspstf09/adultdepression/addeprs.pdf http://www.icsi.org/preventive_services_for_adults/preventive_services_for_adults_4.html

DEVELOPMENTAL DYSPLASIA OF THE HIP

Disease Screening	Organization	Date	Population	Recommendations	Comments	Source
Developmental Dysplasia of the Hip (DDH)	ICSI AAFP	2010 2010	Infants	Evidence is insufficient to recommend routine screening for DDH in infants as a means to prevent adverse outcomes.	1. There is evidence that screening leads to earlier identification; however, 60%–80% of the hips of newborns identified as abnormal or suspicious for DDH by physical exam and >90% of those identified by ultrasound in the newborn period resolve spontaneously, requiring no intervention.	http://www.icsi.org/preventive_services_for_children_guideline_/preventive_services_for_children_and_adolescents_2531.html http://www.guidelines.gov/content.aspx?id=36873
	USPSTF	2006	Infants	Same recommendation as above.	The USPSTF was unable to assess the balance of benefits and harms of screening for developmental dysplasia of hip (DDH) but was concerned about the potential harms associated with treatment, both surgical and nonsurgical, of infants identified by routine screening.	

GESTATIONAL DIABETES

Disease Screening	Organization	Date	Population	Recommendations	Comments	Source
Diabetes Mellitus, Gestational (GDM)	AAFP	2010	Pregnant women	Evidence is insufficient to recommend for or against routine screening.	1. No high-quality evidence is available that shows that screening (vs. testing women with symptoms) for GDM reduces important adverse health outcomes for mothers or their infants. Also, no high-quality evidence is available on the sensitivity or specificity of GDM screening (*Ann Intern Med.* 2008;148(10):766).	http://www.guidelines.gov/content.aspx?id=36873

	DIABETES, TYPE 2				
Disease Screening	Organization	Date	Population	Recommendations	Comments	Source
Diabetes Mellitus (DM), Type 2	ADA	2012	Pregnant women	1. Screen for undiagnosed DM type 2 at first prenatal visit if aged ≥ 45 years or if risk factors for DM are present.[a] 2. For all other women, screen at 24–28 weeks with a 75-g 2-hour oral glucose tolerance test (OGTT) in the morning after an overnight fast of at least 8 hours.	1. Pre-existing diabetes if: a. Fasting glucose ≥ 126 mg/dL b. 2-hour glucose ≥ 200 mg/dL after 75-g glucose load c. Random glucose ≥ 200 mg/dL with classic hyperglycemic symptoms d. Hemoglobin A1c ≥ 6.5% 2. Criteria for GDM by 75-g 2-hour OGTT if any of the following are abnormal: a. Fasting ≥ 92 mg/dL (5.1 mmol/L) b. 1 hour ≥ 180 mg/dL (10.0 mmol/L) c. 2 hour ≥ 153 mg/dL (8.5 mmol/L)	http://care.diabetesjournals.org/content/35/Supplement_1/S11.full
	ADA	2011	Children at start of puberty or aged ≥ 10 years	1. Screen all children at risk for DM type 2[b]		

Disease Screening	Organization	Date	Population	Recommendations	Comments	Source
Diabetes Mellitus (DM), Type 2 (continued)	ADA	2011	Adults	1. Screen asymptomatic adults aged ≥ 45 years or if risk factors for DM are present.[a]	1. Australian Carbohydrate Intolerance Study in Pregnant Women (ACHOIS): Treatment of a screening-detected population with mild gestational diabetes reduced serious neonatal and maternal outcomes (*Ann Intern Med.* 2008;148(10):766).	http://www.guidelines.gov/content.aspx?id=36873
	AAFP USPSTF	2010 2010	Hypertensive adults	Screen asymptomatic adults with sustained BP (either treated or untreated) > 135/80 mm Hg.	2. Fasting plasma glucose ≥ 126 mg/dL or a casual plasma glucose ≥ 200 mg/dL, or confirmed on a subsequent day, *and precludes the need for glucose challenge.* (ADA).	http://www.ahrq.gov/clinic/pocketgd1011/pocketgd1011.pdf
	AAFP USPSTF	2010 2010	Adults	Evidence is insufficient to recommend for or against routinely screening asymptomatic adults with a BP < 135/80 mm Hg.	Screen at least every 3 years in asymptomatic adults.	

[a]DM risk factors: overweight (BMI ≥ 25 kg/m²) AND an additional risk factor: physical inactivity; first-degree relative with DM; high-risk ethnicity (eg, African American, Latino, Native American, Asian American, Pacific Islander); history of GDM; prior baby with birth weight > 9 lb; hypertension (HTN) on therapy or with BP ≥ 140/90 mm Hg; HDL-C level < 35 mg/dL (0.90 mmol/L) and/or a triglyceride level > 250 mg/dL (2.82 mmol/L); polycystic ovary syndrome; history of impaired glucose tolerance or HgbA1c ≥ 5.7%; *Acanthosis nigricans*; or cardiovascular disease.

[b]Test asymptomatic children if BMI > 85% for age/gender, weight for height > 85th percentile, or weight > 120% of ideal for height PLUS ANY TWO of the following: family history of DM in first- or second-degree relative; high-risk ethnic group (eg, Native American, African American, Latino, Asian American, or Pacific Islander); *Acanthosis nigricans*; HTN; dyslipidemia, polycystic ovary syndrome; small-for-gestational-age birth weight; maternal history of DM or GDM during the child's gestation.

DIABETES, TYPE 2

FALLS IN THE ELDERLY

Disease Screening	Organization	Date	Population	Recommendations	Comments	Source
Falls in the Elderly	NICE	2004	All older persons	Ask at least yearly about falls.[a,b,c]	1. Individuals are at increased risk if they report at least two falls in the previous year, or one fall with injury.	http://www.nice.org.uk
	AAOS	2001				*JAGS.* 2001;49:664–672
	AGS	2001			2. Calcium and vitamin D supplementation reduces falls by 45% over 3 years in women, but no effect is seen in men. (*Arch Intern Med.* 2006;166:424)	http://www.americangeriatrics.org/files/documents/health_care_pros/JAGS.Falls.guidelines.pdf
	British Geriatrics Society	2001			3. A fall prevention clinic appears to reduce the number of falls among the elderly (*Am J Phys Med Rehabil.* 2006;85:882)	http://www.bgs.org.uk/
	CTF	2005	All persons admitted to long-term care facilities	Recommend programs that target the broad range of environmental and resident-specific risk factors to prevent falls and hip fractures.[d]	4. See also page 109 for fall prevention and Appendix II. 5. 15.9% of U.S. adults aged ≥ 65 years fell in the preceding 3 months; of these, 31.3% sustained an injury that resulted in a doctor visit or restricted activity for a least 1 day. (*MMWR Morb Mortal Wkly Rep.* 2008;57(9):225)	http://www.ctfphc.org

[a]All who report a single fall should be observed as they stand up from a chair without using their arms, walk several paces, and return (see Appendix II). Those demonstrating no difficulty or unsteadiness need no further assessment. Those who have difficulty or demonstrate unsteadiness, have ≥ 1 fall, or present for medical attention after a fall should have a fall evaluation (see Fall Prevention, page 109).

[b]Risk factors: Intrinsic: lower-extremity weakness, poor grip strength, balance disorders, functional and cognitive impairment, visual deficits. Extrinsic: polypharmacy (≥ 4 prescription medications), environment (poor lighting, loose carpets, lack of bathroom safety equipment).

[c]"Free "Tip Sheet" for patients from AGS (http://www.healthinaging.org/public_education/falls_tips.php).

[d]Post-fall assessments may detect previously unrecognized health concerns.

FAMILY VIOLENCE AND ABUSE

Disease Screening	Organization	Date	Population	Recommendations	Comments	Source
Family Violence and Abuse	AAFP	2010	Children, women, and older adults	Insufficient evidence to recommend for or against routine screening of parents or guardians for the physical abuse or neglect of children, of women for intimate partner violence, or of older adults or their caregivers for elder abuse.	1. Recent studies show that screening for intimate partner violence in emergency departments and pediatric clinics shows high prevalence (10%–20%) and does not increase harm. (*Ann Emerg Med.* 2008;51:433. *Pediatrics.* 2008;121:e85) 2. In screening for intimate partner violence, women prefer self-completed approaches (written or computer-based) over face-to-face questioning. (*JAMA.* 2006;296:530) 3. All providers should be aware of physical and behavioral signs and symptoms associated with abuse and neglect, including burns, bruises, and repeated suspect trauma.	http://www.uspreventiveservicestaskforce.org/uspstf/uspsfamv.htm http://www.guidelines.gov/content.aspx?id=36873

GONORRHEA						

Disease Screening	Organization	Date	Population	Recommendations	Comments	Source
Gonorrhea	CDC	2010	Sexually active women	Annually screen all women at risk for gonorrhea.[a]	Gonorrhea is a reportable illness to state Public Health Department.	http://www.cdc.gov/mmwr/pdf/rr/rr5912.pdf
	CDC	2010	Women aged ≤ 35 years who are sexually active and in juvenile detention or jail	Screen at intake and then annual screenings.		http://www.cdc.gov/mmwr/pdf/rr/rr5912.pdf
	CDC	2010	Homosexual men	Annual testing for men who have had insertive or receptive intercourse in the past year.		http://www.cdc.gov/mmwr/pdf/rr/rr5912.pdf

[a]Women aged < 25 years are at highest risk for gonorrhea infection. Other risk factors that place women at increased risk include a previous gonorrhea infection, the presence of other sexually transmitted diseases (STDs), new or multiple sex partners, inconsistent condom use, commercial sex work, and drug use.

GROUP B STREPTOCOCCAL DISEASE

Disease Screening	Organization	Date	Population	Recommendations	Comments	Source
Group B Streptococcal (GBS) Disease	CDC	2010	Pregnant women	Universal screening of all women at 35–37 gestational weeks for GBS colonization with a vaginal-rectal swab.	Women who are colonized with GBS should receive intrapartum antibiotic prophylaxis to prevent neonatal GBS sepsis.	http://www.cdc.gov/mmwr/preview/mmwrhtml/rr5910a1.htm?s_cid=rr5910a1_w

GROWTH ABNORMALITIES, INFANT

Disease Screening	Organization	Date	Population	Recommendations	Comments	Source
Growth Abnormalities, Infant	CDC	2010	Children 0–59 months	Use the 2006 World Health Organization (WHO) international growth charts for children aged < 24 months.	1. The Centers for Disease Control and Prevention (CDC) and American Academy of Pediatricians (AAP) recommend the WHO as opposed to the CDC growth charts for children aged < 24 months. 2. The CDC growth charts should still be used for children aged 2–19 years. 3. This recommendation recognizes that breast-feeding is the recommended standard of infant feeding and therefore the standard against which all other infants are compared.	www.cdc.gov/mmwr/preview/mmwrhtml/rr5909a1.htm

Disease Screening	Organization	Date	Population	Recommendations	Comments	Source
HEARING IMPAIRMENT						
Hearing Impairment	AAFP USPSTF	2010 2008	Newborns	Routine screening of all newborn infants for hearing loss.	1. Screening involves either a one-step or a two-step process. 2. The two-step process includes otoacoustic emissions (OAEs) followed by auditory brainstem response (ABR) in those who fail the OAE test. 3. The one-step process uses either OAE or ABR testing.	http://www.guidelines.gov/content.aspx?id=36873 http://www.uspreventiveservicestaskforce.org/uspstf08/newbornhear/newbhearrs.htm
	ICSI	2010	Newborns	Universal screening of infants for congenital hearing loss should be performed during the first month of life.		http://www.icsi.org/preventive_services_for_children_guideline_/preventive_services_for_children_and_adolescents_2531.html
	AAFP ICSI USPSTF	2010 2010 2011	Adults aged >50 years	Question older adults periodically about hearing impairment, counsel about availability of hearing aid devices, and make referrals for abnormalities when appropriate. See also Appendix II: Functional Assessment Screening in the Elderly.	1. 20%–40% of adults aged > 50 years and > 80% of adults aged ≥80 years have some degree of hearing loss. 2. Additional research is required to determine if hearing loss screening can lead to improved health outcomes. 3. No harm from hearing loss screening. 4. No harm related to hearing aid use.	http://www.guidelines.gov/content.aspx?id=36873 http://www.icsi.org/preventive_services_for_adults/preventive_services_for_adults_4.html http://www.uspreventiveservicestaskforce.org/uspstf11/adulthearing/adulthearart.pdf

HEMOCHROMATOSIS

Disease Screening	Organization	Date	Population	Recommendations	Comments	Source
Hemochromatosis (hereditary)	AASLD	2011	Adults	Screen people with iron studies and a serum HFE mutation analysis if they have first-degree relatives with HFE-related hemochromatosis.	1. There is fair evidence that clinically significant disease due to hereditary hemochromatosis is uncommon in the general population. Male homozygotes for C282Y gene mutation have a 2-fold increase in the incidence of iron overload-related symptoms compared with females.	http://www.aasld.org/practiceguidelines/Practice%2)Guideline%20Archive/Diagnosis%20and%20Management%20of%20Hemochromatosis.pdf
	AAFP USPSTF	2008 2006	Asymptomatic adults	Recommends against routine genetic screening for hereditary hemochromatosis in asymptomatic adults. Patients with a family history should be counseled with further testing based on clinical considerations. (*Arch Int Med.* 2006;166:269. *Blood.* 2008;111:5375)	2. There is poor evidence that early therapeutic phlebotomy improves morbidity and mortality in screening-detected versus clinically detected individuals.	http://www.aafp.org/online/en/home/clinical/exam.html http://www.ahrq.gov/clinic/uspstf/uspshemoch.htm

HEMOCHROMATOSIS

Disease Screening	Organization	Date	Population	Recommendations	Comments	Source
Hemochromatosis (hereditary) (continued)	ACP	2005	Adults	Insufficient evidence to recommend for or against screening.[a] In case-finding for hereditary hemochromatosis, serum ferritin and transferrin saturation tests should be performed.	1. If testing is performed, cut-off values for serum ferritin levels > 200 µg/L in women and > 300 µg/L in men and transferrin saturation > 45% may be used as criteria for case-finding, but there is no general agreement about diagnostic criteria. 2. For clinicians who choose to screen, one-time screening of non-Hispanic white men with serum ferritin level and transferrin saturation has highest yield.	*Am Intern Med.* 2005;143:517–521 http://www.acponline.org/clinical/guidelines/ *N Engl J Med.* 2004;350:2383

[a]Discuss the risks, benefits, and limitations of genetic testing in patients with a positive family history of hereditary hemochromatosis or those with elevated serum ferritin levels or transferrin saturation.

HEMOGLOBINOPATHIES

Disease Screening	Organization	Date	Population	Recommendations	Comments	Source
Hemoglobinopathies	AAFP USPSTF	2010 2007	Newborns	Recommend screening all newborns for hemoglobinopathies (including sickle cell disease).	Newborn screen tests for phenylketonuria (PKU), hemoglobinopathies, and hypothyroidism.	http://www.guidelines.gov/ content.aspx?id=36873 http://www. uspreventiveservicestaskforce. org/uspstf07/sicklecell/s cklers. htm

HEPATITIS B VIRUS INFECTION, CHRONIC

Disease Screening	Organization	Date	Population	Recommendations	Comments	Source
Hepatitis B Virus (HBV) Infection, Chronic	USPSTF ACOG AAP AAFP CDC	2009 2007 2006 2010 2010	Pregnant women	Screen all women with HBsAg at their first prenatal visit.	1. Breast-feeding is not contraindicated in women with chronic HBV infection if the infant has received hepatitis B immunoglobulin (HBIG)–passive prophylaxis and vaccine-active prophylaxis. 2. All pregnant women who are HBsAg-positive should be reported to the Local Health Department to ensure proper follow-up. 3. Immunoassays for HBsAg have sensitivity and specificity > 98% (*MMWR*. 1993;42:707).	http://www.annals.org/content/150/12/1-36.full http://www.guidelines.gov/content.aspx?id=36873 http://www.cdc.gov/mmwr/pdf/rr/rr5912.pdf
	NIH AASLD	2009 2009	Adults and children	1. Recommend routine screening for HBV infection of newly arrived immigrants from countries where the HBV prevalence rate is > 2%.[a] 2. Screen all patients with chronically elevated alanine transaminase (ALT), homosexual men, persons with multiple sexual partners, injection drug users, jail inmates, dialysis patients, household contacts of persons with chronic HBV infection, and persons infected with either hepatitis C virus (HCV) or HIV.		http://www.guidelines.gov/content.aspx?id=14240 http://www.guidelines.gov/content.aspx?id=15475

[a]Immigrants from Asia, Africa, South Pacific, Middle East (except Israel), Eastern Europe (except Hungary), the Caribbean, Malta, Spain, Guatemala, and Honduras.

HEPATITIS C VIRUS INFECTION, CHRONIC

Disease Screening	Organization	Date	Population	Recommendations	Comments	Source
Hepatitis C Virus (HCV) Infection, Chronic	ACOG CDC	2007 2010	Pregnant women at increased risk[a]	Perform routine counseling and testing at the first prenatal visit.	1. Route of delivery has not been shown to influence rate of vertical transmission of HCV infection. Cesarean section should be reserved for obstetric indications only. 2. Breast-feeding is not contraindicated in women with chronic HCV infection.	www.guidelines.gov/content.aspx?id=12627 http://www.cdc.gov/mmwr/pdf/rr/rr5912.pdf
	AASLD	2009	Persons at increased risk for HCV infection[a]	Recommend HCV antibody testing by enzyme immunoassay in all high-risk adults.	1. HCV RNA testing should be performed for: a. Positive HCV antibody test result in a patient b. When antiviral treatment is being considered c. Unexplained liver disease in an immunocompromised patient with a negative HCV antibody test result d. Suspicion of acute HCV infection 2. HCV genotype should be determined in all HCV-infected persons prior to interferon treatment. 3. Seroconversion may take up to 3 months. 4. 15%–25% of persons with acute hepatitis C resolve their infection; of the remaining, 10%–20% develop cirrhosis within 20–30 years after infection, and 1%–5% develop hepatocellular carcinoma. 5. Patients testing positive for HCV antibody should receive a nucleic acid test to confirm active infection. A quantitative HCV RNA test and genotype test can provide useful prognostic information prior to initiating antiviral therapy. (*JAMA*. 2007;297:724)	www.bccdc.ca/NR/rdonlyes/9F6B2AE8-D8A9-4DCB-A83D-710045A62B3A/0/AASLD_guidelines_HEP_C_2009.pdf

HEPATITIS C VIRUS INFECTION, CHRONIC

Disease Screening	Organization	Date	Population	Recommendations	Comments	Source
Hepatitis C Virus (HCV) Infection, Chronic (continued)	AAFP	2010	General asymptomatic adults	Recommends against routine screening for HCV infection in adults who are not at increased risk.[a]		http://www.guidelines.gov/content.aspx?id=34005

[a]HCV risk factors: HIV infection; sexual partners of HCV-infected persons; persons seeking evaluation or care for STDs, including HIV; history of injection drug use; persons who have ever been on hemodialysis; intranasal drug use; history of blood or blood component transfusion or organ transplant prior to 1992; hemophilia; multiple tatooes; children born to HCV-infected mothers; and healthcare providers who have sustained a needle stick injury.

HERPES SIMPLEX VIRUS, GENITAL

Disease Screening	Organization	Date	Population	Recommendations	Comments	Source
Herpes Simplex Virus (HSV), Genital	AAFP CDC	2010 2010	Adolescents and adults	Recommends against routine serological screening for HSV.		http://www.guidelines.gov/content.aspx?id=36873 http://www.cdc.gov/mmwr/pdf/rr/rr5912.pdf
	AAFP CDC	2010 2010	Pregnant women	Recommends against routine serological screening for HSV to prevent neonatal HSV infection.	1. In women with a history of genital herpes, routine serial cultures for HSV are not indicated in the absence of active lesions. 2. Women who develop primary HSV infection during pregnancy have the highest risk for transmitting HSV infection to their infants.	http://www.guidelines.gov/content.aspx?id=36873 http://www.cdc.gov/mmwr/pdf/rr/rr5912.pdf

HUMAN IMMUNODEFICIENCY VIRUS

Disease Screening	Organization	Date	Population	Recommendations	Comments	Source
Human Immunodeficiency Virus (HIV)	AAFP USPSTF	2010 2005	Pregnant women	Clinicians should screen all pregnant women for HIV.	Rapid HIV antibody testing during labor identified 34 HIV-positive women among 4849 women with no prior HIV testing documented (prevalence, 7 in 1000). Eighty-four percent of women consented to testing. Sensitivity was 100%, specificity was 99.9%, positive predictive value was 90%. (*JAMA.* 2004;292:219).	http://www.guidelines.gov/content.aspx?id=36873 http://www.ahrq.gov/clinic/uspstf/uspshivi.htm
	CDC	2010	Pregnant women	Include HIV testing in panel of routine prenatal screening tests. Retest high-risk women at 36 weeks' gestation. Rapid HIV testing of women in labor who have not received prenatal HIV testing.		http://www.cdc.gov/mmwr/pdf/rr/rr5912.pdf
	CDC	2010	Adolescents and adults who seek evaluation and treatment for STDs	HIV screening should be offered to all people who seek evaluation for STDs and all adolescents who are sexually active or who engage in injection drug use.	1. HIV testing should be voluntary and must have a verbal consent to test. Patients may "opt out" of testing. 2. Educate and counsel all high-risk patients regarding HIV testing, transmission, risk-reduction behaviors, and implications of infection.	http://www.cdc.gov/mmwr/pdf/rr/rr5912.pdf

HUMAN IMMUNODEFICIENCY VIRUS

Disease Screening	Organization	Date	Population	Recommendations	Comments	Source
Human Immunodeficiency Virus (HIV) (continued)	AAFP	2010	Adolescents and adults at increased risk	Strongly recommends screening.	1. If acute HIV is suspected, also use plasma RNA test. 2. False-positive results with electroimmunoassay (EIA): nonspecific reactions in persons with immunologic disturbances (eg, systemic lupus erythematosus or rheumatoid arthritis), multiple transfusions, recent influenza, or rabies vaccination. 3. Confirmatory testing is necessary using Western blot or indirect immunofluorescence assay. 4. Awareness of HIV positively reduces secondary HIV transmission risk and high-risk behavior and viral load if on highly active antiretroviral therapy HAART. (CDC, 2006)	http://www.guidelines.gov/content.aspx?id=36873
	AAFP USPSTF	2010 2005	Adolescents and adults who are not at increased risk	Insufficient evidence to recommend for or against routine screening.		http://www.guidelines.gov/content.aspx?id=36873 http://www.uspreventiveservicestaskforce.org/uspstf/uspshivi.htm

aRisk factors for HIV: men who have had sex with men after 1975; multiple sexual partners; history of intravenous drug use; prostitution; history of sex with an HIV-infected person; history of sexually transmitted disease; history of blood transfusion between 1978 and 1985; or persons requesting an HIV test.

HYPERTENSION, CHILDREN & ADOLESCENTS

Disease Screening	Organization	Date	Population	Recommendations	Comments	Source
Hypertension (HTN), Children & Adolescents	AAFP Pediatrics	2006 2004 2011	Age 3–20 years[a]	Children aged ≥ 3 years should have BP measured as part of routine evaluation.	1. Hypertension: average systolic blood pressure (SBP) or diastolic blood pressure (DBP) ≥ 95th percentile for gender, age, and height on ≥ 3 occasions. See Appendices. 2. Prehypertension: average SBP or DBP 90th–95th percentile. 3. Adolescents with BP ≥ 120/80 mm Hg are prehypertensive. 4. Evaluation of hypertensive children: assess for additional risk factors. Follow-up BP: if normal, repeat in 1 year; if prehypertensive, repeat BP in 6 months; if stage 1, repeat in 2 weeks; if symptomatic or stage 2, refer or repeat in 1 week. 5. Indications for antihypertensive drug therapy in children: symptomatic HTN, secondary HTN, target-organ damage, diabetes, persistent HTN despite nonpharmacologic measures. 6. Accumulating evidence suggests that ambulatory BP monitoring is a more accurate method for diagnosis of HTN in children and allows better assessment for therapy.	http://www.aafp.org/afp/2006/0501/p.1558.html *Pediatrics.* 2004;114: 555–576 www.nhlbi.nih.gov/guidelines/cvd_ped/index.htm. Accessed 12/9/2011 *Am Fam Physician.* 2006;73 (9):1558–1568.
	NHLBI	2004	Aged 3–20 years[a]			http://www.nhlbi.nih.gov/ *Contemp Pediatr.* Oct 14, 2008
	Bright Futures	2008	Aged 3–21 years[a]	Annual screening.		http://www.brightfutures.org *Hypertension.* 2008; 52:433–451

[a]In children aged < 3 years, conditions that warrant BP measurement: prematurity; very low-birth-weight, or neonatal complications; congenital heart disease; recurrent urinary tract infections (UTIs), hematuria, or proteinuria; renal disease or urologic malformations; family history of congenital renal disease; solid-organ transplant; malignancy or bone marrow transplant; drugs known to raise BP; systemic illnesses; increased intracranial pressure.

HYPERTENSION, ADULTS						
Disease Screening	Organization	Date	Population	Recommendations	Comments	Source
Hypertension, (HTN), Adults	USPSTF AAFP USPSTF	2009 2008 2007	Adults aged >18 years	1. Screen for HTN 2. HTN > 140/90 mm Hg 3. Diagnosis after two or more BP readings obtained at least two visits over several weeks		*Am Fam Physician.* 2009;79(12):1087–1088 http://www.aafp.org/online/en/home/clinical/exam.html http://www.ahrq.gov/clinic/uspstf/uspshtype.htm
	ESH ESC	2007	Adults	The diagnosis of HTN is usually based on at least two BP readings at least two visits, although in cases of *severe BP elevation*, especially if associated with end-organ damage, the diagnosis can be based on measurements taken at a single visit.		*J Hypertens.* 2007;25:1105 http://www.escardio.org/knowledge/guidelines/Guidelines_list.htm?hit=quick
	JNC VII (NHLBI)	2003	Aged > 18 years	Normal: recheck in 2 years (see Comments). Pre-HTN: recheck in 1 year. Stage 1 HTN: confirm within 2 months. Stage 2 HTN: evaluate or refer to source of care within 1 month (evaluate and treat immediately if BP > 180/110).	1. Pre-HTN: SBP 120–139 or DBP 80–89. 2. Stage 1 HTN: SBP 140–159 or DBP 90–99. 3. Stage 2 HTN: SBP ≥ 160 or DBP ≥ 100 (based on average of ≥ 2 measurements on ≥ 2 separate office visits). 4. Perform physical exam and routine labs.[a] 5. Pursue secondary causes of HTN.[b]	*JAMA.* 2003;289:2560 *Hypertension.* 2003;42:1206

	HYPERTENSION, ADULTS				
Disease Screening	**Organiza-tion**	**Date**	**Population**	**Recommendations**	**Comments**	**Source**
Hypertension, (HTN), Adults (continued)					6. Treatment goals are for BP < 140/90, unless patient has diabetes or renal disease (< 130/80). See JNC VII Management Algorithm, page 148. 7. Ambulatory BP monitoring is a better (and independent) predictor of cardiovascular outcomes compared with office visit monitoring and is covered by Medicare when evaluating white-coat HTN. (*NEJM.* 2006;354:2368)	*J Am Coll Cardiol.* 2011;57(20): 2037–2110
	ACCF/AHA	2011	Aged > 65 years	Identification and treatment of systolic and diastolic HTN in the very elderly is beneficial in reduction in all-cause mortality and stroke death.	Increased frequency of systolic HTN compared with younger patients. HTN is more likely associated with end-organ damage and more often associated with other risk factors.	

[a]Physical exam should include: measurements of height, weight, and waist circumference; funduscopic exam (retinopathy); carotid auscultation (bruit); jugular venous pulsation; thyroid gland (enlargement); cardiac auscultation (left ventricular heave, S3 or S4, murmurs, clicks); chest auscultation (rales, evidence of chronic obstructive pulmonary disease); abdominal exam (bruits, masses, pulsations); exam of lower extremities (diminished arterial pulsations, bruits, edema); and neurologic exam (focal findings). Routine labs include urinalysis, complete blood count, electrolytes (potassium, calcium), creatinine, glucose, fasting lipids, and 12-lead electrocardiogram.

[b]Pursue secondary causes of HTN when evaluation is suggestive (clues in parentheses) of: (1) pheochromocytoma (labile or paroxysmal HTN accompanied by sweats, headaches, and palpitations); (2) renovascular disease (abdominal bruits); (3) autosomal dominant polycystic kidney disease (abdominal or flank masses); (4) Cushing syndrome (truncal obesity with purple striae); (5) primary hyperaldosteronism (hypokalemia); (6) hyperparathyroidism (hypercalcemia); (7) renal parenchymal disease (elevated serum creatinine, abnormal urinalysis); (8) poor response to drug therapy; (9) well-controlled HTN with an abrupt increase in BP; (10) SBP > 180 or DBP > 110 mm Hg; or (11) sudden onset of HTN.

	ILLICIT DRUG USE				

Disease Screening	Organization	Date	Population	Recommendations	Comments	Source
Illicit Drug Use	AAFP USPSTF ICSI	2010 2008 2010	Adults, adolescents, and pregnant women	Insufficient evidence to recommend for or against routine screening for illicit drug use		http://www.guidelines.gov/content.aspx?id=36873 http://www.uspreventiveservicestaskforce.org/uspstf08/druguse/drugrs.htm http://www.icsi.org/preventive_services_for_adults/preventive_services_for_adults_4.html

	KIDNEY DISEASE, CHRONIC					

Disease Screening	Organization	Date	Population	Recommendations	Comments	Source
Kidney Disease, Chronic (CKD)	NICE	2008	Adults	1. Monitor glomerular filtration rate (GFR) at least annually in people prescribed drugs known to be nephrotoxic.[a] 2. Screen renal function in people at risk for CKD.[b]		http://www.nice.org.uk/nicemedia/live/12069/42117/42117.pdf

[a]Examples: calcineurin inhibitors, lithium, or nonsteroidal anti-inflammatory drugs (NSAIDs).

[b]DM, HTN, cardiovascular disease, structural renal disease, nephrolithiasis, benign prostatic hyperplasia (BPH), multisystem diseases with potential kidney involvement (eg, systemic lupus erythematosus [SLE]), family history of stage 5 CKD or hereditary kidney disease, or personal history of hematuria or proteinuria.

LEAD POISONING						
Disease Screening	**Organization**	**Date**	**Population**	**Recommendations**	**Comments**	**Source**

Lead Poisoning	AAFP	2010	Children aged 1–5 years	1. Insufficient evidence to or against routine screening in asymptomatic children at increased risk.
				2. Recommends against screening in asymptomatic children at average risk.
					1. Risk assessment should be performed during prenatal visits and continue until aged 6 years.
					2. CDC personal risk questionnaire:
					  a. Does your child live in or regularly visit a house (or other facility, e.g. daycare) that was built before 1950?
					  b. Does your child live in or regularly visit a house built before 1978 with recent or ongoing renovations or remodeling (within the last 6 months)?
					  c. Does your child have a sibling or playmate who has or did have lead poisoning? (http://www.cdc.gov/nceh/lead/publications/screening.htm)
						http://www.guidelines.gov/content.aspx?id=36873

	AAFP	2010	Pregnant women	Recommends against screening in asymptomatic pregnant women.		http://www.guidelines.gov/content.aspx?id=36873

LEAD POISONING

Disease Screening	Organization	Date	Population	Recommendations	Comments	Source
Lead Poisoning (continued)	CDC	2010	Pregnant women	Routine blood lead testing of pregnant women is recommended in clinical settings that serve populations with specific risk factors for lead exposure.[a]		http://www.cdc.gov/nceh/lead/publications/LeadandPregnancy2010.pdf
	CDC	2009	Children aged 1–5 years	Recommend blood lead screening in Medicaid-eligible children at increased risk for lead exposure.[b]	Screen at ages 1 and 2 years, or by age 3 years if a high-risk child has never been screened.	http://www.cdc.gov/mmwr/preview/mmwrhtml/rr5809a1.htm

[a]Important risk factors for lead exposure in pregnant women include recent immigration, pica practices, occupational exposure, nutritional status, culturally specific practices such as the use of traditional remedies or imported cosmetics, and the use of traditional lead-glazed pottery for cooking and storing food.

[b]Child suspected by parent, healthcare provider, or Health Department to be at risk for lead exposure; sibling or playmate with elevated blood lead level; recent immigrant, refugee, or foreign adoptee; child's parent or caregiver works with lead; household member uses traditional folk or ethnic remedies or cosmetics or who routinely eats food imported informally from abroad; residence near a source of high lead levels.

MOTOR VEHICLE SAFETY						
Disease Screening	Organization	Date	Population	Recommendations	Comments	Source
Motor Vehicle Safety	ICSI	2010	Children and adolescents	Recommend that all health-care providers ask about: 1. Car seats 2. Booster seats 3. Seat belt use 4. Helmet use while riding motorcycles	One study demonstrated a 21% reduction in mortality with the use of child restraint systems versus seat belts in children aged 2–6 years involved in motor vehicle collisions. (*Arch Ped Adolesc Med.* 2006;160:617–521)	http://www.icsi.org/preventive_services_for_children._guidel ne_/preventive_services_for_children_and_adolescents_2531.html

	NEWBORN SCREENING				
Disease Screening	Organization	Date	Population	Recommendations	Comments	Source
Newborn Screening	ICSI	2010	Newborns	All newborns should receive a newborn metabolic screening test prior to hospital discharge.	The newborn screen should be performed after 24 hours of age. Infants who receive their newborn screen before 24 hours of age should have it repeated before two weeks of age.	http://www.icsi.org/ preventive_services_for_ children__guideline_/ preventive_services_for_ children_and_adolescents_ 2531.html

OBESITY					
Disease Screening	Organization	Date	Population	Recommendations	Comments	Source
Obesity	AAFP USPSTF	2010 2010	Children aged ≥ 6 years	The AAFP recommends that clinicians screen children aged 6 years and older for obesity.	Obese children should be offered intensive counseling and behavioral interventions to promote improvement in weight status.	http://www.guidelines.gov/content.aspx?id=36873 http://www.uspreventiveservicestaskforce.org/uspstf/uspschobes.htm
	ICSI	2010	Children aged ≥ 2 years	Height, weight, and body mass index (BMI) should be recorded annually starting at age 2 years.	1. Children with a BMI ≥ 25 are five times more likely to be overweight as adults compared with their normal-weight counterparts. 2. Overweight children should be counseled about wholesome eating, 30–60 minutes of daily physical activity, and avoiding soft drinks.	http://www.icsi.org/preventive_services_for_children_guideline_/preventive_services_for_children_and_adolescents_2531.html

OBESITY

Disease Screening	Organization	Date	Population	Recommendations	Comments	Source
Obesity (continued)	AAFP	2010	Adults aged > 18 years	Recommends screening all adults and offering intensive counseling and behavioral interventions to promote sustained weight loss in obese adults.	Intensive counseling involves more than 1 session per month for at least 3 months.	http://www.guidelines.gov/content.aspx?id=36873
	ICSI	2010	Adults aged > 18 years	Height, weight, and BMI should be measured at least annually.	Intensive intervention to promote weight loss should be offered to all obese adults (BMI ≥ 30 or waist circumference ≥ 40 in [men] or ≥ 35 in [women]).	http://www.icsi.org/preventive_services_for_adults/preventive_services_for_adults_4.html
	VA/DoD	2006	Adults	1. Height, weight, and BMI should be measured at least annually. 2. Waist circumference should be measured at least annually.	1. Intensive intervention to promote weight loss should be offered to: a. Obese adults (BMI ≥ 30 or waist circumference ≥ 40 in [men] or ≥ 35 in [women]) b. Overweight adults (BMI 25–29.9) with an obesity-associated condition[a]	http://www.healthquality.va.gov/obesity/obe06_final1.pdf

[a]HTN, DM type 2, dyslipidemia, obstructive sleep apnea, degenerative joint disease, or metabolic syndrome.

	OSTEOPOROSIS				
Disease Screening	Organization	Date	Population	Recommendations	Comments	Source
Osteoporosis	USPSTF ACPM	2011 2009	Women aged ≥ 65 years or younger women whose fracture risk is ≥ that of a 65-year-old white woman	Routine screening for women using either dual-energy x-ray absorptiometry (DXA) of the hip and lumbar spine or quantitative ultrasonography of the calcaneus.	1. The optimal screening interval is unclear. 2. Screening should not be performed more frequently than every 2 years. 3. Ten-year risk for osteoporotic fractures can be calculated for individuals by using the FRAX tool (http://www.shef.ac.uk/FRAX/). 4. Quantitative ultrasonography of the calcaneus predicts fractures of the femoral neck, hip, and spine as effectively as does DXA. 5. The criteria for treatment of osteoporosis rely on DXA measurements.	http://www.uspreventiveservicestaskforce.org/uspstf10/osteoporosis/osteors.htm http://www.guideline.gov/content.aspx?id=1527)
	AAFP	2010	Women aged ≥ 65 years or aged ≥ 60 years at an increased risk for osteoporotic fracture	Routine screening for osteoporosis.		http://www.guidelines.gov/content.aspx?id=36873
	USPSTF	2011	Older men	Insufficient evidence to recommend for or against routine osteoporosis screening.		http://www.uspreventiveservicestaskforce.org/uspstf10/osteoporosis/osteors.htm
	ICSI	2010	Women aged ≥ 65 years	Routine screening for osteoporosis.		http://www.icsi.org/preventive_services_for_adults/preventive_services_for_adults_4.html
	NOF ACPM	2008 2009	Men aged ≥ 70 years	Recommends routine screening via bone mineral density (BMD).	Repeat every 3–5 years if "normal" baseline score; if high risk, then every 1–2 years.	http://www.guideline.gov/content.aspx?id=15270

PHENYLKETONURIA

Disease Screening	Organization	Date	Population	Recommendations	Comments	Source
Phenylketonuria (PKU)	AAFP USPSTF	2010 2007	Newborns	Recommend screening all newborns for PKU.	Newborn screen tests for PKU, hemoglobinopathies, and hypothyroidism.	http://www.guidelines.gov/content.aspx?id=36873 http://www.uspreventiveservicestaskforce.org/uspstf07/sicklecell/sicklers.htm

RH (D) INCOMPATIBILITY

Disease Screening	Organization	Date	Population	Recommendations	Comments	Source
Rh (D) Incompatibility	AAFP USPSTF	2010 2007	Pregnant women	1. Recommend blood typing and Rh (D) antibody testing for all pregnant women at their first prenatal visit. 2. Repeat Rh (D) antibody testing for all unsensitized Rh (D)-negative women at 24–28 weeks' gestation.	Rh (D) antibody testing at 24–28 weeks can be skipped if the biological father is known to be Rh (D)-negative.	http://www.guidelines.gov/content.aspx?d=36873 http://www.uspreventiveservicestaskforce.org/3rduspstf/rh/rhrs.htm

						SCOLIOSIS

Disease Screening	Organization	Date	Population	Recommendations	Comments	Source
Scoliosis	AAFP USPSTF	2010 2004	Adolescents	Recommend against routine screening of asymptomatic adolescents for idiopathic scoliosis.		http://www.guidelines.gov/content. aspx?id=36873 http://www. uspreventiveservicestaskforce. org/3rduspstf/scoliosis/scoliors. htm

SPEECH & LANGUAGE DELAY

Disease Screening	Organization	Date	Population	Recommendations	Comments	Source
Speech & Language Delay	AAFP	2008	Preschool children	Evidence is insufficient to recommend for or against routine use of brief, formal screening instruments in primary care to detect speech and language delay in children up to age 5 years.	1. Fair evidence suggests that interventions can improve the results of short-term assessments of speech and language skills; however, no studies have assessed long-term consequences. 2. In a study of 9000 toddlers in the Netherlands, two-time screening for language delays reduced the number of children who required special education (2.7% vs. 3.7%) and reduced deficient language performance (8.8% vs. 9.7%) at age 3 years. (*Pediatrics.* 2007;120:1317.) 3. Studies have not fully addressed the potential harms of screening or interventions for speech and language delays, such as labeling, parental anxiety, or unnecessary evaluation and intervention.	http://www.aafp.org/online/en/home/clinical/exam.html http://www.ahrq.gov/clinic/uspstf/uspschdv.htm
	USPSTF	2006				

SYPHILIS

Disease Screening	Organization	Date	Population	Recommendations	Comments	Source
Syphilis	CDC AAFP USPSTF	2010 2010 2009	Pregnant women	Strongly recommends routine screening of all pregnant women at the first prenatal visit.	1. A nontreponemal test (Venereal Disease Research Laboratory [VDRL] or rapid plasma reagent [RPR] test) should be used for initial screening. 2. All reactive nontreponemal tests should be confirmed with a fluorescent treponemal antibody absorption (FTA-ABS) test. 3. Women at high risk for syphilis or who are previously untested should be tested again at 28 gestational weeks. Consider testing a third time at the time of delivery. 4. Syphilis is a reportable disease in every state.	http://www.cdc.gov/mmwr/pdf/rr/rr5912.pdf http://www.guidelines.gov/content.aspx?id= 36873 http://www.uspreventiveservicestaskforce.org/uspstf/uspssyphpg.htm
	AAFP CDC USPSTF	2010 2010 2004	Persons at increased risk[a]	Recommends screening high-risk persons.		http://www.guidelines.gov/content.aspx?id= 36873 http://www.cdc.gov/mmwr/pdf/rr/rr5912.pdf

[a]High-risk includes commercial sex workers, persons who exchange sex for money or drugs, persons with other STDs (including HIV), sexually active homosexual men, and sexual contacts of persons with syphilis, gonorrhea, chlamydia, or HIV infection.

THYROID DISEASE					
Disease Screening	Organization	Date	Population	Recommendations	Comments	Source
Thyroid Disease	AAFP ICSI	2010 2010	Adults	Insufficient evidence to recommend for or against routine screening for thyroid disease.	Individuals with symptoms and signs potentially attributable to thyroid dysfunction and those with risk factors for its development may require thyroid-stimulating hormone (TSH) testing.	http://www.guidelines.gov/content.aspx?id=36873 http://www.icsi.org/preventive_services_for_adults/ preventive_services_for_adults_4.html
	ICSI	2010	Newborns	Recommends screening for congenital hypothyroidism in newborns.		http://www.icsi.org/preventive_services_for_children_guideline_/preventive_services_for_children_and_adolescents_2531.html

THYROID DISEASE, PREGNANCY AND POSTPARTUM						
Disease Screening	Organization	Date	Population	Recommendations	Comments	Source
Thyroid Disease, Pregnancy and Postpartum	ATA	2011	Women who are pregnant or immediately postpartum	TSH levels should be obtained in first trimester for: • History of thyroid dysfunction or prior thyroid surgery • Age >30 years • Symptoms of thyroid dysfunction • Goiter • TPO antibody+ • Autoimmune disorder • History of miscarriage • History of preterm delivery • History of head or neck radiation • Family history of thyroid disease • Morbid obesity • Use of amiodarone or lithium use • Infertility • Lives in an area of severe iodine deficiency		http://thyroidguidelines.net/sites/thyroidguidelines.net/files/file/thy.2011.0087.pdf

TOBACCO USE					
Disease Screening	Organization	Date	Population	Recommendations	Comments	Source
Tobacco Use	AAFP USPSTF ICSI	2010 2009 2010	Adults	Recommends screening all adults for tobacco use and provide tobacco cessation interventions for those who use tobacco products.	The "5-A" framework is helpful for smoking cessation counseling: a. Ask about tobacco use. b. Advise to quit through clear, individualized messages. c. Assess willingness to quit d. Assist in quitting. e. Arrange follow-up and support sessions.	http://www.guidelines.gov/content.aspx?id=36873 http://www.uspreventiveservicestaskforce.org/uspstf/uspstbac2.htm http://www.icsi.org/preventive_services_for_adults/preventive_services_for_adults_4.html
	AAFP USPSTF ICSI	2010 2009 2010	Pregnant women	Recommends screening all pregnant women for tobacco use and provide pregnancy-directed counseling and literature for those who smoke		http://www.guidelines.gov/content.aspx?id=36873 http://www.uspreventiveservicestaskforce.org/uspstf/uspstbac2.htm http://www.icsi.org/preventive_services_for_adults/preventive_services_for_adults_4.html

	TOBACCO USE				
Disease Screening	Organization	Date	Population	Recommendations	Comments	Source
Tobacco Use (continued)	AAFP	2010	Children and adolescents	Evidence is insufficient to recommend for or against routine screening.	The avoidance of tobacco products by children and adolescents is desirable. It is uncertain whether advice and counseling by healthcare professionals in this area is effective.	http://www.guidelines.gov/content.aspx?id=36873
	ICSI	2010	Children and adolescents aged ≥ 10 years	Screen for tobacco use and reassess at every opportunity.	Provide ongoing cessation services to all tobacco users at every opportunity.	http://www.icsi.org/preventive_services_for_children_guideline_/preventive_services_for_children_and_adolescents_2531.html

TUBERCULOSIS, LATENT

Disease Screening	Organization	Date	Population	Recommendations	Comments	Source
Tuberculosis, Latent	CDC	2010	Persons at increased risk of developing tuberculosis (TB)	Screening by tuberculin skin test (TST) or interferon-gamma release assay (IGRA) is recommended. Frequency of testing is based on likelihood of further exposure to Tb and level of confidence in the accuracy of the results.	1. Typically, a TST is used to screen for latent Tb. 2. IGRA is preferred if: a. Testing persons who have a low likelihood of returning to have their TST read b. Testing persons who have received a Bacille Calmette-Guérin (BCG) vaccination	http://www.cdc.gov/mmwr/pdf/rr/rr5905.pdf

VISUAL IMPAIRMENT, GLAUCOMA, OR CATARACT

Disease Screening	Organization	Date	Population	Recommendations	Comments	Source
Visual Impairment, Glaucoma, or Cataract	USPSTF AAFP	2009 2010	Older adults	Insufficient evidence to recommend for or against visual acuity screening or glaucoma screening in older adults.		http://www.uspreventiveservicestaskforce.org/uspstf09/visualscr/viseldrs.htm http://www.guidelines.gov/content.aspx?id=36873
	ICSI	2010	Older adults	Objective vision testing (Snellen chart) recommended for adults aged ≥65 years.		http://www.icsi.org/preventive_services_for_adults/preventive_services_for_adults_4.html
	AAO	2011	Adults	Avoid routine genetic testing for genetically complex disorders like age-related macular degeneration and late-onset primary open-angle glaucoma.	Genotyping of such individuals should be confined to research studies until more definitive data are available.	http://one.aao.org/CE/PracticeGuidelines/ClinicalStatements_Content.aspx?cid=f84ff8ef-9772-42ea-a168-8e096ac24d00#section7
	ICSI	2010	Children ≤4 years	Vision screening recommended for children aged ≤4 years.	Screen for amblyopia, strabismus, or decreased visual acuity.	http://www.icsi.org/preventive_services_for_children__guideline_/preventive_services_for_children_and_adolescents_2531.html
	USPSTF	2011	Children 3–5 years	Vision screening for all children 3–5 years at least once to detect amblyopia.	May screen with a visual acuity test, a stereoacuity test, a cover-uncover test, and the Hirschberg light reflex test.	http://www.uspreventiveservicestaskforce.org/uspstf11/vischildren/vischildrs.htm
	USPSTF	2011	Children <3 years	Insufficient evidence for vision screening in children <3 years of age.		

2
Disease Prevention

	PRIMARY PREVENTION OF CANCER (CA): NCI EVIDENCE SUMMARY 2012		
CA Type	Minimize Risk Factor Exposure	Strength of Evidence That Modifying or Avoiding Risk Factor Will Reduce CA	Therapeutic	Strength of Evidence
Breast[a,b]	Hormone replacement therapy —About 26% increased incidence of invasive breast CA with combination hormone replacement therapy (HRT) (estrogen and progesterone) —Estrogen alone with mixed evidence—unlikely to increase risk significantly	Solid	Tamoxifen (postmenopausal and high-risk premenopausal women) —Treatment with tamoxifen for 5 years reduced breast CA risk by 40%–50% —Meta-analysis shows relative risk (RR) = 2.4 (95% confidence interval [CI], 1.5–4.0) for endometrial CA and 1.9 (95% CI, 1.4–2.6) for venous thromboembolic events	Solid
	Ionizing radiation —Increased risk occurs about 10 years after exposure. Risk depends on dose and age at exposure	Solid	Raloxifene (postmenopausal women) —Similar effect as tamoxifen in reduction of invasive breast CA but does not reduce the incidence of noninvasive tumors—studied only in postmenopausal women —Similar risks as tamoxifen for venous thrombosis, but no risk of endometrial CA or cataracts	Solid
	Obesity —In WHI, RR = 2.85 for breast CA for women > 82.2 kg compared with women < 58.7 kg	Solid	Aromatase inhibitors —Anastrozole reduces the incidence of new primary breast CAs by 50% compared with tamoxifen; similar results have been reported with letrozole and exemestane treatment	Fair
	Alcohol —RR for intake of four alcoholic drinks/day is 1.32 —RR increases about 7% for each drink per day	Solid	—There is a 65% reduction in the risk of breast CA occurrence in postmenopausal women treated with exemestane for 5 years. (*N Engl J Med.* 2011;364:2381) —Harmful effects of aromatase inhibitors include decreased bone mineral density, hot flashes, increased falls, and decreased cognitive function, fibromyalgia, and carpal tunnel syndrome	Fair

PRIMARY PREVENTION OF CANCER (CA): NCI EVIDENCE SUMMARY 2012 (CONTINUED)

CA Type	Minimize Risk Factor Exposure	Strength of Evidence That Modifying or Avoiding Risk Factor Will Reduce CA	Therapeutic	Strength of Evidence

Breast[a,b] (continued)	Factors of unproven or disproven association
	—Abortions
	—Environmental factors
	—Diet and vitamins
	  *epidemiologic studies suggest vit. D may decrease risk of breast CA—more studies needed. (*N Engl J Med.* 2011;364:1385)
	—Active and passive cigarette smoking
	—Use of statin drugs
	—Use of low-dose daily aspirin
	  *population based studies have shown reduction in breast CA risk but more data needed. (*J Clin Oncol.* 2010;25:1467. *Lancet Oncol.* 2012;13:518)
			—Fracture rate for women being treated with anastrozole was 5.9% compared with 3.7% for those being treated with tamoxifen
			Prophylactic bilateral mastectomy (high-risk women)
			—Reduces risk as much as 90%
			—About 6% of women were dissatisfied with their decision; regrets about mastectomy were less among women who opted not to have reconstruction
				Solid

			Prophylactic salpingo-oophorectomy among *BRCA*-positive women —Breast CA incidence decreased as much as 50% —Nearly all women experience some sleep disturbances, mood changes, hot flashes, and bone demineralization, but the severity of these symptoms varies greatly	Fair
			Exercise —Exercising >4 hours/week results in average risk reduction of 30%–40% The effect may be greatest for premenopausal women of normal or low body weight Breast-feeding —The RR of breast CA is decreased 4.3% for every 12 months of breast-feeding, in addition to 7% for each birth Pregnancy before age 20 years —About 50% decrease in breast CA compared with nulliparous women or those who give birth after age 35 years Bisphosphonates —Far data suggest use of bisphosphonates will reduce risk of breast CA (*Anti Cancer Agents Med Chem.* 2012 12:144)	Solid

		PRIMARY PREVENTION OF CANCER (CA): NCI EVIDENCE SUMMARY 2012 (CONTINUED)			
CA Type	Minimize Risk Factor Exposure	Strength of Evidence That Modifying or Avoiding Risk Factor Will Reduce CA	Therapeutic	Strength of Evidence
Cervical	Human papillomavirus (HPV) infection[c] —Abstinence of sexual activity; condom and/or spermicide use (RR, 0.4)	Solid	HPV-16/HPV-18 vaccination[d] —Reduces incident and persistent infections with efficacy of 91.6% (95% CI, 64.5–98.0) and 100% (95% CI, 45–100), respectively; duration of efficacy is not yet known; impact on long-term cervical CA rates also unknown but likely to be significant	Solid Solid
	Cigarette smoke (active or passive) —Increases risk of high-grade cervical intraepithelial neoplasia (CIN) or invasive CA 2- to 3-fold among HPV-infected women	Solid	Screening with Pap smears —Estimates from population studies suggest that screening may decrease CA incidence and mortality by more than 80%. Adding screening for HPV after age 30 years increases sensitivity	Fair
	High parity —HPV-infected women with seven or more full-term pregnancies have a 4-fold increased risk of squamous cell CA of the cervix compared with nulliparous women	Solid		Solid
	Long-term use of oral contraceptives —Increases risk by 3- to 4-fold —Longer use related to higher risk	Solid		

	PRIMARY PREVENTION OF CANCER (CA): NCI EVIDENCE SUMMARY 2012 (CONTINUED)			
CA Type	**Minimize Risk Factor Exposure**	**Strength of Evidence That Modifying or Avoiding Risk Factor Will Reduce CA**	**Therapeutic**	**Strength of Evidence**
Colorectal[b,c]	Excessive alcohol use, RR is 1.41 for >45 g/day (>4.5 drinks/day)	Solid	—Based on solid evidence, nonsteroidal anti-inflammatory drugs (NSAIDs) reduce the risk of adenomas, but how much this reduces the risk of CRC is uncertain. Harms include upper gastrointestinal (UGI) bleeding (4–5/1000 people/year), chronic kidney disease (CKD), and cardiovascular (CV) events[f]	Solid
	Cigarette smoking—RR for current smokers versus never smokers, 1.18	Solid	—Based on solid evidence, daily aspirin use for at least 5 years reduces CRC incidence and mortality (37%) with an absolute risk reduction from 3.1% to 1.9%. Harm of low-dose aspirin use includes about 10–30 extra cases of UGI complications per 1000 users over a 1-year period. Risk increases with age. Benefit shown in other GI cancers as well (*Lancet*. 2011;377:31;	
	Obesity—RR for woman with a body mass index (BMI) > 29 is 1.45. Similar increase seen in colorectal CA (CRC) mortality	Solid	Postmenopausal combination hormone replacement (not estrogen alone)	
	Regular physical activity—a meta-analysis of 52 studies showed a 24% reduction in incidence of CRC	Solid	—Based on solid evidence (WHI), 44% reduction seen in CRC incidence among HRT users	Solid
			—Based on solid evidence (WHI), combination HRT users have a 26% increased invasive breast CA risk, a 29% increase in coronary heart disease (CHD) events, and a 41% increase in stroke rates. These risks obviate use of HRT for CRC prevention.	
			Polyp removal	
			—Based on fair evidence, removal of adenomatous polyps reduces the risk of CRC, especially polyps > 1 cm (*Ann Intern Med*. 2011;154:22)	

PRIMARY PREVENTION OF CANCER (CA): NCI EVIDENCE SUMMARY 2012 (CONTINUED)

CA Type	Minimize Risk Factor Exposure	Strength of Evidence That Modifying or Avoiding Risk Factor Will Reduce CA	Therapeutic	Strength of Evidence
Colorectal[b,e] (continued)			—Based on fair evidence, complications of polyp removal include perforation of the colon and bleeding estimated at 7–9 events per 1000 procedures Low-fat, high-fiber diet does not reduce the risk of CRC to a significant degree Statins do not reduce the incidence or mortality of CRC Data are inadequate to show a reduction in the risk of CRC from calcium or vitamin D supplementation. Fair data that calcium intake > 1000 mg/day will increase risk of MI. (*BMJ.* 2010;341:3691)	
Endometrial	Unopposed estrogen —Use in postmenopausal women (≥ 5 years of use = 10-fold higher risk) —Obesity—risk increases 1.59-fold for each 5 kg/m^2 change in body mass —Lack of exercise—regular exercise (2 hrs/week) with 38%–48% decrease in risk —Tamoxifen—used for > 2 years has a 2.3–7.5-fold increased risk of endometrial CA (usually stage I—95% cure rate with surgery). Nulliparous women have a 35% increased risk of endometrial CA	Solid Solid Solid Solid	Oral contraception (estrogen and progesterone containing) —Use of oral contraceptions for 4 years reduces the risk of endometrial CA by 56%; 8 years, by 67%; and 12 years, by 72% Increasing parity and lactation —35% reduction vs. nulliparous women–increasing length of breast feeding with decreasing risk	Fair Fair Inadequate Solid

		Strength of Evidence That Modifying or Avoiding Risk Factor Will Reduce CA	Therapeutic	Strength of Evidence
CA Type	**Minimize Risk Factor Exposure**			
Gastric	*Helicobacter pylori* infection	Solid	Anti-*H. pylori* therapy may reduce risk but effect on mortality unclear	Inadequate
	Excessive salt intake	Fair	Dietary interventions	Inadequate
	Deficient consumption of fruits/vegetables	Fair	Smoking cessation will reduce risk by 20%–30%	
Liver	Avoidance of cirrhosis (hepatitis B and C, excessive alcohol use, hepatic steatosis in diabetes mellitus)	Fair	Hepatitis B virus (HBV) vaccination: (newborns of mothers infected with HBV) —HBV vaccination of newborns of Taiwanese mothers reduced the incidence of hepatocellular carcinoma (HCC) from 0.7 to 0.36 per 100,000 children after about 10 years	Solid
Lung	Cigarette smoking (20-fold increased risk) and second-hand exposure to tobacco smoke (20% increased risk)	Solid	No evidence that vitamin E/tocopherol, retinoids, vitamin C, or beta-carotene in any dose reduces the risk of lung CA	
	Beta-carotene, pharmacologic doses, actually increases the risk of lung CA, especially in high-intensity smokers	Solid	Minimize indoor exposure to radon, especially if smoker. Avoid occupational exposures (asbestos, arsenic, nickel, chromium)	
	Radon gas exposure	Solid		
Oral	Tobacco (in any form, including smokeless) Alcohol & dietary factors—double the risk for people who drink 3–4 drinks/day vs. nondrinkers	Solid	Oropharyngeal squamous cell CAs (tonsil and base of tongue) are related to HPV infection (type 16 and 18) in 60% of patients—related to sexual practices, number of partners, and may be prevented by HPV vaccine. (*N Engl J Med.* 2010;363:24) Inadequate evidence to suggest change in diet will reduce risk	
	Oral HPV infection—found in 6.9% of general population	Inadequate		

PRIMARY PREVENTION OF CANCER (CA): NCI EVIDENCE SUMMARY 2012 (CONTINUED)

PRIMARY PREVENTION OF CANCER (CA): NCI EVIDENCE SUMMARY 2012 (CONTINUED)

CA Type	Minimize Risk Factor Exposure	Strength of Evidence That Modifying or Avoiding Risk Factor Will Reduce CA	Therapeutic	Strength of Evidence
Ovarian	Postmenopausal use of HRT (estrogen replacement only) with a 3.2-fold increased risk after ≥ 20 years of use	Fair	Oral contraceptives —5%–10% reduction in ovarian CA per year of use, up to 80% maximum RR reduction	Solid
	Obesity —Elevated BMI including during adolescence associated with increased mortality from ovarian CA (*J Natl Cancer Inst.* 2003;95:1244)	Fair	—Increased risk of deep venous thrombosis (DVT) with oral contraceptive pill (OCP) use of about three events per 10,000 women per year; increased breast CA risk among long-term OCP users of about one extra case per 100,000 women per year	Solid
	Talc exposure and use of fertility drugs with inadequate data to show increased risk of ovarian CA		Prophylactic salpingo-oophorectomy—in high-risk women (eg, *BRCA1* or *BRCA2*) —Ninety percent reduction in ovarian CA risk and 50% reduction in breast cancer —When prior to menopause, about 50% of women experience vasomotor symptoms; 4.5-fold increased RR of heart disease	
Prostate	Family history of prostate CA in men aged < 60 years defines risk. One first-degree relative with prostate CA increases the risk 3-fold, two first-degree relatives increase the risk 5-fold. —Incidence of prostate CA in African Americans increased, occurs at a younger age, and is more virulent	Cannot be modified	Finasteride —Decreased 7-year prostate CA incidence from 25% (placebo) to 18% (finasteride), but no change in mortality —Trial participants report reduced ejaculate volume (47% → 60%); increased erectile dysfunction (62% → 67%); increased loss of libido (60% → 65%); increased gynecomastia (3% → 4.5%) Dutasteride —Absolute risk reduction of 22.8%. —No difference in prostate CA-specific or overall mortality. Increase in more aggressive CA (Gleason 7–10) in dutasteride group	Solid

PRIMARY PREVENTION OF CANCER (CA): NCI EVIDENCE SUMMARY 2012 (CONTINUED)

CA Type	Minimize Risk Factor Exposure	Strength of Evidence That Modifying or Avoiding Risk Factor Will Reduce CA	Therapeutic	Strength of Evidence
Prostate (continued)	—High dietary fat intake does not increase risk for prostate CA but is associated with aggressive cancers and shorter survivals	Fair	Vitamin E/alpha-tocopherol—inadequate data—one study showed a 17% increase in prostate CA with vit. E alone. (*JAMA*. 2011;306:1549) Selenium —No study shows benefit in reducing risk of prostate CA	Inadequate
			Lycopene—larges: trials to date show no benefit (*Am J Epidemiol*. 2010;172:566)	Inadequate
Skin	Sunburns (melanoma) Tanning booths[g]	Inadequate	Sunscreen, protective clothing, limited time in the sun, avoid blistering sunburn in adolescence and young adults (squamous cell, basal cell carcinoma of the skin and malignant melanoma)	Inadequate

[a]National Surgical Adjuvant Breast and Bowel Project (NSABP) Study of Tamoxifen and Raloxifene (STAR) trial: raloxifene is as effective as tamoxifen in reducing the risk of invasive breast CA among postmenopausal women with at least a 5-year predicted breast CA risk of 1.66% based on the Gail model (http://bcra.nci.nih.gov/brc). Raloxifene does not reduce the risk of noninvasive CA and is not associated with endometrial CA.

[b]Women's Health Initiative (WHI): alternate-day use of low-dose aspirin (100 mg) for an average of 10 years of treatment does not lower the risk of total, breast, colorectal or other site-specific CAs. There was a trend toward reduction in risk for lung CA (*JAMA*. 2005;294:47–55).

[c]Methods to minimize risk of HPV infection include abstinence from sexual activity and the use of barrier contraceptives and/or spermicidal gel during sexual intercourse.

[d]On June 8, 2006, the U.S. Food and Drug Administration (FDA) announced approval of Gardasil, the first vaccine developed to prevent cervical CA, precancerous genital lesions, and genital warts due to HPV types 6, 11, 16, and 18. The vaccine is approved for use in females aged 9–26 years. (http://www.fda.gov). A bivalent vaccine, Cervarix, is also FDA approved with activity against HPV subtypes 16 and 18 (*N Engl J Med.* 2006;354:1109–1112).

[e]Cereal fiber supplementation and diets low in fat and high in fiber, fruits, and vegetables do not reduce the rate of adenoma recurrence over a 3- to 4-year period.

[f]There is solid evidence that NSAIDs reduce the risk of adenomas, but the extent to which this translates into a reduction in CRC is uncertain.

[g]28 million Americans/year use indoor tanning salons—increased risk of squamous cell and basal cell cancers greater than melanoma.

Source: http://www.cancer.gov/cancertopics/pdq/prevention.

CATHETER-RELATED BLOODSTREAM INFECTION

Disease Prevention	Organization	Date	Population	Recommendations	Comments	Source
Catheter-Related Bloodstream Infections	IDSA	2011	Adults and children requiring intravascular catheters	1. Educate staff regarding proper procedures for insertion and maintenance of intravascular catheters. 2. Use the arm preferentially over the leg for catheter insertion. 3. Use a central venous catheter (CVC) when the duration of IV therapy is likely to exceed 6 days. 4. Avoid the femoral vein for central venous access in adult patients. 5. Subclavian vein is preferred over femoral or internal jugular vein to minimize infection risk for nontunneled CVC. 6. Use ultrasound guidance to place CVCs to minimize mechanical complications. 7. Promptly remove a CVC that is no longer essential. 8. Wash hands before and after catheter insertion, replacement, accessing, or dressing an intravascular catheter. 9. Use maximal sterile barrier precautions including a cap, mask, sterile gown, sterile gloves, and a sterile full-body drape for the insertion of CVCs. 10. Chlorhexidine skin antisepsis preferred over povidone-iodine. 11. Avoid antibiotic ointments on insertion sites.	Clean gloves should be worn when changing the catheter dressings.	http://www.cdc.gov/hicpac/BSI/01-BSI-guidelines-2011.html

DENTAL CARIES

Disease Prevention	Organization	Date	Population	Recommendations	Comments	Source
Dental Caries	AAFP	2010	Children and adolescents	Recommends fluoride supplementation to prevent dental caries for infants and children aged 6 months through 16 years residing in areas with inadequate fluoride in the water supply (< 0.6 ppm).		http://www.guidelines.gov/content.aspx?id=36873

DIABETES MELLITUS (DM), TYPE 2

Disease Prevention	Organization	Date	Population	Recommendations	Comments	Source
Diabetes Mellitus (DM), Type 2	ADA	2012	Persons with impaired glucose tolerance (IGT)[a]	1. Recommend initiation of an effective ongoing program targeting weight loss. Program should emphasize moderate activity most days of the week. 2. Consider initiation of metformin for patients at highest risk for developing diabetes (eg, HgbA1c 5.7%–6.4%, BMI 35 kg/m², those aged 60 years or older, and those with prior GDM).	1. Goal of program is weight loss of at least 7% of body weight and to encourage at least 30 minutes of moderate activity a minimum of 5 days/week. 2. Program should include follow-up counseling.	http://care.diabetesjournals.org/content/35/Supplement_1/S11.full.pdf+html

[a]IGT if fasting glucose 110–125 mg/dL, 2-hour glucose after 75-g anhydrous glucose load 140–199 mg/dL, or HgbA1c 5.7%–6.4%.

DOMESTIC VIOLENCE

Disease Prevention	Organization	Date	Population	Recommendations	Comments	Source
Domestic Violence	WHO	2010	Adolescents and adult women	Recommend school-based programs that emphasize preventing dating violence.	1. Interventions of possible, but not proven, efficacy include: a. School-based programs that teach children to recognize and avoid sexually abusive situations. b. Empowerment and relationship skills training for women. c. Programs that change social and cultural gender norms.	http://www.who.int/violence_injury_prevention/publications/violence/9789241564007_eng.pdf

Disease Prevention	Organization	Date	Population	Recommendations	Comments	Source
Driving Risk	AAN	2010	Adults with dementia	Assess patients with dementia for the following characteristics that place them at increased risk for unsafe driving: 1. Caregiver's assessment that the patient's driving ability is marginal or unsafe. 2. History of traffic citations. 3. History of motor vehicle collisions. 4. Reduced driving mileage. 5. Self-reported situational avoidance. 6. Mini-Mental Status Exam score ≤ 24. 7. Aggressive or impulsive personality.		http://www.guidelines.gov/content.aspx?id=15853

ENDOCARDITIS

Disease Prevention	Organization	Date	Population	Recommendations	Comments	Source
Endocarditis	AHA ESC	2007 2009	Endocarditis is more likely a result of random exposure to bacteremia rather than associated with procedures. Certain persons are at highest risk for adverse sequelae from endocarditis.[a]	1. Give antibiotic prophylaxis[b] before certain dental[c] as well as certain other procedures only to those patients at highest risk.[d] 2. Antibiotic prophylaxis is no longer indicated for native valvular heart disease unless previous endocarditis is present.	1. Emphasis is on providing prophylaxis to patients at greatest risk of endocarditis. 2. General consensus suggests few cases of infective endocarditis can be prevented by preprocedure prophylaxis with antibiotics.	*Circulation.* 2007;116 1736 *Eur Heart J.* 2009;30:2359–2413 *Circulation.* 2008;52:676–685

[a] Patients with prosthetic valves; previous endocarditis; selected patients with congenital heart disease (unrepaired cyanotic congenital heart disease [CHD]; completely repaired congenital heart defect with prosthetic material or device during first 6 months after procedure; repaired cyanotic CHD with residual defects at or near-repair site); and cardiac transplant recipients who develop valvulopathy.

[b] Standard prophylaxis regimen: amoxicillin (adults 2.0 g; children 50 mg/kg orally 1 hour before procedure). If unable to take oral medications, give ampicillin (adults 2.0 g IM or IV; children 50 mg/kg IM or IV within 30 minutes of procedure). If penicillin-allergic, give clindamycin (adults 600 mg; children 20 mg/kg orally 1 hour before procedure) or azithromycin or clarithromycin (adults 500 mg; children 15 mg/kg orally 1 hour before procedure). If penicillin-allergic and unable to take oral medications, give clindamycin (adults 600 mg; children 20 mg/kg IV within 30 minutes before procedure). If allergy to penicillin is not anaphylaxis, angioedema, or urticaria, options for nonoral treatment also include cefazolin (1 g IM or IV for adults, 50 mg/kg IM or IV for children); and for penicillin-allergic, oral therapy includes cephalexin 2 g PO for adults or 50 mg/kg PO for children (IM, intramuscular; IV, intravenous; PO, by mouth, orally).

[c] All dental procedures that involve manipulation of gingival tissue or the periapical region of teeth or perforation of oral mucosa only in high-risk patients.

[d] Antibiotic prophylaxis is recommended for procedures in the respiratory tract or infected skin, skin structures, or musculoskeletal tissue in high-risk patients. Antibiotic prophylaxis for genitourinary (GU) or gastrointestinal (GI) procedures is indicated with ongoing infection.

	FALLS IN THE ELDERLY				
Disease Prevention	Organization	Date	Population	Recommendations	Comments	Source
Falls in the Elderly	USPSTF	2010	Older adults	1. Recommends vitamin D supplementation (800 international units [IUs] orally daily). 2. Recommends home-hazard modification (eg, adding nonslip tape to rugs and steps, provision of grab bars, etc.) for all homes of persons aged ≥ 65 years. 3. Recommends exercise or physical therapy interventions targeting gait and balance training. 4. Insufficient evidence to recommend a multifactorial assessment and management approach for all elderly persons.	1. 30%–40% of all community-dwelling persons aged ≥ 65 years fall at least once a year. 2. Falls are the leading cause of fatal and nonfatal injuries among persons aged ≥ 65 years. 3. A review and modification of chronic medications, including psychotropic medications, is important although not proven to reduce falls.	http://www. uspreventiveservicestaskforce. org/uspstf11/fallsprevention/ fallspreves.pdf

GONORRHEA, OPHTHALMIA NEONATORUM

Disease Prevention	Organization	Date	Population	Recommendations	Comments	Source
Gonorrhea, Ophthalmia Neonatorum	AAFP USPSTF	2010 2005	Newborns	Recommend prophylactic ocular topical medication against gonococcal ophthalmia neonatorum for all newborns.		http://www.guidelines.gov/content.aspx?id=36873 http://www.uspreventiveservicestaskforce.org/uspstf/uspsgono.htm

GROUP B STREPTOCOCCAL INFECTION

Disease Prevention	Organization	Date	Population	Recommendations	Comments	Source
Group B Streptococcal (GBS) Infection	CDC	2010	Pregnant women	1. Intrapartum antibiotic prophylaxis (IAP) to prevent early-onset invasive GBS disease in newborns is indicated for high-risk pregnancies.[a] • IAP is **not** indicated for GBS colonization or GBS bacteriuria **during a previous pregnancy,** negative vaginal-rectal GBS culture, or if a cesarean delivery is performed with intact membranes and before the onset of labor (regardless of GBS screening culture status).	1. Penicillin G is the agent of choice for IAP. 2. Ampicillin is an acceptable alternative to penicillin G. 3. Cefazolin may be used if the patient has a penicillin allergy that does not cause anaphylaxis, angioedema, urticaria, or respiratory distress. 4. Clindamycin or erythromycin may be used if the patient has a penicillin allergy that causes anaphylaxis, angioedema, urticaria, or respiratory distress.	http://www.cdc.gov/mmwr/preview/mmwrhtml/rr5910a1.htm?s_cid=rr5910a1_w

[a]Indications for IAP: previous infant with invasive GBS disease; history of GBS bacteriuria during current pregnancy; positive GBS vaginal-rectal screening culture within 5 weeks of delivery; unknown GBS status with any of the following: preterm labor at < 37 gestational weeks, amniotic membrane rupture ≥ 18 hours, intrapartum fever ≥ 100.4°F (≥ 38°C); intrapartum nucleic acid amplification test positive for GBS.

HUMAN IMMUNODEFICIENCY VIRUS (HIV), OPPORTUNISTIC INFECTIONS

Disease Prevention	Organization	Date	Population	Recommendations	Comments	Source
Human Immunodeficiency Virus (HIV), Opportunistic Infections	CDC	2009	HIV—infected adults and adolescents	See table below (from the clinical practice guidelines at http://www.cdc.gov/mmwr/preview/mmwrhtml/rr5804a1.htm)		http://www.cdc.gov/mmwr/preview/mmwrhtml/rr5804a1.htm
	CDC	2009	HIV—infected children	See table below (from the clinical practice guidelines at http://www.cdc.gov/mmwr/preview/mmwrhtml/rr5811a1.htm)		http://www.cdc.gov/mmwr/preview/mmwrhtml/rr5811a1.htm

PROPHYLAXIS TO PREVENT FIRST EPISODE OF OPPORTUNISTIC DISEASE AMONG HIV-INFECTED ADULTS

Pathogen	Indication	First Choice	Alternative
Pneumocystis carinii pneumonia (PCP)	CD4+ count < 200 cells/μL (AII) or oropharyngeal candidiasis (AII) CD4 < 14% or history of AIDS-defining illness (BII) CD4+ count > 200 but < 250 cells/μL if monitoring CD4+ count every 1–3 months is not possible (BIII)	Trimethoprim-sulfamethoxazole (TMP-SMX), 1 DS PO daily (AII); or 1 SS daily (AII)	• TMP-SMX 1 DS PO tiw (BI); or • Dapsone 100 mg PO daily or 50 mg PO bid (BI); or • Dapsone 50 mg PO daily + pyrimethamine 50 PO weekly + leucovorin 25 mg PO weekly (BI); or • Aerosolized pentamidine 300 mg via Respigard III nebulized every month (BI); or • Atovaquone 1500 mg PO daily (BI); or • Atovaquone 1500 mg + pyrimethamine 25 mg + leucovorin 10 mg PO daily (CIII)
Toxoplasma gondii encephalitis	Toxoplasma IgG postive patients with CD4+ count < 100 cells/μL (AII) Seronegative patients receiving PCP prophylaxis not active against toxoplasmosis should have toxoplasma serology retested if CD4+ count decline to < 100 cells/μL (CIII) Prophylaxis should be initiated if seroconversion occurred (AII)	TMP-SMX 1 DS PO daily (AII)	• TMP-SMX 1 DS OI tiw (BIII); or • TMP-SMX 1 SS PO daily (BIII); • Dapsone 50 mg PO daily + pyrimethamine 50 mg PO weekly + leucovorin 25 mg PO weekly (BI); or • (Dapsone 200 mg + pyrimethamine 75 mg + leucovorin 25 mg) PO weekly (BIII); • (Atovaquone 1500 mg +/– pyrimethamine 25 mg + leucovorin 10 mg) PO daily (CIII)
Mycobacterium tuberculosis infection (TB) (Treatment of latent TB infection or LTBI)	(+) diagnostic test for LTBI, no evidence of active TB, and no prior history of treatment for active or latent TB (AII); (−) diagnostic test for LTBI and no evidence of active TB, but close contact with a person with infectious pulmonary TB (AII); A history of untreated or inadequately treated healed TB (ie, old fibrotic lesions) regardless of diagnostic tests for LTBI and no evidence of active TB (AII)	Isoniazid (INH) 300 mg PO daily (AII) or 900 mg PO biw (BII) for 9 months—both plus pyridoxine 50 mg PO daily (BIII); or For persons exposed to drug-resistant TB, selection of drugs after consultation with public health authorities (AII)	• Rifampin (RIF) 600 mg PO daily × 4 months (BIII); or • Rifabutin (RFB) (dose adjusted based on concomitant ART) × 4 months (BIII)

PROPHYLAXIS TO PREVENT FIRST EPISODE OF OPPORTUNISTIC DISEASE AMONG HIV-INFECTED ADULTS (CONTINUED)			
Pathogen	Indication	First Choice	Alternative
Disseminated *Mycobacterium axiom* complex (MAC) disease	CD4+ count < 50 cells/μL—after ruling out active MAC infection (AI)	Azithromycin 1200 mg PO once weekly (AI); or Clarithromycin 500 mg PO bid (AI); or azithromycin 600 mg PO twice weekly (BIII)	• RFB 300 mg PO dai y (BI) (dosage adjustment based on drug-drug interactions with ART); rule out active TB before starting RFB
Streptococcus pneumonia infection	CD4+ count > 200 cells/μL and no receipt of pneumococcal vaccine in the past 5 years (AII) CD4+ count < 200 cells/μL—vaccination can be offered (CIII) In patients who received polysaccharide pneumococcal vaccination (PPV) when CD4+ count < 200 cells/μL but has increased to > 200 cells/μL in response to ART (CIII)	23-valent PPV 0.5 mL IM × 1 (BII) Revaccination every 5 years may be considered (CIII)	
Influenza A and B virus infection	All HIV-infected patients (AI)	Inactivated influenza vaccine 0.5 mL IM annually (AIII)	
Histoplasma capsulatum infection	CD4+ count ≥ 150 cells/μL and at high risk because of occupational exposure or live in a community with a hyperendemic rate of histoplasmosis (> 10 cases/100 patient-years) (CI)	Itraconazole 200 mg PO daily (CI)	
Coccidioidomycosis	Positive IgM or IgG serologic test in a patient from a disease-endemic area; and CD4+ count < 250 cells/μL (CIII)	Fluconazole 400 mg PO daily (CIII) Itraconazole 200 mg PO bid (CIII)	

PROPHYLAXIS TO PREVENT FIRST EPISODE OF OPPORTUNISTIC DISEASE AMONG HIV-INFECTED ADULTS (CONTINUED)

Pathogen	Indication	First Choice	Alternative
Varicella-zoster virus (VZV) infection	*Pre-exposure prevention:* Patient with CD4+ count ≥ 200 cells/μL who have not been vaccinated, have no history of varicella or herpes zoster, or who are seronegative for VZV (CIII) Note: Routine VZV serologic testing in HIV-infected adults is not recommended *Postexposure–close contact with a person who has active varicella or herpes zoster:* For susceptible patients (those who have no history of vaccination or infection with either condition, or are known to be VZV seronegative [AIII])	*Pre-exposure prevention:* Primary varicella vaccination (Varivax), two doses (0.5 mL SQ) administered 3 months apart (CIII) If vaccination results in disease because of vaccine virus, treatment with acyclovir is recommended (AIII) *Postexposure therapy:* Varicella-zoster immune globulin (VariZIG) 125 IU per 10 kg (maximum of 625 IU) IM, administered within 96 hours after exposure to a person with active varicella or herpes zoster (AIII) Note: As of June 2007, VariZIG can be obtained only under a treatment IND (1-800-843-7477, FFF Enterprises)	• VZV-susceptible household contacts of susceptible HIV-infected persons should be vaccinated to prevent potential transmission of VZV to their HIV-infected contacts (BIII) *Alternative postexposure therapy:* • Postexposure varicella vaccine (Varivax) 0.5 mL, SO × 2 doses, 3 months apart if CD4+ count >200 cells/μL (CIII); or • Preemptive acyclovir 800 mg PO 5x/day for 5 days (CIII) • These two alternatives have not been studied in the HIV population
Human papillomavirus (HPV) infection	Women aged 15–26 years (CIII)	HPV quadrivalent vaccine 0.5 mL IM months 0, 2, and 6 (CIII)	
Hepatitis A virus (HAV) infection	HAV-susceptible patients with chronic liver disease, or who are injection-drug users, or men who have sex with men (AII). Certain specialists might delay vaccination until CD4+ count > 200 cells/μL (CIII)	Hepatitis A vaccine 1 mL IM × 2 doses—at 0 & 6–12 months (AII) IgG antibody response should be assessed 1 month after vaccination: nonresponders should be revaccinated (BIII)	

PROPHYLAXIS TO PREVENT FIRST EPISODE OF OPPORTUNISTIC DISEASE AMONG HIV-INFECTED ADULTS (CONTINUED)

Pathogen	Indication	First Choice	Alternative
Hepatitis B virus (HBV) infection	All HIV patients without evidence of prior exposure to HBV should be vaccinated with HBV vaccine, including patients with CD4+ count < 200 cells/µL (AII) *Patients with isolated anti-HBc:* (BII) (consider screening for HBV DNA before vaccination to rule out occult chronic HBV infection)	Hepatitis B vaccine IM (Engerix-B 20 µg/mL or Recombivax HB® 10 µg/mL) at 0, 1, and 5 months (AII) Anti-HBs should be obtained 1 month after receipt of the vaccine series (BIII)	Some experts recommend vaccinating with 40-µg doses of either vaccine (CIII)
	Vaccine nonresponders: Defined as anti-HBs < 10 IU/mL 1 month after a vaccination series. For patients with low CD4+ count at the time of first vaccination series, certain specialists might delay revaccination until after a sustained increase in CD4+ count with ART.	Revaccinate with a second vaccine series (BIII)	Some experts recommend revaccinating with 40 µg doses of either vaccine (CIII)
Malaria	Travel to disease-endemic area	Recommendations are the same for HIV-infected and noninfected patients. One of the following three drugs is usually recommended depending on location: atovaquone/proguanil, doxycycline, or mefloquine. Refer to the following website for the most recent recommendations based on region and drug susceptibility. http://www.cdc.gov/malaria/(AII)	

DS, double strength; PO, by mouth; SS, single strength; bid, twice daily; tiw, three times weekly; SQ, subcutaneous; IM, intramuscular

PROPHYLAXIS TO PREVENT FIRST EPISODE OF OPPORTUNISTIC INFECTIONS AMONG HIV-EXPOSED AND HIV-INFECTED INFANTS AND CHILDREN, UNITED STATES[a,b]

Pathogen	Indication	Preventive Regimen	
		First Choice	Alternative
		STRONGLY RECOMMENDED AS STANDARD OF CARE	
Pneumocystis pneumonia[c]	HIV-infected or HIV-indeterminate infants aged 1–12 months; HIV-infected children aged 1–5 years with CD4 count of < 500 cells/mm³ or CD4 percentage of < 15%; HIV-infected children aged 6–12 years with CD4 count of < 200 cells/mm³ or CD4 percentage of < 15%	• TMP-SMX 150/750 mg/m² body surface area per day (max: 320/1600 mg) orally divided into two doses daily and administered three times weekly on consecutive days (AI) • Acceptable alternative dosage schedules for same dose (AI): single dose orally three times weekly on consecutive days; two divided doses orally daily; or two divided doses orally three times weekly on alternate days	• Dapsone: children aged ≥ 1 month, 2 mg/kg body weight (max 100 mg) orally daily; or 4 mg/kg body weight (max 200 mg) orally weekly (BI) • Atovaquone: children aged 1–3 months and > 24 months, 30 mg/kg body weight orally daily; children aged 4–24 months, 45 mg/kg body weight orally daily (BI) • Aerosolized pentamidine: children aged ≥ 5 years, 300 mg every month by Respirgard I (Marquest, Englewood, CO) nebulizer (BI) • Doxycycline 100 mg orally daily for children > 8 years (2.2 mg/kg/day).

Malaria	Travel to area in which malaria is endemic	• Recommendations are the same for HIV-infected and HIV-uninfected children. Refer to http://www.cdc.gov/malaria/ for the most recent recommendations based on region and drug susceptibility
		• Mefloquine 5 mg/kg body weight orally 1 time weekly (max 250 mg)
		• Atovaquone/proguanil (Malarone) 1 time daily
		  11–20 kg = 1 pediatric tablet (62.5 mg/25 mg)
		  21–30 kg = 2 pediatric tablets (125 mg/50 mg)
		  31–40 kg = 3 pediatric tablets (187.5 mg/75 mg)
		  > 40 kg = 1 adult tablet (250 mg/100 mg)
			• Chloroquine base 5 mg/kg base orally up to 300 mg weekly for sensitive regions only (7.5 mg/kg chloroquine phosphate)

PROPHYLAXIS TO PREVENT FIRST EPISODE OF OPPORTUNISTIC INFECTIONS AMONG HIV-EXPOSED AND HIV-INFECTED INFANTS AND CHILDREN, UNITED STATES[a,b] (CONTINUED)

Pathogen	Indication	Preventive Regimen	
		First Choice	Alternative
		STRONGLY RECOMMENDED AS STANDARD OF CARE	
Mycobacterium tuberculosis	TST reaction ≥ 5 mm or prior positive TST result without treatment or regardless of current	• Isoniazid 10–15 mg/kg body weight (max 300 mg) orally daily for 9 months (AII) or 20–30 mg/kg body weight (max 900 mg) orally 2 times weekly for 9 months (BII)	• Rifampin 10–20 mg/kg body weight (max 600 mg) orally daily for 4–6 months (BIII)
Isoniazid-sensitive	TST result and previous treatment, close contact with any person who has contagious TB. TB disease must be excluded before start of treatment		
Isoniazid-resistant	Same as previous pathogen; increased probability of exposure to isoniazid-resistant TB	• Rifampin 10–20 mg/kg body weight (max 600 mg) orally daily for 4–6 months (BIII)	• Uncertain
Multidrug-resistant (isoniazid and rifampin)	Same as previous pathogen; increased probability of exposure to multidrug-resistant TB	• Choice of drugs requires consultation with public health authorities and depends on susceptibility of isolate from source patient	
Mycobacterium avium complex[d]	For children aged ≥ 6 years with CD4 count of < 50 cells/mm³; aged 2–5 years with CD4 count of < 75 cells/mm³; aged 1–2 years with CD4 count of < 500 cells/mm³; aged < 1 year with CD4 count of < 750 cells/mm³	• Clarithromycin 7.5 mg/kg body weight (max 500 mg) orally 2 times daily (AII), or azithromycin 20 mg/kg body weight (max 1200 mg) orally weekly (AII)	• Azithromycin 5 mg/kg body weight (max 250 mg) orally daily (AII); children aged ≥ 6 years, rifabutin 300 mg orally daily (BI)

PROPHYLAXIS TO PREVENT FIRST EPISODE OF OPPORTUNISTIC INFECTIONS AMONG HIV-EXPOSED AND HIV-INFECTED INFANTS AND CHILDREN, UNITED STATES[a,b] (CONTINUED)

Pathogen	Indication	Preventive Regimen	
		First Choice	Alternative
	STRONGLY RECOMMENDED AS STANDARD OF CARE		
Varicella-zoster virus[c]	Substantial exposure to varicella or shingles with no history of varicella or zoster or seronegative status for VZV by a sensitive, specific antibody assay or lack of evidence for age-appropriate vaccination	• Varicella-zoster immune globulin (VariZIG) 125 IU per 10 kg (max 625 IU) IM, administered within 96 hours after exposure[c] (AIII)	• If VariZIG is not available or > 96 hours have passed since exposure, some experts recommend prophylaxis with acyclovir 20 mg/kg body weight (max 800 mg) per dose orally 4 times a day for 5–7 days. Another alternative to VariZIG is intravenous immune globulin (IVIG), 400 mg/kg, administered once. IVIG should be administered within 96 hours after exposure (CIII)
Vaccine-preventable pathogens	Standard recommendations for HIV-exposed and HIV-infected children	Routine vaccinations	
Toxoplasma gondii[g]	Immunoglobulin G (IgG) antibody to *Toxoplasma* and severe immunosuppression: HIV-infected children aged < 6 years with CD4 < 15%; HIV-infected children aged ≥ 6 years with CD4 < 100 cells/mm³ (BIII)	• TMP-SMX, 150/750 mg/m² body surface area daily orally in 2 divided doses (BIII) • Acceptable alternative dosage schedules for same dosage (AI): single dose orally 3 times weekly on consecutive days; 2 divided doses orally daily; or 2 divided doses orally 3 times weekly on alternate days	• Dapsone (children aged ≥ 1 month) 2 mg/kg body weight or 15 mg/m² body surface area (max 25 mg) orally daily; PLUS pyrimethamine 1 mg/kg body weight (max 25 mg) orally daily; PLUS leucovorin 5 mg orally every 3 days (BI) • Atovaquone (children aged 1–3 months and > 24 months, 30 mg/kg body weight orally daily; children aged 4–24 months, 45 mg/kg body weight orally daily) with or without pyrimethamine 1 mg/kg body weight or 15 mg/m² body surface area (max 25 mg) orally daily; PLUS leucovorin 5 mg orally every 3 days (CIII)

PROPHYLAXIS TO PREVENT FIRST EPISODE OF OPPORTUNISTIC INFECTIONS AMONG HIV-EXPOSED AND HIV-INFECTED INFANTS AND CHILDREN, UNITED STATES[a,b] (CONTINUED)

Pathogen	Indication	Preventive Regimen	
		First Choice	Alternative
		STRONGLY RECOMMENDED AS STANDARD OF CARE	
		NOT RECOMMENDED FOR MOST CHILDREN; INDICATED FOR USE ONLY IN UNUSUAL CIRCUMSTANCES	
Invasive bacterial infections	Hypogammaglobulinemia (ie, IgG < 400 mg/dL)	• IVIG (400 mg/kg body weight every 2–4 weeks) (AI)	
Cytomegalovirus (CMV)	CMV antibody positivity and severe immunosuppression (CD4 < 50 cells/mm³)	• Valganciclovir 900 mg oral 1 time daily with food for older children who can receive adult dosing (CIII)	

[a] Abbreviations: HIV, human immunodeficiency virus; PCP, *Pneumocystis* pneumonia; TMP-SMX, trimethoprim-sulfamethoxazole; TST, tuberculin skin test; TB, tuberculosis; IM, intramuscularly; IVIG, intravenous immune globulin; IgG immunoglobulin G; CMV, cytomegalovirus; VZV, varicella-zoster virus; FDA, Food and Drug Administration.

[b] Information in these guidelines might not represent FDA approval or FDA-approved labeling for products or indications. Specifically, the terms "safe" and "effective" might not be synonymous with the FDA-defined legal standards for product approval. Letters and roman numerals in parentheses after regimens indicate the strength of the recommendation and the quality of the evidence supporting it.

[c] Daily trimethoprim-sulfamethoxazole (TMP-SMX) reduces the frequency of certain bacterial infections. TMP-SMX, dapsone-pyrimethamine, and possibly atovaquone (with or without pyrimethamine) protect against toxoplasmosis; however, data have not been prospectively collected. Compared with weekly dapsone, daily dapsone is associated with lower incidence of PCP but higher hematologic toxicity and mortality. Patients receiving therapy for toxoplasmosis with sulfadiazine-pyrimethamine are protected against PCP and do not need TMP-SMX.

[d] Substantial drug interactions can occur between rifamycins (ie, rifampin and rifabutin) and protease inhibitors and nonnucleoside reverse transcriptase inhibitors. A specialist should be consulted.

[e] Children routinely being administered intravenous immune globulin (IVIG) should receive VariZIG if the last dose of IVIG was administered > 21 days before exposure.

[f] As of 2007, VariZIG can be obtained only under a treatment Investigational New Drug protocol.

[g] Protection against toxoplasmosis is provided by the preferred anti-*Pneumocystis* regimens and possibly by atovaquone.

					HYPERTENSION (HTN)	
Disease Prevention	Organization	Date	Population	Recommendations	Comments	Source
Hypertension (HTN)	Canadian CHEP Program JNC VII ICSI 13th Edition	2012 2003 2010	Persons at risk for developing HTN[a]	Recommend weight loss, reduced sodium intake, moderate alcohol consumption, increased physical activity, potassium supplementation, and modification of eating patterns.[b]	1. A 5-mm Hg reduction in systolic blood pressure in the population would result in a 14% overall reduction in mortality due to stroke, a 9% reduction in mortality due to CHD, and a 7% decrease in all-cause mortality.	www.hypertension.ca http://www. hypertension.ca *JAMA.* 2003;289:2560–2572
	ESC	2012			2. Weight loss of as little as 10 lb (4.5 kg) reduces blood pressure and/or prevents HTN in a large proportion of overweight patients.	eurheartj.oxfordjournals. org. Joint ESC Guidelines Acquired May 15, 2012
	ACCF/AHA	2011	Patients aged >65 years	Lifestyle management is effective in all ages.		*J Am Coll Cardiol.* 2011;57(20): 2037–2114
		2010	Patients ages >80 years	A higher target SBP and DBP at >140/70 mm Hg.		*J Am J Med.* 2010;123:71–726

[a]Family history of HTN; African American (black race) ancestry; overweight or obesity; sedentary lifestyle; excess intake of dietary sodium; insufficient intake of fruits, vegetables, and potassium; excess consumption of alcohol.
[b]See Lifestyle Modifications for Primary Prevention of Hypertension on page 122.

LIFESTYLE MODIFICATIONS FOR PRIMARY PREVENTION OF HYPERTENSION

- Maintain healthy body weight for adults (BMI, 18.5–24.9 kg/m^2; waist circumference < 102 cm for men and < 88 cm for women).
- Reduce dietary sodium intake to no more than 100 mmol/day (approximately 6 g of sodium chloride or 2.4 g of sodium/day).
- Engage in regular aerobic physical activity, such as brisk walking, jogging, cycling, or swimming (30–60 minutes/day, 4–7 days/week), in addition to the routine activities of daily living. Higher intensities of exercise are not more effective.
- Limit alcohol consumption to no more than 2 drinks (eg, 24 oz [720 mL] of beer, 10 oz [300 mL] of wine, or 3 oz [90 mL] of 100-proof whiskey) per day in most men and to no more than one drink per day in women and lighter-weight persons.
- Maintain adequate intake of dietary potassium (> 90 mmol [3500 mg]/day).
- Consume a diet that is rich in fruits and vegetables and in low-fat dairy products with a reduced content of saturated and total fat (Dietary Approaches to Stop Hypertension [DASH] eating plan).
- Maintain a smoke-free environment.

Sources: http://www.hypertension.ca and *Hypertension.* 2003;42:1206–1252.
Trials of Hypertension Prevention (TDHP) long-term follow-up: risk of CV event 25% lower in sodium-reduction group (RR, 0.75; 95% CI, 0.57–0.99) (*BMJ.* 2007;334:885–892).

IMMUNIZATIONS, ADULTS						
Disease Prevention	**Organization**	**Date**	**Population**	**Recommendations**	**Comments**	**Source**
Immunizations, Adults	CDC ICSI	2011 2010	Adults	Recommend immunizing adults according to the Centers for Disease Control and Prevention (CDC) recommendations unless contraindicated (see Appendix IX).		http://www.cdc.gov/vaccines/recs/schedules/downloads/adult/mmwr-adult-schedule.pdf http://www.icsi.org/preventive_services_for_adults/preventive_services_for_adults_4.html

IMMUNIZATIONS, INFANTS AND CHILDREN

Disease Prevention	Organization	Date	Population	Recommendations	Comments	Source
Immunizations, Infants and Children	CDC ICSI	2011 2010	Infants and children aged 0–6 years	Recommend immunizing infants and children according to the CDC recommendations unless contraindicated. (See Appendix IX)		http://www.cdc.gov/vaccines/recs/schedules/downloads/child/0-6yrs-schedule-pr.pdf http://www.cdc.gov/vaccines/recs/schedules/downloads/child/catchup-schedule-pr.pdf http://www.icsi.org/preventive_service_for_children_guideline_/preventive_services_for_children_and_adolescents_2531.html

IMMUNIZATIONS, CHILDREN AND ADOLESCENTS

Disease Prevention	Organization	Date	Population	Recommendations	Comments	Source
Immunizations, Children and Adolescents	CDC ICSI	2011 2010	Children and adolescents aged 7–18 years	Recommend immunizing children and adolescents according to the CDC recommendations unless contraindicated (see Appendix IX)		http://www.cdc.gov/vaccines/recs/schedules/downloads/child/7-18yrs-schedule-pr.pdf http://www.cdc.gov/vaccines/recs/schedules/downloads/child/catchup-schedule-pr.pdf http://www.icsi.org/preventive_services_for_children_guideline_/preventive_services_for_children_and_adolescents_2531.html

INFLUENZA, CHEMOPROPHYLAXIS

Disease Prevention	Organization	Date	Population	Recommendations	Comments	Source

Influenza, Chemoprophylaxis	IDSA CDC	2009 2011	Children and adults	1. Consider antiviral chemoprophylaxis for adults and children aged ≥ 1 year at high risk of influenza complications (see Influenza, Vaccination section) when any of the following conditions are present:
				  a. Influenza vaccination is contraindicated.[a]
				  b. Unvaccinated adults or children when influenza activity has been detected in the community. Vaccinate simultaneously.
				  c. Unvaccinated adults and children in close contact with people diagnosed with influenza.
				  d. Residents of extended-care facilities with an influenza outbreak.
					1. Influenza vaccination is the best way to prevent influenza.
					2. Antiviral chemoprophylaxis is not a substitute for influenza vaccination.
					3. Duration of chemoprophylaxis is 2 weeks postvaccination in most persons but is indicated for 6 weeks in children who were not previously vaccinated or who require two vaccine doses.
					4. Chemoprophylaxis for 10 days in a household in which a family member has influenza.
					5. Agents for chemoprophylaxis of influenza A (H1N1) and B: zanamivir or oseltamivir.
						http://www.guidelines.gov/content.aspx?id=14173
						
						http://www.cdc.gov/mmwr/preview/mmwrhtml/rr60)1a1.htm?s_cid=rr6001a1_w

[a]Contraindications for influenza vaccination: anaphylactic hypersensitivity to eggs, acute febrile illness, history of Guillain-Barré syndrome within 6 weeks of a previous influenza vaccination.

Disease Prevention	Organization	Date	Population	Recommendations	Comments	Source
INFLUENZA, VACCINATION						
Influenza, Vaccination	CDC	2010	All persons aged ≥ 6 months	1. All persons aged ≥ 6 months should receive the seasonal influenza vaccine annually. 2. All children aged 6 months–8 years should receive two doses of the 2011–2012 seasonal influenza vaccine (≥ 4 weeks apart) if: a. Vaccination status is unknown. b. Persons have never received the influenza vaccine before. c. Those who did not receive the 2009 H1N1 vaccine.	1. Highest-risk groups for influenza complications are: a. Pregnant women b. Children aged 6 months–4 years c. Adults aged ≥ 50 years d. Persons with chronic medical conditions[a] e. Residents of extended-care facilities f. Morbidly obese (BMI ≥ 40) persons h. Healthcare personnel j. Household contacts or caregivers of children aged < 5 years or adults aged ≥ 50 years	http://www.cdc.gov/mmwr/preview/mmwrhtml/rr59e0729a1.htm?s_cid=rr59e0729a1_w
Influenza, Prevention	AAP	2011	Children and adolescents ≥ 6 months	Annual trivalent seasonal influenza immunization for all children and adolescents ≥ 6 months.	High-risk children include infants born prematurely, children with chronic heart disease, lung disease, kidney disease, neurologic disorders, diabetes, HIV infection, immunosuppression, sickle cell anemia, or chronic metabolic disorders.	http://pediatrics.aappublications.org/content/128/4/813.full

[a]Chronic heart, lung, renal, liver, hematologic, cancer, neuromuscular, or seizure disorders, severe cognitive dysfunction, diabetes, HIV infection, or immunosuppression.

MOTOR VEHICLE INJURY					
Disease Prevention	Organization	Date	Population	Recommendations	Comments	Source
Motor Vehicle Injury	ICSI	2010	Infants, children, and adolescents	1. Providers should ask the family about the use of car seats, booster seats, and seat belts. 2. Ask children and adolescents about helmet use in recreational activities.	1. Head injury rates are reduced by about 75% in motorcyclists who wear helmets compared with those who do not. 2. Properly used child restraint systems can reduce mortality up to 21% compared with seat belt usage in children aged 2–6 years.	http://www.icsi.org/ preventive_services_for_ children_guideline_/ preventive_services_for_ children_and_ adolescents_2531.html

MYOCARDIAL INFARCTION (MI)					
Disease Prevention	Organization	Date	Population	Recommendations	Comments	Source

In a report showing a 50% reduction in the population's CHD mortality rate, 81% was attributable to primary prevention of CHD through tobacco cessation and lipid- and blood pressure-lowering activities. Only 19% of CHD mortality reduction occurred in patients with existing CHD (secondary prevention).

Disease Prevention	Organization	Date	Population	Recommendations	Comments	Source
Myocardial Infarction (MI)	ASPC (American Society for Preventive Cardiology) USPSTF ESC	2011 2009 2012	Establish risk factors by the Framingham Heart Study in all men and women. Aspirin therapy in adults	Similar risk factors occur in men and women; although unique conditions in women; such as polycystic ovaries and pregnancy complications occur, they act through traditional risk factors 1. Recommends aspirin (ASA) usage for MI prevention in men aged 45–79 years when the potential benefit outweighs the risk. 2. Recommends against ASA usage for MI prevention in men aged < 45 years. 3. Recommends aspirin (ASA) usage for MI prevention in women aged 55–79 years when the potential benefit outweighs the risk. 4. Insufficient evidence to recommend ASA usage for CV disease prevention in men and women aged ≥ 80 years.	1. Meta-analysis concludes ASA prophylaxis reduces ischemic stroke risk in women (−17%) and MI events in men (−32%). No mortality benefit is seen in either group. Risk of bleeding is increased in both groups to a similar degree as the event rate reduction. *Initiation of therapy based on a case by case basis. (JAMA. 2006; 295:306–313. Arch Intern Med. 2012:172:209–216).*	*Clin Cardiol.* 2011:34: 658-662 http://www. uspreventiveservicestaskforce. org/uspstf/uspsasmi.htm eurheartj.oxfordjournals.org. Joint ESC Guidelines Acquired May 15, 2012
	ADA	2011 2012	Aspirin therapy in diabetes type 1 or 2	Consider ASA (75–162 mg/day) if at increased CV risk (10-year > 10% based on Framingham risk score (see Appendix VI and VII), and in men aged > 50 years or women aged > 60 years with one additional risk factor.		*Diabetes Care.* 2011:34(S1): S11–S61 *Diabetes Care.* 2012:35(1): S4–S110.

BMJ. 2005; 331(7517):614

MYOCARDIAL INFARCTION (MI)

Disease Prevention	Organization	Date	Population	Recommendations	Comments	Source
Myocardial Infarction (MI) (continued)	AHA ESC AHA/ACCF	2006 2012 2011	Dietary therapy in all children and adults	*Dietary guidelines:* (1) Balance calorie intake and physical activity to achieve or maintain a healthy body weight. (2) Consume a diet rich in vegetables and fruit. (3) Choose whole grain, high-fiber foods. (4) Consume fish, especially oily fish, at least twice a week. (5) Limit intake of saturated fats to < 7% energy, trans fats to < 1% energy, and cholesterol to < 300 mg per day by: • Choosing lean meats and vegetable alternatives • Selecting fat-free (skim), 1% fat, and low-fat dairy products • Minimizing intake of partially hydrogenated fats. (6) Minimize intake of beverages and foods with added sugars. (7) Choose and prepare foods with little or no salt. (8) If you consume alcohol, do so in moderation. (9) Follow these recommendations for food consumed/prepared inside *and* outside of the home. *Avoid use of and exposure to tobacco products.*		*Circulation.* 2006;114:82–96 eurheartj.oxfordjournals.org. Joint ESC Guidelines Acquired May 15, 2012 *J Am Coll Cardiol.* 2011: 58(23):2432–2446

Disease Prevention	Organization	Date	Population	Recommendations	Comments	Source
MYOCARDIAL INFARCTION (MI)						
Myocardial Infarction (MI) (continued)	AHA NCEP III	2002 2002	Hyperlipidemia[a]	For screening recommendations, see page 40; also see NCEP III screening and management (page 133) recommendations.	1. Short-term reduction in low-density lipoprotein (LDL) using dietary counseling by dietitians is superior to that achieved by physicians (*Am J Med.* 2000;109:549). 2. Lowest rate of recurrent events related to absolute LDL reduction (*Lancet.* 2005;366(9493): 1267–1278).	*Circulation.* 2002;106:338 *Circulation.* 2004;110: 227–239
	Cochrane	2011		Statin therapy should be employed in primary prevention only in high-risk patients (Framingham risk > 20%). Restraint should be exercised in patients at low or intermediate 10-years risk, < 10%; 10%–20%). If low or intermediate 10-year risk, calculate *lifetime risk* to better assess benefit of statin therapy.		*Cochrane Database Syst Rev.* 2011 (1): CD004816 *Am J Med.* 2012;125: 440–446 *Circulation.* 2006;113: 791–798 *N Engl J Med.* 2012;366: 321–329

MYOCARDIAL INFARCTION (MI)

Disease Prevention	Organization	Date	Population	Recommendations	Comments	Source
Myocardial Infarction (MI) (continued)	ACP	2004		Statins should be used for primary prevention of macrovascular complications if patient has type 2 DM and other CV risk factors (ages > 55 years, left ventricular hypertrophy, previous cerebrovascular disease, peripheral arterial disease, smoking, or HTN).		*N Engl J Med.* 2012;366:321–329 *Ann Intern Med.* 2004;140:644–649
	FDA Warning	2012		Statins may cause nonserious reversible cognitive side effects as well as increased blood sugar and HbA1c levels.	No longer required to monitor liver enzymes.	
	JNC VII	2003	HTN	See page 148 for JNC VI treatment algorithms.		*Hypertension.* 2003;42:1206–1252
	AHA AHA/ACCF	2007 2011		Goal: Blood pressure (BP) < 140/90 mm Hg for general population.		*Circulation.* 2007;115:2761–2788 *Am Coll Cardiol* 58:58(23):2432–2446
	ESC	2012		< 130/80 mm Hg goal in diabetics and other high-risk patients has not been supported by trials. No benefit and possible harm is suggested with SBP < 130 mm Hg. Elderly patients goal is < 160 mm Hg.		eurheartj.oxfordjournals. org. Joint ESC Guidelines Acquired May 15, 2012

	MYOCARDIAL INFARCTION (MI)					
Disease Prevention	Organization	Date	Population	Recommendations	Comments	Source
Myocardial Infarction (MI) (continued)	ADA	2012	Diabetes mellitus	Goals: Normal fasting glucose (≤126 mg/dL) and HbA1c (<6.5%), BP <130/80 mm Hg; low-density-lipoprotein cholesterol (LDL–C) <100 mg/dL (or <70 for high risk), high-density-lipoprotein cholesterol (HDL–C) >50 mg/dL and triglycerides <150 mg/dL.	1. Intensive glucose lowering should be avoided in patients with a history of hypoglycemic spells, advanced microvascular or macrovascular complications, long-standing DM, or if extensive comorbid conditions are present.	*Diabetes Care.* 2012;35 (S11–S71) *Diabetes Care.* 2009;32(1):187–192 *Circulation.* 2006;114: 82–96
	AHA ADA	2006 2012		Advise all patients not to smoke.	2. DM with BP readings of 130–139/80–89 mm Hg that persist after lifestyle and behavioral therapy should be treated with ACE inhibitor or ARB agents. Multiple agents are often needed. *Administer at least one agent at bedtime.* No advantage of combining ACE inhibitor and ARB in HTN Rx (ONTARGET Trial). *N Engl J Med.* 2008;358:1547–1559.	*Circulation.* 2006;114: 82–96 *N Engl J Med.* 2008;358:1547–1559 *N Engl J Med.* 2008;358:2545–2559 *N Engl J Med.* 2008;358:2560–2572

Disease Prevention	Organization	Date	Population	Recommendations	Comments	Source
MYOCARDIAL INFARCTION (MI)						
Myocardial Infarction (MI) (continued)	AHA	2011	Women	Standard CVD lifestyle recommendations, PLUS: Waist circumference ≤35 in Omega-3 fatty acids if high risk (EPA 1800 mg/d).[a] BP < 120/80 mm Hg. Lipids: LDL-C < 100 mg/dL, HDL-C > 50 mg/dL, triglycerides < 150 mg/dL. ASA (75–325 mg/day) indicated only in high-risk women.[a] In women aged ≥ 65 years, *consider* ASA (81 mg daily or 100 mg every other day) if BP is controlled and the benefit of ischemic stroke and MI prevention is likely to outweigh the risk of a GI bleed and hemorrhagic stroke.	Estrogen plus progestin hormone therapy should not be used or continued. Antioxidants (vitamin E, C, and beta-carotene), folic acid, and B_{12} supplementation are not recommended to prevent CHD. ASA is not indicated to prevent MI in low-risk women aged < 65 years.	*J Am Coll Cardiol.* 2011;57(12):1404–1423
	ESC	2007 2012	Adults at risk of CV disease	Smoking cessation. Weight reduction if BMI ≥ 25 kg/m² or waist circumference ≥ 88 cm in women and ≥ 102 cm in men. No further weight gain if waist circumference 80–88 cm in women and 94–102 cm in men. Thirty minutes of moderately vigorous exercise on most days of the week.	European Society of Cardiology recommends using the SCORE Risk System to estimate risk of atherosclerotic CV disease.	*Euro Heart J.* 2007;28:2375 eurheartj.oxfordjournals. org. Joint ESC Guidelines Acquired May 15, 2012

MYOCARDIAL INFARCTION (MI)

Disease Prevention	Organization	Date	Population	Recommendations	Comments	Source
Myocardial Infarction (MI) (continued)				Healthy diet. Antihypertensives when BP ≥ 140/90 mm Hg. Statins when total cholesterol ≥ 190 mg/dL or LDL ≥ 115 mg/dL. In patients with known CV disease: ASA and statins. In patients with DM: glucose-lowering drugs.		

[a]High risk: CHD or risk equivalent or 10-year absolute CHD risk > 20% based on Framingham risk score (see Appendix VI and VII).

	NEURAL TUBE DEFECTS				
Disease Prevention	Organization	Date	Population	Recommendations	Comments	Source

Disease Prevention	Organization	Date	Population	Recommendations	Comments	Source
Neural Tube Defects	AAFP USPSTF ICSI	2010 2009 2010	Women planning or capable of pregnancy	Recommend that all women of childbearing age take a daily supplement containing 400–800 mcg of folic acid.	1. Women planning a pregnancy should start folic acid supplementation at least 1 month before conception and continue through the first 2–3 months of pregnancy. 2. The ACOG and AAFP recommend 4 mg/day folic acid for women with a history of a child affected by a neural tt be defect.	http://www.guidelines.gov/content.aspx?id=36873 http://www.uspreventiveservicestaskforce.org/uspstf09/folicacid/folicacidrs.htm http://www.icsi.org/preventive_services_for_adults/preventive_services_for_adults_4.html

Disease Prevention	Organization	Date	Population	Recommendations	Comments	Source
					OBESITY	

Obesity	ICSI	2009	Adolescents and adults	1. Recommends a team approach for weight management in all persons of normal weight (BMI 18.5–24.9) or overweight (BMI 25–29.9) including:
				  a Nutrition
				  b. Physical activity
				  c. Lifestyle changes
				  d. Screen for depression
				  e. Screen for eating disorders
				  f. Review medication list and assess if any medications can interfere with weight loss
				2. Recommend regular follow-up to reinforce principles of weight management.
					1. Recommend 30–60 minutes of moderate physical activity on most days of the week.
					2. Nutrition education focused on decreased caloric intake, encouraging healthy food choices, and managing restaurant and social eating situations.
					3. Weekly weight checks
					4. Encourage non-food rewards for positive reinforcement.
					5. Stress management techniques.
						http://www.guidelines.gov/content.aspx?id=14178

	Endocrine Society	2008	Children	1. Recommends exclusive breast-feeding for at least 6 months. 2. Educate children and parents about healthy diets and the importance of regular physical activity. 3. Encourage school systems to promote healthy eating habits and provide health education courses. 4. Clinicians should help to educate communities about healthy dietary and activity habits.	1. Avoid the consumption of calorie-dense, nutrient-poor foods (eg, juices, soft drinks, "fast food" items, and calorie-dense snacks). 2. Control calorie intake by portion control. 3. Reduce saturated dietary fat intake for children aged > 2 years. 4. Increase dietary fiber, fruits, and vegetables. 5. Eat regular, scheduled meals and avoid snacking. 6. Limit television, video games, and computer time to 2 hours daily.	http://www.guidelines.gov/content.aspx?id=13572

OSTEOPOROTIC HIP FRACTURES

Disease Prevention	Organization	Date	Population	Recommendations	Comments	Source
Osteoporotic Hip Fractures	AAFP USPSTF	2010 2005	Postmenopausal women	Recommend against the routine use of combined estrogen and progestin for the prevention of osteoporotic fractures	The results of studies including the WHI and the Heart and Estrogen/Progestin Replacement Study reveal that HRT probably reduces osteoporotic hip and vertebral fractures and may decrease the risk of colon CA; however, HRT may lead to an increased risk of breast CA, stroke, cholecystitis, dementia, and venous thromboembolism. HRT does not decrease the risk of coronary artery disease.	http://www.guidelines.gov/content.aspx?id=36873 http://www.uspreventiveservicestaskforce.org/uspstf/uspspmho.htm
	AAFP USPSTF	2010 2005	Postmenopausal women who have had a hysterectomy	Recommend against the routine use of estrogen for the prevention of osteoporotic fractures in postmenopausal women who have had a hysterectomy.		http://www.guidelines.gov/content.aspx?id=36873 http://www.uspreventiveservicestaskforce.org/uspstf/uspspmho.htm

Disease Prevention	Organization	Date	Population	Recommendations	Comments	Source
					PRESSURE ULCERS	
Pressure Ulcers	ICSI WONCA	2010 2010	Adults or children with impaired mobility	1. Recommend a risk assessment of all persons in both outpatient and inpatient settings (eg, the Braden Scale in adults and Braden Q Scale in children). 2. Recommend education of patient, family, and caregivers regarding the causes and risk factors of pressure ulcers. 3. Recommend caution when using compression stockings with lower-extremity arterial disease. 4. Avoid thigh-high stockings when compression stockings are used. a. Avoid dragging patient when moving. b. Pad skin-to-skin contact. c. Lubricate or powder bed pans prior to placing under patient. d. Keep skin moisturized.	1. Outpatient risk assessment for pressure ulcers: a. Is the patient bed- or wheelchair-bound? b. Does the patient require assistance for transfers? c. Is the patient incontinent of urine or stool? d. Any history of pressure ulcers? e. Does the patient have a clinical condition placing him/her at risk for pressure ulcers? i. DM ii. Peripheral vascular disease iii. Stroke iv. Polytrauma v. Musculoskeletal disorders (fractures or contractures)	http://www. guidelines.gov/ content. aspx?id=16004 http://www. guidelines.gov/ content. aspx?id=23868

	PRESSURE ULCERS				
Disease Prevention	Organization	Date	Population	Recommendations	Comments

Pressure Ulcers (continued)				5. Recommend minimizing pressure on skin, especially areas with bony prominences.
				  a. Turn patient side-to-side every 2 hours.
				  b. Pad areas over bony prominences
				  c. Use heel protectors or place pillows under calves.
				  d. Consider a bariatric bed for patients weighing over 500 lb.
				6. Recommend managing moisture.
				  a. Moisture barrier protectant on skin
				  b. Frequent diaper changes
				  c. Scheduled toileting
				  d. Treat candidiasis if present
				  e. Consider a rectal tube for stool incontinence with diarrhea
				7. Recommend maintaining adequate nutrition and hydration.
				8. Recommend keeping the head of the bed at or less than 30° elevation.
					vi. Spinal cord injury
					  vii. Guillain-Barré syndrome
					  viii. Multiple sclerosis
					  ix. CA
					  x. Chronic obstructive pulmonary disease
					  xi. Coronary heart failure
					  xii. Dementia
					  xiii. Preterm neonate
					  xiv. Cerebral palsy
					f. Does the patient appear malnourished?
					g. Is equipment in use that could contribute to ulcer development (eg, oxygen tubing, prosthetic devices, urinary catheters)?

Source

SEXUALLY TRANSMITTED INFECTIONS						
Disease Prevention	Organization	Date	Population	Recommendations	Comments	Source
Sexually Transmitted Infections (STIs)	AAFP USPSTF	2010 2008	Sexually active adolescents and high-risk adults	Recommend high-intensity behavioral counseling to prevent sexually transmitted infections for all sexually active adolescents and for adults at increased risk for STIs.		http://www.guidelines.gov/content.aspx?id=36873 http://www.uspreventiveservicestaskforce.org/uspstf/uspsstds.htm

Disease Prevention	Organization	Date	Population	Recommendations	Comments	Source
STROKE						
Stroke[a]	AHA/ASA	2011	Treat all known CV risk factors	Screen and treat BP to < 140/90 mm Hg.	1. Strokes and nonfatal strokes are reduced in diabetic patients by lower BP targets (< 130/80 mm Hg). In the absence of harm, this benefit appears to justify the lower BP goal.	*Stroke.* 2011;42: 517–584
	AHA/ASA	2006	HTN	If HTN with diabetes or renal disease, treat to < 130/80 mm Hg.		*Stroke.* 2006;37: 1583–1633 *Chest.* 2004;126: 429S–456S
			Atrial fibrillation	1. Prioritize rate control; consider rhythm control if this is the first event, if it occurs in a young patient with minimal heart disease, or if symptomatic. 2. Rate control goal is < 110 beats per minute (bpm) in patient with stable ventricular function (ejection fraction [EF] > 40%). 3. Antithrombotic therapy is required. Anticoagulation or antiplatelet therapy is determined by ACC/AHA or CHASD2 (nonvalvular atrial fibrillation) Guidelines.	2. Average stroke rate in patients with risk factors is about 5% per year. 3. Adjusted-dose warfarin and antiplatelet agents reduce absolute risk of stroke.	*J Am Coll Cardiol.* 2011;57(2):e22–242 *J Am Coll Cardiol.* 2006;48:e149–e246

					STROKE
Disease Prevention	Organization	Date	Population	Recommendations	Comments	Source
Stroke[a] (continued)				4. Patients with prior CV accident, mitral stenosis, a mechanical valve, or two risk factors require warfarin.[b] 5. Patients with one risk factor may receive either ASA or warfarin.[c] 6. Therapeutic warfarin International Normalized Ratio (INR) goal is 2.5 (+/- 0.5).		*Circulation.* 2006;114: e257–e354 *N Engl J Med.* 2009:360: 2066–2078.
	ECS	2010		ESC recommends the CHA_2DS_2 VASc score as more predictive for stroke risk, especially with a low CHADS2 score In high-risk patient unsuitable for anticoagulation, dual antiplatelet therapy (ASA plus clopidogrel) is reasonable.	Absolute cerebrovascular accident (CVA) risk reduction with dual antiplatelet Rx is 0.8%/year balanced by increased bleeding risk 0.7% ACTIVE Trial.	*Eur Heart J.* 2010:31: 2369–2429
	FDA Warning	2011		Dronedarone should not be used in chronic atrial fibrillation See Management algorithm, page 122–125, for pharmacologic and antithrombotic recommendations	Dronedarone doubles rate of CV death, strike and HF in patients with chronic atrial fibrillation.	*Lancet.* 2006;367: 1903–212

						STROKE

Disease Prevention[a]	Organization	Date	Population	Recommendations	Comments	Source
Stroke[a] (Continued)	AHA/ASA	2011	DM	1. Six-fold increase of stroke. 2. Short-term glycemic control does not lower macrovascular events. 3. HgA1c goal is < 6.5%. 4. BP goal is < 130/80 mm Hg. 5. Statin therapy. 6. Consider ACE inhibitor or ARB therapy for further stroke risk reduction.		*Eur Heart J.* 2010;31: 2369–2429 *Stroke.* 2011;42:517–584
					Consensus statement on treatment of asymptomatic CAS is controversial.[d]	
	USPSTF	2007 2011	Asymptomatic carotid artery stenosis (CAS)	1. No indication for general screening for CAS with ultrasonograph. 2. Screen for other stroke risk factors and treat aggressively. 3. ASA unless contraindicated. 4. Prophylactic carotid endarterectomy (CEA) for patients with high-grade (> 70%) CAS by ultrasonography when performed by surgeons with low (<3%) morbidity/mortality rates may be useful in selected cases depending on life expectancy, age, sex, and comorbidities.	Medical treatment of asymptomatic CAS should be aggressive. Surgical intervention should be individualized guided by comparing comorbid medical conditions, life expectancy to the surgical morbidity and mortality. Atherosclerotic intracranial stenosis: ASA should be used in preference to warfarin. Warfarin—significantly higher rates of adverse events with no benefit over ASA. (*N Engl J Med.* 2005 Mar 31;352(13):1305–1316)	*J Am Coll Cardiol.* 2011;57(8):1002–1038 *Ann Intern Med.* 2007;147:860–870 *Neurology.* 2005;65:6): 794–801 *Stroke. 2011;42:517–584* *Neurology.* 2011;77: 751–758 *Neurology.* 2011;77: 744–750

STROKE						
Disease Prevention[a]	Organization	Date	Population	Recommendations	Comments	Source
Stroke[a] **(continued)**	AHA/ASA			5. However, recent studies have demonstrated that "best" medical therapy results in a stroke rate ≤ 1%. 6. The number needed to treat (NNT) in published trials to prevent one stroke in 1 year in this asymptomatic group varies from 84 up to 2000. (*JACC.* 2011;57;e16–e94)	Qualitative findings (embolic signals and plaque ulceration) may identify patients who would benefit form asymptomatic CEA.	*J Am Coll Cardiol.* 2011;57(8):997–1001. *Stroke.* 2011;42:227–276
	ASA/ACCF/ AHA/AANN AANS/ACR CNS ASA/ACCF/ AHA/AANN AANS/ACR CNS		Symptomatic CAS	Optimal timing for CEA is within 2 weeks post-transient ischemic attack. CEA plus medical therapy is effective within 6 months of symptom onset with > 70% CAS. Intense medical therapy alone is indicated if the occlusion is <50%. Intensive medical therapy plus CEA may be considered with obstruction 50%–69%. Surgery should be *limited* to male patients with a low perioperative stroke/death rate (< 6%) and should have a life expectancy of at least 5 years.		

Disease Prevention	**Organization**	**Date**	**Population**	**Recommendations**	**Comments**	**Source**

STROKE

Disease Prevention	Organization	Date	Population	Recommendations	Comments	Source
Stroke[a] (continued)			Cryptogenic CVA	Carotid artery stenting is associated with increased nonfatal stroke frequency but this is offset by decreased risk of MI post CEA. Cryptogenic CVA with patent foramen ovale should receive ~ASA 81 mg/day. See screening recommendations on page 40.	Consider referral to tertiary center for enrollment in randomized trial to determine optimal Rx. Closure I Trial demonstrated no benefit at 2 years of PFO closure device over medical therapy.	*Arch Intern Med.* 2011;171(20): 1794–1795 *J Am Coll Cardiol.* 2009;53(21):2014–2018 *N Engl J Med.* 2012;366:991–999 *Stroke.* 2011;42:517–584
			Hyperlipidemia	See Cholesterol and Lipid Management (pages 133–135). Statin therapy post-CVA with intensive lipid-lowering goal after an ischemic stroke or transient ischemic attack with or without CHD reduced the risk of stroke and CV events (SPARCL Trial).		*Stroke.* 2006;37:1583–1633
			Sickle cell disease	Begin screening with transcranial Doppler (TCD) at age 2 years.	Transfusion therapy decreased stroke rates from 10% to < 1% per year (*N Engl J Med.* 1998;339:5). Transfusion therapy decreased stroke rates from 10% to < 1% per year (*N Engl J Med.* 1998;339:5).	*Stroke.* 2008;39:16-7–1652 *Stroke.* 2006;37:1583–1633 *Stroke.* 2011;42:517–584
			Smoking	Transfusion therapy is recommended for patients at high-stroke risk per TCD (high cerebral blood flow velocity > 200 cm/s). Frequency of screening not determined.		

[a]Assess risk of stroke in all patients. See Appendix VIII and IX for risk assessment tool.
[b]High-risk factors for stroke in patients with atrial fibrillation include previous transient ischemic attack or stroke or embolus, HTN, poor left ventricular function, age > 75 years, DM, rheumatic mitral valve disease, and prosthetic heart valves.
[c]Moderate risk factors for stroke are ages 65–75 years, DM, and coronary artery disease with preserved left ventricular function.

	SUDDEN INFANT DEATH SYNDROME					
Disease Prevention	Organization	Date	Population	Recommendations	Comments	Source
Sudden Infant Death Syndrome (SIDS)	ICSI	2010	Newborns and infants	Counsel all parents to place their infants on their backs to sleep.	Stomach and side sleeping have been identified as major risk factors for SIDS.	http://www.icsi.org/preventive_services_for_children__guideline_/preventive_services_for_children_and_adolescents_2531.html

	TOBACCO USE				

Disease Prevention	Organization	Date	Population	Recommendations	Comments	Source
Tobacco Use	AAFP	2010	Children and adolescents	Recommends counseling that avoidance of tobacco products is desirable.	The efficacy of counseling to prevent tobacco use in children and adolescents is uncertain.	http://www.guidelines.gov/content. as>x?id=36873

						VENOUS THROMBOEMBOLISM
Disease Prevention	Organization	Date	Population	Recommendations	Comments	Source
VTE Prophylaxis in Nonsurgical Patients	ACCP ACP	2012 2011	Medical patients with low risk (**Padua Prediction score—see Table I**) Medical patients with high risk (*JAMA* 2012; 307:306) (**Padua Prediction score—see Table I**)	Recommend against the use of pharmacologic prophylaxis or mechanical prophylaxis. Recommend for anticoagulant thromboprophylaxis with low molecular weight heparin (LMWH)—equivalent of enoxaparin 40 mg SQ daily, low dose unfractionated heparin (UFH) 5000 units BID or TID or fondaparinux 2.5 mg SQ daily. If patient bleeding or high risk of bleeding (see Table II), mechanical prophylaxis with graduated compression stockings (GCS) or intermittent pneumatic compression (IPC) recommended. When bleeding risk decreases substitute pharmacologic thromboprophylaxis for mechanical prophylaxis—continue thromboprophylaxis for duration of hospital stay—extended prophylaxis after discharge not recommended for medical patients.	Routine ultrasound screening for DVT is not recommended in any group. 150–200,000 deaths from VTE in U.S./year. Hospitalized patients VTE risk 130-fold greater than community residents. (*Mayo Clin Proc.* 2001; 76:1102) Neither heparin or warfarin is recommended prophylactically for patients with central venous catheters. In higher risk long-distance travelers, frequent ambulation, calf muscle exercises, aisle seat, and below-the-knee GCS gradual compression stockings is recommended over aspirin or anticoagulants. Inpatients with solid tumors and additional risk factors for VTE (history of DVT, thrombophilic drugs, immobilization), prophylactic dose LMWH or VFH is recommended. Be cautious in patients with Ccr < 30 ml/min—UFH or dalteparin preferred.	*Ann Intern Med.* 2011; 155:625–632 http://Chest Journal. chestpubs. org/content/ suppl/2012

VENOUS THROMBOEMBOLISM					
Disease Prevention	Organization	Date	Population	Recommendations	Comments	Source
VTE Prophylaxis in Nonsurgical Patients (continued)					Consider adjusted heparin dose in patients < 50 kg or > 110 kg in weight. IVC filter indicated in patients with diagnosed DVT or PE who cannot be anticoagulated because of bleed— IVC filter should not be used prophylactically. Although several studies have shown survival benefit for VTE prophylaxis in surgical patients, this has not been proven in medical patients. (*N Engl J Med.* 2011;365:2-63; *N Engl J Med.* 2007;356:1438)	

TABLE I RISK FACTORS FOR VTE IN HOSPTALIZED MEDICAL PATIENTS PADUA PREDICTIVE SCALE	
RISK FACTOR	**POINTS**
Active cancer[a]	3
Previous VTE	3
Reduced mobility[b]	3
Underlying thrombophilic disorder [c]	3
Recent (< 1 month) trauma or surgery	2
Age (≥ 70 years)	1
CHF or respiratory failure	1
Acute MI or stroke	1
Acute infection or inflammatory disorder	1
Obesity (BMI ≥ 30)	1
Thrombophilic drugs (hormones, tamoxifen, erythroid stimulating agents, lenalidomide, bevacizumab)	1
High risk: ≥ 4 points—11% risk of VTE without prophylaxis	
Low risk: ≤ 3 points—0.3% risk of VTE without prophylaxis	
a. Local or distant metastasis, chemotherapy or radiation within last 6 months	
b. Bedrest for ≥ 3 days	
c. Hereditary thrombophilia (see **Table III**) and antiphospholipid antibody syndrome, nephrotic syndrome, hemolytic anemia	

TABLE II RISK FACTORS FOR BLEEDING (*CHEST*. 2011;134:69–79)		
Risk Factor[c,d]	**N=10,866% of Patients**	**Overall Risk**
Active gastroduodenal ulcer	2.2	4.15
GI bleed ≤ 3 months previous	2.2	3.64
Platelet count < 50 K	1.7	3.37
Age ≥ 85 year (vs. 40 year)	10	2.96
Hepatic failure (INR[a] > 1.5)	2	2.18
Renal failure (GFR[b] < 30 mL/min)	11	2.14
ICU admission	8.5	2.10
Current cancer	10.7	1.78
Male sex	49.4	1.48
a. International normalized ratio		
b. Glomerular filtration		
c. Although not studied in medical patients, anti-platelet rate therapy would be expected to increase risk of bleeding		
d. Go to www.outcomesumassmed.org/IMPROVE/riskscore/bleeding/index.html to calculate risk of bleed for individual patients.		

TABLE III HEREDITARY THROMBOPHILIC DISORDERS		
Disorder	% of U.S. Population	Increase in Lifetime of Risk of Clot
Resistance to activated protein C (Factor V Leiden mut)	5–6	3X
Prothrombin gene mutation	2–3	2.5X
Elevated Factor 8 (> 175% activity)	6–8	2-3X
↑ Homocysteine	10–15	1.5–2X
Protein C deficiency	0.37	10X
Protein S deficiency	0.5	10X
Antithrombin deficiency	0.1	25X
Homozygous Factor V Leiden	0.3	60X

	VENOUS THROMBOEMBOLISM (VTE)				
Disease Prevention	**Organization**	**Date**	**Population**	**Recommendations**	**Comments**	**Source**
Venous Thromboembolism (VTE) in Surgical Patients	ACCP	2012	SURGICAL —Low risk (<40 year, minor surgery[a], no risk factor[b], Caprini score ≤2) (see Table IV)	Early ambulation—consider mechanical prophylaxis (intermittent pneumatic compression—IPC or GCS)	1. 75–90% of surgical bleeding is structural. VTE prophylaxis adds minimally to risk 2. With creatinine clearance <30 cc/min UFH with PTT monitoring is preferred 3. Patients with liver disease and prolonged INR are still at risk for clot. Risk-benefit ratio of VTE prophylaxis should be individualized 4. Epidural anesthesia —wait 10–12 hours after bid prophylactic dose of LMWH, 18 hours after daily prophylactic dose of LMWH and 24 hours after prophylactic dose of fondaparinux 5. Prophylactic inferior vena cava (IVC) filter for high risk surgery NOT recommended	http://chestjournal.Chestpubs.Org/Content/Suppl/2012
			—Intermediate risk (minor surgery plus risk factors, age 40–60 year, major surgery with no risk factors; Caprini score 3–4)	Unfractionated heparin (UFH) 5000 u SC q8h starting 2 hour pre-op Low molecular weight heparin (LMWH) equivalent to enoxaparin 40 mg SQ 2 hour before surgery then daily or 30 mg q 12h SQ starting 8–12h post-op. —Fondaparinux 2.5 mg SQ daily starting 8–12h post-op		

Disease Prevention	Organization	Date	Population	Recommendations	Comments	Source
Venous Thromboembolism (VTE) in Surgical Patients (continued)	ACCP	2012	—High risk (Major surgery plus risk factors, high risk medical patient, major trauma, spinal cord injury, craniotomy, total hip or knee arthroplasty (THA, TKA) thoracic, abdominal, pelvic cancer surgery	UFH 5000 u SQ q8h starting 2 hour pre-op—LMWH—equivalent to enoxaparin 40 mg SQ 2 hour pre-op than daily or 30 mg SQ q12h starting 8–12 h post-op, mechanical prophylaxis with IPC or GCS —Extend prophylaxis for as long as 28–35 days in high risk patients. In THA, TKA ortho patients acceptable VTE prophylaxis also includes rivaroxaban 10 mg/day, dabigatran 225 mg/d, adjusted dose warfarin and aspirin although LMWH is preferred. If high risk of bleeding use IPC alone (*Ann Int Med.* 2012; 156:710, *Ann Int Med.* 2012; 156:720, *JAMA.* 2012:307:294.)	6. For cranial and spinal surgery at low risk for VTE use mechanical prophylaxis —high risk patients should have pharmacologic prophylaxis added to mechanical once hemostasis is established and bleeding risk decreased 7. Patients at high risk of bleeding [c] with major surgery should have mechanical prophylaxis (IPC, GCS) — initiate anticoagulant prophylaxis if risk lowered	

[a] Eye, ear, laparoscopy, cystoscopy, arthroscopic operations
[b] Prior VTE, cancer, stroke, obesity, CHF, pregnancy, thrombophilic medications (tamoxifen, raloxifene, lenolidamide, thalidomide, erythroid stimulating agents)
[c] **SELECTED RISK FACTORS RAISING RISK OF MAJOR BLEEDING COMPLICATIONS.**
General Risk Factors
Active bleeding, previous major bleed, known untreated bleeding disorder, renal or liver failure, thrombocytopenia, acute stroke, uncontrolled HBP, concomitant use of anticoagulants, or anti-platelet therapy
Procedure-Specific Risk Factors
Major abdominal surgery—extensive cancer surgery, pancreatico-duodenectomy, hepatic resection, cardiac surgery, thoracic surgery (pneumonectomy or extended resection)
Procedures where bleeding complications have especially severe consequences—craniotomy, spinal surgery, spinal trauma

TABLE IV CAPRINI RISK ASSESSMENT MODEL			
1 Point	**2 Points**	**3 Points**	**5 Points**
• Age 41–60 year. • Minor surgery • BMI >251 g/m² • Swollen legs • Varicose veins • Pregnancy or post partum • History of recurrent spontaneous abortion • Sepsis (<1 month) • Lung disease • History of acute MI • CHF (<1 month) • History of inflammatory bowel disease • Medical patient at bed rest	• Age 61–74 years • Arthroscopic surgery • Major open surgery >45 min • Laparoscopic surgery • Malignancy • Confined to bed • Immobilizing cast • Central venous cath.	• Age ≥ 75 years • History VTE • Family history of VTE • Factor V Leiden • Prothrombin gene mutation • Lupus anticoagulant • Elevated homocysteine • Other congenital or acquired thrombophilia	• Stroke (<1 month) • Elective arthroplasty hip, pelvis or leg fracture • Acute spinal cord injury (<1 month)
		Caprini Score <3: low risk Caprini Score 3–4: intermediate risk Caprini Score ≥ 5: high risk	

3
Disease Management

ADRENAL INCIDENTALOMAS					
Disease Management	Organization	Date	Population	Recommendations	Comments	Source
Adrenal Incidentalomas	AACE	2009	Adults	1. Recommends clinical, biochemical, and radiographic evaluation for evidence of hypercortisolism, aldosteronism, the presence of pheochromocytoma, or a malignant tumor. 2. Patients who will be managed expectantly should have reevaluation at 3–6 months and then annually for 1–2 years.	1. A 1-mg overnight dexamethasone suppression test can be used to screen for hypercortisolism. 2. Measure plasma fractionated metanephrines and normetanephrines to screen for pheochromocytoma. 3. Measure plasma renin activity and aldosterone concentration to assess for primary or secondary aldosteronism.	https://www.aace.com/files/adrenal-guidelines.pdf

ALCOHOL USE DISORDERS

Disease Management	Organization	Date	Population	Recommendations	Comments	Source

Alcohol Use Disorders	ICSI
	NICE
	VA/DoD
		2010
		2010
		2009
			Adults	1. For patients icertified with alcohol dependence, schedule a referral to a substance use disorders specialist before the patient has left the office.
				2. Refer all patients with alcohol abstinence syndrome to a hospital for admission.
				3. Recommend prophylactic thiamine for all harmful alcohol use or alcohol dependence.
				4. Refer suitable patients with decompensated cirrhosis for consideration of liver transplantation once they have been sober from alcohol for ≥ 3 months.
				5. Recommend pancreatic enzyme supplementation for chronic alcoholic pancreatitis with steatorrhea and malnutrition.
					1. Assess all patients for a coexisting psychiatric disorder (dual diagnosis).
					2. Addiction-focused psychosocial intervention is helpful for patients with alcohol dependence.
					3. Consider adjunctive pharmacotherapy under close supervision for alcohol dependence:
					  a. Naltrexone
					  b. Acamprosate
						http://www.icsi.org/chronic_disease_risk_factors__primary_prevention_of__guideline_23506/
						chronic_disease_risk_factors__primary_prevention_of__guideline_23508.html
						http://www.guidelines.gov/content.aspx?id=23784
						http://www.guidelines.gov/content.aspx?id=15576

Disease Management	Organization	Date	Population	Recommendations	Comments	Source
ANAPHYLAXIS						
Anaphylaxis	NICE	2011	Children and adults	• Blood samples for mast cell tryptase testing should be obtained at onset and after 1–2 hours • All people 16 years or older suspected of having an anaphylactic reaction should be observed for at least 6–12 hours before discharge • All children under age 16 suspected of having an anaphylactic reaction should be admitted for observation • Patients treated for an anaphylactic reaction should be referred to an allergy specialist • Treat anaphylaxis with epinephrine (1:1,000) 0.01 mg/kg (max 0.5 mg) SC, may repeat as necessary every 15 min • Patients should be prescribed an epinephrine injector (eg, EpiPen)	Anaphylaxis is defined as a severe, life-threatening, generalized hypersensitivity reaction. It is characterized by the rapid development of: • Airway edema • Bronchospasm • Circulatory dysfunction	http://www.nice.org.uk/nicemedia/live/13626/57474/57474.pdf

ANDROGEN DEFICIENCY SYNDROME

Disease Management	Organization	Date	Population	Recommendations	Comments	Source
Androgen Deficiency Syndrome	Endocrine Society	2010	Adult men	1. Recommends an AM total testosterone level for men with symptoms and signs of androgen deficiency.[a] 2. Measure a serum luteinizing hormone (LH) and follicular stimulating hormone (FSH) in all men with testosterone deficiency. 3. Recommends a dual-energy x-ray absorptiometry scan for all men with testosterone deficiency. 4. Testosterone therapy indicated for androgen deficiency syndromes unless contraindications exist.[b]	1. Testosterone therapy options: a. Testosterone enanthate or cypionate 150–200 mg IM every 2 weeks b. Testosterone patch 5–10 mg qhs c. 1% testosterone gel 5–10 gm daily d. Testosterone 30 mg to buccal mucosa q12h	http://www.guidelines.gov/content.aspx?id=16326

[a]Lethargy, easy fatigue, lack of stamina or endurance, reduced libido, mood changes, irritability, and loss of libido and motivation.
[b]Breast CA, prostate CA, hematocrit > 50%, untreated severe obstructive sleep apnea, severe obstructive urinary symptoms, or uncontrolled heart failure.

	ANXIETY	

Disease Management	Organization	Date	Population	Recommendations	Comments	Source
Anxiety	NICE	2011	Adults	1. Recommends cognitive behavioral therapy for generalized anxiety disorder (GAD). 2. Recommends sertraline if drug treatment is needed. 3. If sertraline is ineffective, recommend a different selective serotonin reuptake inhibitor (SSRI) or (SNRI). 4. Avoid long-term benzodiazepine use or antipsychotic therapy for GAD.		http://www.nice.org.uk/nicemedia/live/13314/52599/52599.pdf

ASTHMA

Disease Management	Organization	Date	Population	Recommendations	Comments	Source

Asthma	VA/DoD
	GINA
		2009
		2009
			Children aged > 5 years, adolescents, and adults	1. Recommend classification of asthma by level of control.
				2. Recommend a chest radiograph at the initial visit to exclude alternative diagnoses.
				3. Recommend assessing for tobacco use and strongly advise smokers to quit
				4. Recommend spirometry with bronchodilators to determine the severity of airflow limitation and its reversibility.
				  a. Repeat spirometry at least every 1–2 years for asthma monitoring.
				5. Consider allergy testing for history of atopy, rhinitis, rhinorrhea, and seasonal variation or specific extrinsic triggers.
				6. Recommend an asthma action plan based on peak expiratory flow (PEF) monitoring for all patients.
					1. Controlled asthma defined by:
					  a. Daytime symptoms ≤ 2/week
					  b. No limitations of daily activities
					  c. No nocturnal symptoms
					  d. Need for reliever medicines ≤ 2×/week
					  e. Normal or near-normal lung function
					  f. No exacerbations
					2. Partially controlled asthma if:
					  a. Daytime symptoms > 2×/week
					  b. Any limitations of daily activities or any nocturnal symptoms
					  c. Need for reliever medicines > 2×/week
					  d. < 80% predicted PEF or forced expiratory volume at 1 second (FEV_1)
					  e. Any exacerbations
					3. Uncontrolled asthma if there are ≥ 3 features of partially controlled asthma in any week.
						http://www.guidelines.gov/content.aspx?id=15706
						
						http://www.guidelines.gov/content.aspx?id=15556

					ASTHMA	
Disease Management	Organization	Date	Population	Recommendations	Comments	Source
Asthma (continued)				7. Recommend allergen and environmental trigger avoidance. 8. Physicians should help educate patients, assist them in self-management, create an asthma action plan, and regularly monitor asthma control. 9. Recommend systemic glucocorticoids for asthma exacerbations. 10. Develop a chronic medication regimen for patients adjusted based on their asthma action plan.	4. Recommend an inhaled corticosteroid for partially controlled or uncontrolled asthma. 5. Add a long-acting beta-agonist or leukotriene inhibitor for incomplete control with inhaled corticosteroid alone. 6. Short-acting beta-agonists should be used as needed for relief of acute asthma symptoms or 20 minutes prior to planned exertion in exercise-induced asthma.	

ATRIAL FIBRILLATION: MANAGEMENT OVERVIEW
HEART RATE CONTROL
Source: **AMERICAN COLLEGE OF CARDIOLOGY/AMERICAN HEART**
ASSOCIATION/EUROPEAN SOCIETY OF CARDIOLOGY

Classification of Atrial Fibrillation (AF)
Paroxysmal = Self-terminating
Recurrent = Two or more episodes
Persistent = Lasts > 7 days
Silent = Detected by monitor
Lone = Unassociated with/heart disease

Initiate Treatment
Slow the ventricular rate
Establish anticoagulation
Consider rhythm conversion

Determine Etiology
Hypertension/coronary artery disease
Cardiomyopathy/heart valve disease
Pulmonary disease/hyperthyroidism
Sinus node disease

- Expected ventricular heart rate (HR) in untreated AF is between 110–210 beats per minute (bpm).
  If HR < 110 bpm, atrioventricular (AV) node disease present; If HR > 220 bpm, preexcitation syndrome (WPW) present
- Initial choice of AV nodal slowing agent to be determined by:
  Ventricular rate/Blood pressure (BP)
  Presence of heart failure (HF) or asthma
  Associated cardiovascular (CV) symptoms (chest pain/shortness of breath [SOB])

Usual Rx
Beta-blocker
Diltiazem
Verapamil
Digoxin

HF or Low BP
Digoxin
Amiodarone

Preexcitation Syndrome
Amiodarone
Propafenone

- **Urgent electrical cardioversion** should be considered if hemodynamic instability or persistent symptoms of ischemia, HF, or if inadequate HR control with optimal medications.
- **Resting HR goal and exercise HR goal** should be determined. Holter monitor best measures the adequacy of the chronic HR control. In acute medical conditions when the patient has noncardiac illness (ie, pneumonia), the resting HR may be allowed to increase to simulate physiologic demands (mimic HR if sinus rhythm was present).

Lenient Target
Resting HR < 110 bpm
May be considered in
younger or patients
without CV symptoms.

Aggressive Target
Resting HR < 80 bpm/exercise
HR < 110 bpm treatment choice if
decreased ejection fraction (EF) < 40%
if symptoms at higher rates.

ATRIAL FIBRILLATION: MANAGEMENT OVERVIEW
HEART RATE CONTROL (CONTINUED)
Source: AMERICAN COLLEGE OF CARDIOLOGY/AMERICAN HEART ASSOCIATION/EUROPEAN SOCIETY OF CARDIOLOGY

(ESC recommends HR target < 110 bpm; CCS recommends < 100 bpm; ACCF/AHA/HRS recommends HR target < 110 bpm only if EF > 40%)

- **Consider AV nodal ablation** when chronic HR target cannot be achieved with maximal medical therapy with placement of ventricular pacemaker.

ESC, European Society of Cardiology; CCS, Canadian CV Society; ACCF, American College of Cardiology Foundation; AHA, American Heart Association; HRS, Heart Rhythm Society

Sources: ACC/AHA/ESC 2006 Guidelines. *J Am Coll Cardiol.* 2006;48:858–906. ACCF/AHA/HRS. *J Am Coll Cardiol.* 2011;57:223–242. ACC/AHA. *Circulation.* 2008;117:1101–1120. ESC 2010 Guidelines. *Euro Heart J.* 2010;31:2369–2429. Comparing the 2010 NA and European AF Guidelines. *Canadian J Cardiol.* 2011;27:7–13.

ATRIAL FIBRILLATION: MANAGEMENT, ANTITHROMBOTIC THERAPY
Source: AMERICAN COLLEGE OF CARDIOLOGY/AMERICAN HEART ASSOCIATION/EUROPEAN SOCIETY OF CARDIOLOGY

Antithrombotic selection is based on stroke risk versus bleeding risk.

- Antithrombotic therapy is recommended in all atrial fibrillation (AF) or atrial flutter patients except those with LONE AF or contraindications.
- **Moderate risk factors (RF)** for embolization: Aged > 75 years, hypertension (HTN), heart failure (HF), ejection fraction (EF) ≤ 35%, diabetes mellitus (DM).
- **High risk factors (RF)** for embolization: Mechanical heart valve, mitral stenosis, prior embolization (cardiovascular accident [CVA], transient ischemic attack [TIA], systemic embolism).

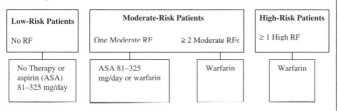

Low-Risk Patients	**Moderate-Risk Patients**		**High-Risk Patients**
No RF	One Moderate RF	≥ 2 Moderate RFs	≥ 1 High RF
No Therapy or aspirin (ASA) 81–325 mg/day	ASA 81–325 mg/day or warfarin	Warfarin	Warfarin

- Warfarin international normalized ratio (INR) goal 2.5 (+/– 0.5) in all patients unless mechanical valve present, in which case INR goal 3 (+/– 0.5).
- INR should be determined weekly during initiation of therapy and then monthly when stable.
- Warfarin reduces the relative risk (RR) of thromboembolism versus placebo by 67%. ASA reduces RR of thromboembolism versus placebo by 19%. Warfarin reduces the RR of thromboembolism versus ASA by 39%. Warfarin reduced the RR over ASA plus clopidogrel by 42%.
- The daily recommended dose of dietary vitamin K is 65–80 mcg/day. If unexplained variations noted in the INR, increase vitamin K dosage to 100–200 mcg daily. www.nal. usda.gov/fnic/foodcomp/Data/Other/IFT2002_VitK.pdf)
- Warfarin resistance should be considered if INR < 2 with a warfarin dose > 15 mg daily. Should exclude dietary and medication interference or patient nonadherence. Check Factor II and Factor X activity. If these factors are < 40% of normal, the INR is inaccurate and the patient is therapeutically anticoagulated. If these factors are > 40%, check warfarin level.
- The ESC recommends the **CHA$_2$DS$_2$-VASc score**, a new risk factor-based approach to be used in nonvalvular AF (high-risk score > 3). It goes beyond the **CHADS$_2$ score** by adjusting the importance of age and adding factors of female gender and vascular disease (coronary artery disease [CAD] or peripheral arterial disease [PAD]). The ACC/AHA and the Canadian Cardiovascular Society recommend the CHADS$_2$ score (high-risk score ≥ 2). Comparative efficacy to the present system awaits further evaluation.
- **HAS-BLED bleeding risk score** is utilized to determine the risk of bleeding while taking warfarin. Risk factors include: **H**ypertension (≥ 160 mm Hg); **A**bnormal kidney function (creatinine ≥ 2, chronic dialysis, transplant); **A**bnormal liver function (cirrhosis, bilirubin > 2×, aspartate transaminase [AST] > 3×); **S**troke; **B**leeding history or anemia; **L**abile INR (< 60% within range); **E**lderly (aged ≥ 65 years); **D**rugs/alcohol (use of ASA or clopidogrel) or alcohol (8 or more alcoholic drinks/week). Each risk factor is assigned 1 point for a total of 9 points. A high risk of bleeding is considered ≥ 3 points.

ATRIAL FIBRILLATION: MANAGEMENT, ANTITHROMBOTIC THERAPY (CONTINUED)
Source: **AMERICAN COLLEGE OF CARDIOLOGY/AMERICAN HEART ASSOCIATION/EUROPEAN SOCIETY OF CARDIOLOGY**

- In high-risk patients unable to take warfarin, may consider dual antiplatelet therapy (ASA + clopidogrel). (*Lancet.* 2006;367:1903–1912) The absolute CVA risk reduction was 0.8%, which was offset by a 0.7% increased risk of bleeding.
- Dabigatran (Pradaxa @ 150 mg bid) maybe a useful alternative to warfarin in high-risk patients who **do not have** a mechanical heart valve, significant valve disease, renal failure (creatinine clearance < 15 mL/min), or advanced liver disease (impaired baseline clotting). Dabigatran required twice-daily dosing, has a higher risk of nonhemorrhagic complications than does warfarin, a higher rate of drug discontinuation, and no difference in mortality. Consider use in patients with labile INR measurements on warfarin or in patients with a high risk of bleeding. (*J Am Coll Cardiol.* 2011;57:1330–1337)

ESC, European Society of Cardiology; ACC, American College of Cardiology; AHA, American Heart Association; CCS, Canadian Cardiovascular Society

Sources: ACC/AHA/ESC 2006 Guidelines. *J Am Coll Cardiol.* 2006;48:858–906. ACCF/AHA/HRS. *J Am Coll Cardiol.* 2011;57:223–242. ACC/AHA. *Circulation.* 2008;117:1101–1120. ESC Guidelines. 2010;31:2369–2429. ACCF/AHA/HRS Focus Update. *J Am Coll Cardiol.* 2011;57(2):223–242. Comparing the 2010 NA and European AF Guidelines. *Can J Cardiol.* 2011;27:7–13.

ANTITHROMBOTIC STRATEGIES FOLLOWING CORONARY ARTERY STENTING IN PATIENTS WITH AF AT MODERATE TO HIGH THROMBO-EMBOLIC RISK (IN WHOM ORAL ANTICOAGULATION THERAPY IS REQUIRED)

Haemorrhagic Risk	Clinical Setting	Stent Implanted	Anticoagulation Regimen
Low or intermediate (eg HAS-BLED score 0–2)	Elective	Bare-metal	1 month: triple therapy of VKA (INR 2.0–2.5) + aspirin ≤100 mg/day + clopidogrel 75 mg/day Up to 12th month: combination of VKA (INR 2.0–2.5) + clopidogrel 75 mg/day[b] (or aspirin 100 mg/day) Lifelong: VKA (INR 2.0–3.0) alone
	Elective	Drug-eluting	3 (-olimus[a] group) to 6 (paclitaxel) months: triple therapy of VKA (INR 2.0–2.5) + aspirin ≤100 mg/day + clopidogrel 75 mg/day Up to 12th month: combination of VKA (INR 2.0–2.5) + clopidogrel 75 mg/day[b] (or aspirin 100 mg/day) Lifelong: VKA (INR 2.0–3.0) alone
	ACS	Bare-metal/drug-eluting	6 months: triple therapy of VKA (INR 2.0–2.5) + aspirin ≤100 mg/day + clopidogrel 75 mg/day Up to 12th month: combination of VKA (INR 2.0–2.5) + clopidogrel 75 mg/day[b] (or aspirin 100 mg/day) Lifelong: VKA (INR 2.0–3.0) alone
High (eg. HAS-BLED score ≥3)	Elective	Bare-metal[c]	2–4 weeks: triple therapy of VKA (INR 2.0–2.5) + aspirin ≤100 mg/day + clopidogrel 75 mg/day Lifelong: VKA (INR 2.0–3.0) alone
	ACS	Bare-metal[c]	4 weeks: triple therapy of VKA (INR 2.0–2.5) + aspirin ≤100 mg/day + clopidogrel 75 mg/day Up to 12th month: combination of VKA (INR 2.0–2.5) + clopidogrel 75 mg/day[b] (or aspirin 100 mg/day) Lifelong: VKA (INR 2.0–3.0) alone

ACS, acute coronary syndrome; AF, atrial fibrillation; INR, international normalized ratio; VKA, vitamin K antagonist.

Gastric protection with a proton pump inhibitor (PPI) should be considered where necessary.

[a]Sirolimus, everolimus, and tacrolimus.

[b]Combination of VKA (INR 2.0–3.0)+aspirin ≤100 mg/day (with PPI, if indicated) may be considered as an alternative.

[c]Drug-eluting stents should be avoided as far as possible, but, if used, consideration of more prolonged (3–6 months) triple antithrombotic therapy is necessary.

Adapted from Lip GY, Huber K, Andreotti F, Amesen H, Airaksinen KJ, Cuisisset T, Kirchhof P, Martin F. Management of antithrombotic therapy in atrial fibrillation patients presenting with acute coronary syndrome and/or undergoing percutaneous coronary intervention/stent. Thromb Haemost 2010.

ATRIAL FIBRILLATION: MANAGEMENT, RHYTHM CONTROL DRUG NONPHARMACOLOGIC THERAPY
Source: AMERICAN COLLEGE OF CARDIOLOGY/AMERICAN HEART ASSOCIATION/EUROPEAN SOCIETY OF CARDIOLOGY

- **AFFIRM, RACE, PIAF,** and **STAF** Trials found no difference in quality of life between rate and rhythm control in atrial fibrillation (AF). The AFFIRM and RACE Trials demonstrated no difference in stroke rate or mortality between rate and rhythm control in AF.

Favors Rate Control	versus	Favors Rhythm Control
Asymptomatic in AF		Continued symptoms in AF
Older patients		Younger patients
Advanced heart disease		LONE or minimal heart disease
Comorbid conditions		Few comorbid conditions
Persistent AF		Recent onset/paroxysmal AF

- **Rhythm Control**
  Fifty percent of patients with new-onset AF spontaneously convert to sinus in 48 hours.
- **2, 3, 4 Cardioversion Rule**
  - New-onset AF **< 2 days** in duration—may be considered for acute electrical or drug conversion to sinus rhythm while on heparin.
  - Onset of AF **> 2 days** or of unknown duration—require either **3 weeks** of therapeutic oral anticoagulation (international normalized ratio [INR] 2–3) or a negative transesophageal echocardiogram (TEE) to exclude clot before conversion while on heparin should be considered.
  - In either approach to conversion, oral anticoagulation (OAC) must be continued at least **4 weeks** postconversion due to the possibility of delayed return of atrial contraction and clot release. In high-risk patients, lifelong OAC should be considered.

- **Pharmacologic Approach:** Choice based on etiology of heart disease
  - LONE: flecainide, propafenone, sotalol, amiodarone
  - HTN: flecainide, propafenone, sotalol, amiodarone (LVH)
  - CAD: sotalol, dofetilide, amiodarone
  - HF: amiodarone, dofetilide

(LONE, no associated disease; HTN, hypertension; CAD, coronary artery disease; HF, heart failure; LVH, left ventricular hypertrophy)
FDA Warning 2011: Dronedarone should not be used in chronic atrial fibrillation; it doubles rate of CV death, stroke, and HF.
- **Nonpharmacologic Approach:**
- AF catheter ablation/MAZE procedure (open surgical approach)

  Consider if antiarrhythmic drug therapy fails or if AF coexists with preexcitation pathway. AF ablation is more effective in younger patients with paroxysmal AF; catheter ablation maintains sinus rhythm ~ 80% as opposed to ~ 40% with drugs @ 5 years.
  May require repeat procedures (average 1.8 procedures).
  Long-term anticoagulation should be continued even after successful ablation in patients at high risk for thromboembolism. In low-embolic-risk patients, warfarin may be converted to aspirin (ASA) therapy after 3 months. (*J Am Coll Cardiol.* 2010;55:735–743)

- Consider MAZE procedure if performing open heart surgery for other reasons or if vascular or cardiac anatomy prevents the less invasive catheter approach.
- Consider implantable atrial defibrillators: least commonly used treatment.

ATRIAL FIBRILLATION: MANAGEMENT, RHYTHM CONTROL DRUG/NONPHARMACOLOGIC THERAPY (CONTINUED)
Source: **AMERICAN COLLEGE OF CARDIOLOGY/AMERICAN HEART ASSOCIATION/EUROPEAN SOCIETY OF CARDIOLOGY**

- **Prevention of Atrial Remodeling**
  - Calcium channel blockers
  - Angiotensin-converting enzyme (ACE) inhibitors
  - Angiotensin receptor blocker (ARB) agents
  - Statins

Sources: ACC/AHA/ESC 2006 Guidelines. *J Am Coll Cardiol.* 2006;48:858–906. ACCF/AHA/HRS. *J Am Coll Cardiol.* 2011;57:223–242. ACC/AHA. *Circulation.* 2008;117:1101–1120. ESC 2010 Guidelines. *Euro Heart J.* 2010;31:2369–2429. *Circulation.* 2009;119:606–618.

HAS-BLED BLEEDING RISK SCORE FOR WARFARIN THERAPY		
Letter	**Clinical Characteristics**	**Points Awarded**
H	**Hypertension** (systolic BP > 160 mm Hg)	1
A	**Abnormal renal function** (presence of chronic dialysis or renal transplantation or serum creatinine ≥ 2.6 mg/mL μmol/L) and **Abnormal liver function** (chronic hepatic disease or biochemical evidence of significant hepatic derangement (bilirubin >2× upper limit of normal, in association with GOT/GPT >3× upper limit normal) *1 point each*	1 or 2
S	**Stroke**	1
B	**Bleeding** (previous bleeding history and/or predisposition to bleeding, eg, bleeding diathesis, anemia)	1
L	**Labile INRs** (unstable/high INRs or poor time in therapeutic range, eg, < 60%)	1
E	*Elderly* (age > 65 years)	1
D	**Drugs or alcohol** (concomitant use of drugs such as antiplatelet agents, nonsteroidal anti-inlammatory drugs or alcohol abuse) *1 point each*	1 or 2
		Maximum 9 points

HAS-BLED BLEEDING RISK SCORE FOR WARFARIN THERAPY (CONTINUED)

Interpretation

The risk of (spontaneous) major bleeding (intracranial, hospitalization, hemoglobin decrease 2 g/L, and/or transfusion) within 1 year in patients with atrial fibrillation enrolled in the Euro Heart Survey, expressed as bleeds per 100 patient years:

- score 0: 1.13
- score 1: 1.02
- score 2: 1.88
- score 3: 3.74
- score 4: 8.70
- score 5: 12.50
- score 6-9: insufficient data to quantify risk

Information adapted from:
- *"2010 Guidelines for the management of atrial fibrillation" European Heart Journal. (2010) 31, 2369-2429. Doi:10.1093/eurheartj/ehq278. Table 10*
- *R. Pisters, D. A. Lane, R. Nieuwlaat, C. B. de Vos, H. J. G. M. Crijns and G. Y. H. Lip "A novel user-friendly score (HAS-BLED) to assess one year risk of major bleeding in atrial fibrillation patients: The Euro Heart Survey." Chest; Prepublished online March 18, 201. Doi: 10.1378/chest.10-0134 Table 5*

THROMBOEMBOLIC RISK SCORES IN NONVALVULAR ATRIAL FIBRILLATION				
	CHADS₂	**Points**	**CHA₂DS₂-VASc**	**Points**
C	Congestive heart failure	1	Congestive heart failure (**or** *left ventricular systolic dysfunction LVEF ≤ 40%*)	1
H	Hypertension (BP consistently > 140/90mm Hg or treated HTN on medication)	1	Hypertension (BP consistently > 140/90mm Hg or treated HTN on medication)	1
A	Age ≥ 75 years	1	Age ≥ 75 years	2
D	Diabetes mellitus	1	Diabetes mellitus	1
S₂	Prior stroke or TIA	2	Prior stroke or TIA or *Thromboembolism*	2
V			*Vascular disease (eg, coronary artery disease, peripheral artery disease, MI, aortic plaque)*	1
A			*Age 65–74*	1
Sc			*Sex category (ie, female gender)*	1
Max.		6		9

RISK FACTORS FOR STROKE AND THROMBOEMBOLISM IN NONVALVULAR AF	
"Major" risk factors	"Clinically relevant non-major" risk factors
Previous • Stroke • TIA • Systemic embolism Age ≥ 75 years	• Heart failure or moderate to severe LV systolic dysfunction (LVEF ≤ 40%) • Hypertension • Diabetes mellitus • Female sex • Age 65–74 years • Vascular disease

Information adapted from:
- *"2010 Guidelines for the management of atrial fibrillation." European Heart Journal. (2010) 31, 2369–2429. Doi:10.1093/eurheartj/ehq278. Table 8 (a) and Table 8 (b)*
- *"Validation of clinical classification schemes for predicting stroke. Results from the national registry of Atrial fibrillation." JAMA, 2001; 285 (22):2864–2870. Doi:10.1001/jama.285.22.2864*

ATTENTION-DEFICIT HYPERACTIVITY DISORDER (ADHD)

Disease Management	Organization	Date	Population	Recommendations	Comments	Source
Attention-Deficit Hyperactivity Disorder (ADHD)	AAP	2011	Children 4–18 years old	• Initiate an evaluation for ADHD in any child who presents with academic or behavioral problems and symptoms of inattention, hyperactivity, or impulsivity. • Consider children with ADHD as children with special health care needs. • For children age 4–5 years parent- or teacher-administered behavior therapy is the treatment of choice. • Methylphenidate is reserved for severe refractory cases. • For children ages 6–18 years, first-line treatment is with FDA-approved medications for ADHD +/– behavior therapy.	• Essential to assess any child with ADHD for concomitant emotional, behavioral, developmental, or physical conditions (eg, mood disorders, tic disorders, seizures, sleep disorders, learning disabilities, or disruptive behavioral disorders) • For children 6–18 years, evidence is best to support stimulant medications and less strong to support atomoxetine, ER guanfacine, and ER clonidine for ADHD	http://pediatrics.aappublications.org/content/early/2011/10/14/peds.2011-2654.full.pdf

Disease Management	Organization	Date	Population	Recommendations	Comments	Source
AUTISM						
Autism	NICE	2011	Children and young adults	• Consider autism for regression in language or social skills in children less than 3 years. • Clinical signs of possible autism have to be seen in the context of a child's overall development, and cultural variation may pertain. • An autism evaluation by a specialist is indicated for any of the following signs of possible autism: ○ Language delay ○ Regression in speech ○ Echolalia ○ Unusual vocalizations or intonations ○ Reduced social smiling ○ Rejection of cuddles by family ○ Reduced response to name being called ○ Intolerance of others entering into their personal space ○ Reduced social interest in people or social play ○ Reduced eye contact ○ Reduced imagination ○ Repetitive movements like body rocking ○ Desire for unchanged routines ○ Immature social and emotional development	• Differential diagnosis of autism includes: ○ Neurodevelopmental disorders ○ Mood disorders ○ ADHD ○ Oppositional defiant disorder ○ Conduct disorder ○ OCD ○ Rett syndrome ○ Hearing or vision impairment ○ Selective mutism	http://www.nice.org.uk/nicemedia/live/13572/56428/56428.pdf

	BARRETT'S ESOPHAGUS					
Disease Management	Organization	Date	Population	Recommendations	Comments	Source
Barrett's Esophagus	AGA	2011	Patients with biopsy diagnosis of Barrett's esophagus (metaplastic columnar epithelium in distal esophagus)	• **No Dysplasia** ○ endoscopic surveillance (ES) every 3–5 years • **Low-Grade Dysplasia** ○ ES every 6–12 months – consider radiofrequency ablation (RFA) —90% complete eradication of dysplasia • **High–Grade Dysplasia** ○ ES every 3 months if no eradication therapy • **Eradication Therapy** ○ RFA, photodynamic therapy (PDT), or endoscopic mucosal resection (EMR) is preferred over ES in high-grade dysplasia (strong recommendation)	- In patients with BE without dysplasia, 0.12% develop esophageal cancer per year compared to 0.5% with low-grade dysplasia -Progression from high grade dysplasia to cancer is 6% per year (*N Engl J Med.* 2011; 365:1375) -Esophagectomy for high-grade dysplasia is an option but less morbidity with ablation therapy (*N Engl J Med;* 2009 360:2277) -40% of patients with BE and esophageal cancer have no history of chronic GERD symptoms -Long-term high-dose proton pump inhibitors (PPI) or anti-reflux therapy has not been proven to decrease risk of esophageal CA in patients with BE	http://download.journals.elsevierhealth.com/pdfs/journals/0016-5085/PIIS0016508511600849.pdf

BENIGN PROSTATIC HYPERPLASIA (BPH)						
Disease Management	Organization	Date	Population	Recommendations	Comments	Source

Benign Prostatic Hyperplasia (BPH)	AUA	2010	Adult men	1. Routine measurement of serum creatinine is not indicated in men with BPH.
				2. Do not recommend dietary supplements or phytotherapeutic agents for lower urinary tract symptoms (LUTS) management.
				3. Patients with LUTS with no signs of bladder outlet obstruction by flow study should be treated for detrusor overactivity.
				  a. Alter fluid intake
				  b. Behavioral modification
				  c. Anticholinergic medications
				4. Options for moderate-severe LUTS from BPH
				  (AUA symptom index score ≥ 8)
				  a. Watchful waiting
				  b. Medical therapies
				    i. Alpha-blockers[a]
				    ii. 5-alpha reductase inhibitors[b]
				    iii. Anticholinergic agents
				    iv. Combination therapy
				  c. Transurethral needle ablation
				  d. Transurethral microwave thermotherapy
					1. Combination therapy with alpha-blocker and 5-alpha reductase inhibitor is effective for moderate-severe LUTS with significant prostate enlargement.
					2. Men with planned cataract surgery should have cataract surgery before initiating alpha-blockers.
					3. 5-alpha reductase inhibitors should not be used for men with LUTS from BPH without prostate enlargement.
					4. Anticholinergic agents are appropriate for LUTS that are primarily irritative symptoms and patient does not have an elevated post-void residual (> 250 mL)
					5. The choice of surgical method should be based on the patient's presentation, anatomy, surgeon's experience, and patient's preference.
						http://www.guidelines.gov/content.aspx?id=256358&search=aua+2010+bph

BENIGN PROSTATIC HYPERPLASIA (BPH)

Disease Management	Organization	Date	Population	Recommendations	Comments	Source
Benign Prostatic Hyperplasia (BPH) (continued)				e. Transurethral laser ablation or enucleation of the prostate f. Transurethral incision of the prostate g. Transurethral vaporization of the prostate h. Transurethral resection of the prostate i. Laser resection of the prostate j. Photoselective vaporization of the prostate k. Prostatectomy 5. Surgery is recommended for BPH causing renal insufficiency, recurrent urinary tract infections (UTIs), bladder stones, gross hematuria, or refractory LUTS.		

[a]Alpha-blockers: alfuzosin, doxazosin, tamsulosin, and terazosin. All have equal clinical effectiveness.
[b]5-alpha reductase inhibitors: dutasteride and finasteride.

	BRONCHITIS, ACUTE					
Disease Management	Organization	Date	Population	Recommendations	Comments	Source
Bronchitis, Acute	Michigan Quality Improvement Consortium	2010	Adults aged ≥ 18 years	1. Recommends against a chest x-ray if all the following are present: a. Heart rate < 100 bpm b. Respiratory rate < 24 breaths/min c. Temperature < 38°C 2. Recommends against antibiotics	1. Consider antitussive agents for short-term relief of coughing. 2. Beta$_2$-agonists or mucolytic agents should not be used routinely to alleviate cough.	http://www.guidelines.gov/content.aspx?id=16317

	CA SURVIVORSHIP: LATE EFFECTS OF CA TREATMENTS	
CA or CA Treatment History	**Late Effect Type**	**Periodic Evaluation**
Any CA experience	Psychosocial disorders[b]	
Any chemotherapy	Oral and dental abnormalities	Dental exam and clearing (every 6 months)
Chemotherapy (alkylating agents)[a]	Gonadal dysfunction	Puberta assessment (yearly) in adults if symptoms of hypogonadism present
	Hematologic disorders[c]	History, exam for bleeding disorder; CBC/differential (yearly)
	Ocular toxicity[d]	Visual acuity, funduscopic exam, evaluation by ophthalmologist (if radiation) yearly if ocular tumors, total body irradiation [TBI], or ≥30 Gy; otherwise, every 3 years)
	Pulmonary toxicity[e]	CXR, PFTs (at entry into long-term follow-up, then as clinically indicated)
	Renal toxicity[f]	Blood pressure (yearly); electrolytes, BUN, creatinine, Ca^+, Mg^{++}, PO_4^-
	Urinary tract toxicity[g]	urinalysis (at entry into long-term follow-up, then clinically as indicated)
Chemotherapy (anthracycline antibiotics)[a]	Cardiac toxicity[h]	ECHO or MUGA; ECG at entry into long-term follow-up, periodic thereafter (↑ frequency if chest radiation); fasting glucose, lipid panel (every 3–5 years)
	Hematologic disorders[c]	See "Chemotherapy (alkylating agents)"
Chemotherapy anti-tumor antibiotics (mitomycin C)[f], bleomycin[e]	Pulmonary toxicity[e]	CXR and PFTs end of exposure then reevaluation as clinically indicated
Chemotherapy-antimetabolites (cytarabine, high-dose IV; MTX, high-dose IV, intrathecal IT)	Clinical leukoencephalopathy[i]	Full neurologic examination (yearly)
	Neurocognitive deficits	Neuropsychological evaluation (at entry into long-term follow-up, then as clinically indicated)
Chemotherapy (epipodophyllotoxins)[a]	Hematologic disorders (causes acute myeloic leukemia [AML] with specific 11q 23 translocation)[c]	See "Chemotherapy (alkylating agents)"

CA SURVIVORSHIP: LATE EFFECTS OF CA TREATMENTS (CONTINUED)

CA or CA Treatment History	Late Effect Type	Periodic Evaluation
Chemotherapy (heavy metals)[a]	Dyslipidemia/hypertension and increased risk of cardiovascular disease	Fasting lipid panel at entry
	Gonadal dysfunction	See "Chemotherapy (alkylating agents)"
	Hematologic disorders[c]	See "Chemotherapy (alkylating agents)"
	Ototoxicity[f]	Complete pure tone audiogram or brainstem auditory-evoked response (yearly × 5 years, then every 5 years)
	Peripheral sensory neuropathy	Examination yearly for 2–3 years
	Renal toxicity[f]	See "Chemotherapy (alkylating agents)"
Chemotherapy—microtubular inhibitors (taxanes, ixabepilone, eribulin)	Peripheral neuropathy	Examination yearly for 2–3 years
Chemotherapy (nonclassical alkylators)[a]	Gonadal dysfunction	See "Chemotherapy (alkylating agents)"
	Reduced CD4 count	
	Hematologic disorders[c]	
Chemotherapy (plant alkaloids)[a]	Peripheral sensory neuropathy	See "Chemotherapy (heavy metals)"
	Raynaud's phenomenon	Yearly history/examination
Chemotherapy (purine agonists)[a]	Hematologic disorders[c]	See "Chemotherapy (alkylating agents)"
	Reduction in CD4 count	Monitor for infection
Corticosteroids (dexamethasone, prednisone)	Ocular toxicity[d]	Musculoskeletal examination (yearly)
	Avascular osteonecrosis	
	Osteopenia/osteoporosis	

CA SURVIVORSHIP: LATE EFFECTS OF CA TREATMENTS (CONTINUED)		
CA or CA Treatment History	**Late Effect Type**	**Periodic Evaluation**
Targeted biological therapy —Trastuzumab (anti-Her-2) —Rituximab (antilymphocyte CD20)	Cardiac dysfunction is usually reversible Reduction in immunoglobulins and increased risk of infection	Monitor 2D echo for ejection fraction every 3 months during therapy and as needed for symptoms Monitor quantitative immunoglobulins if increased frequency of infection
Hematopoietic cell (bone marrow) transplant	Hematologic disorders[c] Oncologic disorders[k] Avascular osteonecrosis Osteopenia/osteoporosis	See "Chemotherapy (alkylating agents)" Inspection/exam targeted to irradiation fields (yearly)[e] See "Corticosteroids (dexamethasone, prednisone)" See "Chemotherapy (antimetabolites)"
Chemotherapy drugs with minimal long-term toxicity effects Topoisomerase I inhibitors (camptosar, topotecan) Antibiotics (actinomycin) Antimetabolites (L-asparaginase, 5 FU, capecitabine, gemcitabine, 6 mercaptopurine)	Mild reduction in bone marrow reserve	Routine monitoring for end-organ dysfunction is not indicated
Radiation therapy (field- and dose-dependent)	Cardiac toxicity[h] Central adrenal insufficiency (pediatric brain tumors) Cerebrovascular complications[l] Chronic sinusitis Functional asplenia	See "Chemotherapy (alkylating agents)" 8 AM serum cortisol (yearly × 15 years, and as clinically indicated) Neurologic exam (yearly) Head/neck exam (yearly) Blood culture when temperature ≥ 101°F, rapid institution of empiric antibiotics

CA SURVIVORSHIP: LATE EFFECTS OF CA TREATMENTS (CONTINUED)

CA or CA Treatment History	Late Effect Type	Periodic Evaluation
	Gonadal dysfunction	See "Chemotherapy (alkylating agents)"
	Growth hormone deficiency (children and adolescents)	Height, weight, BMI (every 6 months until growth completed, then yearly); Tanner staging (every 6 months until sexually mature)
	Hyperthyroidism	TSH, free T_4 (yearly)
	Hyperprolactinemia	Prolactin level (as clinically indicated)
	Hypothyroidism	TSH, free T_4
	Neurocognitive deficits	See "Chemotherapy (cytarabine)"
	Ocular toxicity[d]	See "Chemotherapy (alkylating agents)"
	Oncologic disorders[k]	See "Hematopoietic cell (bone marrow) transplant"
	Oral and dental abnormalities	See "Any chemotherapy"
	Ototoxicity[f]	See "Chemotherapy (heavy metals)"
	Overweight/obesity/metabolic syndrome	Fasting glucose, fasting serum insulin, fasting lipid profile (every 2 years if overweight or obese; every 5 years if normal weight)
	Pulmonary toxicity[e]	See "Chemotherapy (alkylating agents)"
	Renal toxicity[f]	See "Chemotherapy (alkylating agents)"
	Urinary tract toxicity[g]	See "Chemotherapy (alkylating agents)"

CBC, complete blood count; TBI, total body irradiation; MTX, methotrexate; CXR, chest x-ray; PFTs, pulmonary function tests; BUN, blood urea nitrogen; ECHO, echocardiogram; MUGA, multiple-gated acquisition scan; ECG, electrocardiogram; IV, intravenous; IT, intrathecal; AML, acute myelocytic leukemia; BMI, body mass index; TSH, thyroid stimulating hormone

[a]Chemotherapeutic agents, by mechanism of action:

- Alkylating agents: busulfan, carmustine (BCNU), chlorambucil, cyclophosphamide, ifosfamide, lomustine (CCNU), mechlorethamine, melphalan, procarbazine, thiotepa
- Antimetabolites: MTX, cytosine arabinoside, gemcitabine
- Heavy metals: carboplatin, cisplatin, oxaliplatin
- Nonclassical alkylators: dacarbazine (DTIC), temozolomide
- Anthracycline antibiotics: daunorubicin, doxorubicin, epirubicin, idarubicin, mitoxantrone
- Antitumor antibiotics: bleomycin, mitomycin C
- Plant alkaloids: vinblastine, vincristine, vinorelbine
- Purine agonists: fludarabine, pentostatin, cladribine
- Microtubular inhibitors: docetaxel, paclitaxel, cabazitaxel, ixabepilone
- Epipodophyllotoxins: etoposide (VP16), teniposide (VM26)

CA SURVIVORSHIP: LATE EFFECTS OF CA TREATMENTS (CONTINUED)

[b] Psychosocial disorders: mental health disorders, risky behaviors, psychosocial disability due to pain, fatigue, limitations in health care/insurance access, "chemo brain" syndrome.

[c] Hematologic disorders: acute myeloid leukemia, myelodysplasia

[d] Ocular toxicity: cataracts, orbital hypoplasia, lacrimal duct atrophy, xerophthalmia, keratitis, telangiectasias, retinopathy, endophthalmos, chronic painful eye, maculopathy, glaucoma

[e] Pulmonary toxicity: pulmonary fibrosis, interstitial pneumonitis, restrictive lung disease, obstructive lung disease. Increased sensitivity to oxygen toxicity—keep $FiO_2 \leq 28\%$ in patients with bleomycin exposure

[f] Renal toxicity: glomerular and tubular renal insufficiency, hypertension, hemolytic uremic syndrome

[g] Urinary tract toxicity: hemorrhagic cystitis, bladder fibrosis, dysfunctional voiding, vesicoureteral reflux, hydronephrosis, bladder malignancy

[h] Cardiac toxicity: cardiomyopathy, arrhythmias, left ventricular dysfunction, congestive heart failure, pericarditis, pericardial fibrosis, valvular disease, myocardial infarction, atherosclerotic heart disease

[i] Clinical leukoencephalopathy: spasticity, ataxia, dysarthria, dysphagia, hemiparesis, seizures

[j] Ototoxicity: sensorineural hearing loss, tinnitus, vertigo, tympanosclerosis, otosclerosis, eustachian tube dysfunction, conductive hearing loss

[k] Oncologic disorders: secondary benign or malignant neoplasm, especially breast CA after mantle radiation, gastrointestinal malignancy after para-aortic radiation for seminoma of the testis

[l] Cerebrovascular complications: stroke, and occlusive cerebral vasculopathy

Note: Guidelines for surveillance and monitoring for late effects after treatment for adult CAs available via the National Comprehensive Cancer Network, Inc. (NCCN). (http://www. nccn.org/professionals/physician_gls)

Source: Long-Term Follow-Up Guidelines for Survivors of Childhood, Adolescent, and Young Adult Cancers. Children's Oncology Group, Version 2.0, March 2006. (For full guidelines and references, see http://www.survivorshipguidelines.org)

See also: *N Engl J Med.* 2006;355:1722–1782, *J Clin Oncol.* 2007;25:3991–4008.

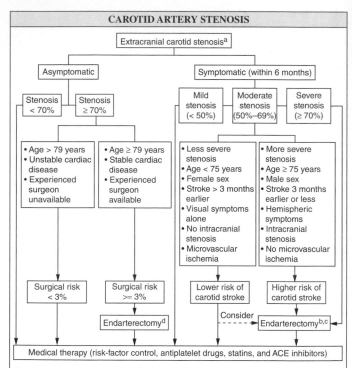

CAROTID ARTERY STENOSIS

[a]Critical stenosis defined as > 70% by noninvasive imaging or > 50% by catheter angiography.

[b]Carotid endarterectomy (CEA) in symptomatic patients with average or low surgical risk should generally be reserved for patients with > 5 years' expectancy, and perioperative stroke/death rate < 6%. When CEA is indicated, it should be performed within 2 weeks after an ischemic central nervous system (CNS) event.

[c]Carotid artery stenting (CAS) with an embolic protection device is an alternative to CEA in symptomatic patients with average or low surgical risk when > 70% obstruction is present, and the periprocedural stroke and mortality rate is < 6%. CAS may be chosen over CEA if the neck anatomy is surgically unfavorable or if comorbid conditions make CEA a very high risk.

[d]The annual rate of stroke in asymptomatic patients treated with optimal medical therapy for carotid artery stenosis has decreased to < 1%. Therefore the benefit of CEA or CAS remains controversial in asymptomatic patients. (*Stroke*. 2010;41:975–979)

Source: AHA/ASA 2005 Guidelines. *Circulation*. 2006;113:e872. *Stroke*. 2006;37:577. ASA/ACCF/AHA/AANN/AANS/ACR/ASNR/CNS/SAIP/SCAI/SIR/SNIS/SVM/SVS 2011 Guidelines. *J Am Coll Cardiol*. 2011;57:e16–e94. ACCF/SCAI/SVMB/SIR/ASITN 2007 Consensus. *J Am Coll Cardiol*. 2007;49(1):126–168.

CATARACT IN ADULTS: EVALUATION & MANAGEMENT ALGORITHM
Source: **AAO & AOA**

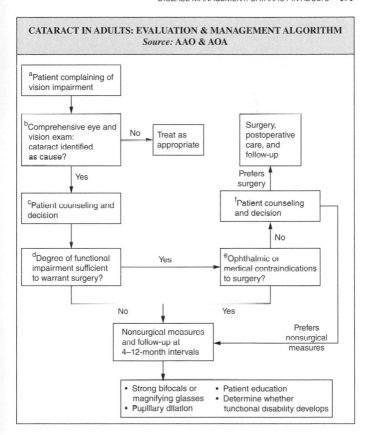

Notes:

[a]Begin evaluation only when patients complain of a vision problem or impairment. Identifying impairment in visual function during routine history and physical exam constitutes sound medical practice.

[b]Essential elements of the comprehensive eye and vision exam:

• *Patient history:* Consider cataract if: acute or gradual onset of vision loss; vision problems under special conditions (eg, low contrast, glare); difficulties performing various visual tasks.

Ask about: refractive history, previous ocular disease, amblyopia, eye surgery, trauma, general health history, medications, and allergies. It is critical to describe the actual impact of the cataract on the person's function and quality of life. There are several instruments available for assessing functional impairment related to cataract, including VF-14, Activities of Daily Vision Scale, and Visual Activities Questionnaire.

• *Ocular exam:* Including: Snellen acuity and refraction; measurement of intraocular pressure; assessment of pupillary function; external exam; slit-lamp exam; and dilated exam of fundus.

• *Supplemental testing:* May be necessary to assess and document the extent of the functional disability and to determine whether other diseases may limit preoperative or postoperative vision.

Most elderly patients presenting with visual problems do not have a cataract that causes functional impairment. Refractive error, macular degeneration, and glaucoma are common alternative etiologies for visual impairment.

[c]Once cataract has been identified as the cause of visual disability, patients should be counseled concerning the nature of the problem, its natural history, and the existence of both surgical and nonsurgical approaches to management. The principal factor that should guide decision making with regard to surgery is *the extent to which the cataract impairs the ability to function in daily life.* The findings of the physical exam should corroborate that the cataract is the major contributing cause of the functional impairment, and that there is a reasonable expectation that managing the cataract will positively impact the patient's functional activity. Preoperative visual acuity is a poor predictor of postoperative functional improvement: The decision to recommend cataract surgery should not be made solely on the basis of visual acuity.

[d]Patients who complain of mild to moderate limitation in activities due to a visual problem, those whose corrected acuities are near 20/40, and those who do not yet wish to undergo surgery may be offered nonsurgical measures for improving visual function. Treatment with nutritional supplements is not recommended. Smoking cessation retards cataract progression. Indications for surgery: cataract-impaired vision no longer meets the patient's needs; evidence of lens-induced disease (eg, phacomorphic glaucoma, phacolytic glaucoma); necessary to visualize the fundus in an eye that has the potential for sight (eg, diabetic patient at risk of diabetic retinopathy).

[e]*Contraindications to surgery:* the patient does not desire surgery; glasses or vision aids provide satisfactory functional vision; surgery will not improve visual function; the patient's quality of life is not compromised; the patient is unable to undergo surgery because of coexisting medical or ocular conditions; a legal consent cannot be obtained; or the patient is unable to obtain adequate postoperative care. Routine preoperative medical testing (12-lead EKG, CBC, measurement of serum electrolytes, BUN, creatinine, and glucose), while commonly performed in patients scheduled to undergo cataract surgery, does not appear to measurably increase the safety of the surgery.

[f]Patients with significant functional and visual impairment due to cataract who have no contraindications to surgery should be counseled regarding the expected risks and benefits of and alternatives to surgery.

Source: American Academy of Ophthalmology Preferred Practice Pattern: Cataract in the Adult Eye. (2006) (http://www.aao.org/PPP)
American Optometric Association Consensus Panel on Care of the Adult Patient with Cataract. Optometric Clinical practice guideline: Care of the Adult Patient with Cataract. (2004) (http://www.aoa.org)

					CERUMEN IMPACTION

Disease Management	Organization	Date	Population	Recommendations	Comments	Source
Cerumen Impaction	AAO-HNS	2008	Children and adults	1. Strongly recommended treating cerumen impaction when it is symptomatic or prevents a needed clinical exam. 2. Clinicians should treat the patient with cerumen impaction with an appropriate intervention: a. Ceruminolytic agents b. Irrigation c. Manual removal	Ceruminolytic agents include Cerumenex, Addax, Debrox, or dilute solutions of acetic acid, hydrogen peroxide, or sodium bicarbonate.	http://www.entnet.org/Practice/upload/FINAL-CerumenImpaction-Journal-2008.pdf

CHOLESTEROL & LIPID MANAGEMENT IN ADULTS

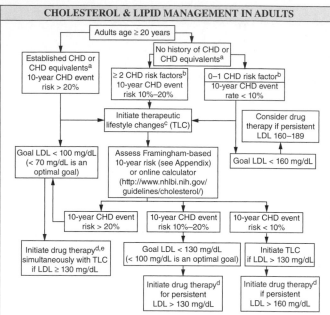

Adults age ≥ 20 years

Established CHD or CHD equivalents[a]
10-year CHD event risk > 20%

No history of CHD or CHD equivalents[a]

≥ 2 CHD risk factors[b]
10-year CHD event risk 10%–20%

0–1 CHD risk factor[b]
10-year CHD event rate < 10%

Initiate therapeutic lifestyle changes[c] (TLC)

Consider drug therapy if persistent LDL 160–189

Goal LDL < 100 mg/dL (< 70 mg/dL is an optimal goal)

Assess Framingham-based 10-year risk (see Appendix) or online calculator (http://www.nhlbi.nih.gov/guidelines/cholesterol/)

Goal LDL < 160 mg/dL

10-year CHD event risk > 20%

10-year CHD event risk 10%–20%

10-year CHD event risk < 10%

Initiate drug therapy[d,e] simultaneously with TLC if LDL ≥ 130 mg/dL

Goal LDL < 130 mg/dL (< 100 mg/dL is an optimal goal)

Initiate TLC if LDL > 130 mg/dL

Initiate drug therapy[d] for persistent LDL > 130 mg/dL

Initiate drug therapy[d] if persistent LDL > 160 mg/dL

[a]CHD risk equivalents carry a risk for major coronary events equal to that of established CHD (ie, > 20% per 10 years) and include: diabetes, other clinical forms of atherosclerotic disease (peripheral arterial disease, abdominal aortic aneurysm, and symptomatic carotid artery disease).

[b]Age (men aged ≥ 45 years, women ≥ 55 years or postmenopausal), hypertension (BP ≥ 140/90 mm Hg or on antihypertensive medication), cigarette smoking, HDL < 40 mg/dL, family history of premature CHD in first-degree relative (males < 55 years, females < 65 years). For HDL ≥ 60 mg/dL, subtract 1 risk factor from above.

[c]Reduce saturated fat (< 7% total calories) and cholesterol (< 200 mg/day intake); increase physical activity; and achieve appropriate weight control. Assess effects of TLC on lipid levels after 3 months.

[d]Drug therapy response should be monitored and modified at 6-week intervals to achieve goal LDL levels; after goal LDL met, monitor response and adherence every 4–6 months.

[e]Addition of fibrate or nicotinic acid is also an option if ↑ TGs or ↓ HDL.

Source: Executive summary of the third report of the National Cholesterol Education Project (NCEP) expert panel on detection, evaluation and treatment of high blood cholesterol in adults (Adult Treatment Panel III). Implications of Recent Clinical Trials for the National Cholesterol Education Program Adult Treatment Panel III Guidelines. *Circulation*. 2004; 110:227–239.

Note: West of Scotland Coronary Prevention Study: 5 years of pravastatin treatment associated with significant reduction in coronary events for subsqunt 10 years in men with hypercholesterolemia and no history of myocardial infarction. *NEJM*. 2007; 357(15):1477–1486.

2004 MODIFICATIONS TO THE ATP III TREATMENT ALGORITHM FOR LDL-C

In high-risk persons (10-year CHD risk > 20%), the recommended LDL-C goal is < 100 mg/dL.

An LDL-C goal of < 70 mg/dL is a therapeutic option, especially for patients at very high risk.

If LDL-C is ≥ 100 mg/dL, an LDL-lowering drug is indicated as initial therapy simultaneously with lifestyle changes.

If baseline LDL-C is < 100 mg/dL, institution of an LDL-lowering drug to achieve an LDL-C level < 70 mg/dL is a therapeutic option.

If a high-risk person has high triglycerides or low HDL-C, consideration can be given to combining a fibrate or nicotinic acid with an LDL-lowering drug. When triglycerides are ≥ 200 mg/dL, non-HDL-C is a secondary target of therapy, with a goal 30 mg/dL higher than the identified LDL-C goal.

For **moderately high-risk persons** (2+ risk factors and 10-year risk 10%–20%), the recommended LDL-C goal is < 130 mg/dL; an LDL-C goal < 100 mg/dL is a therapeutic option. When LDL-C level is 100–129 mg/dL, at baseline or on lifestyle therapy, initiation of an LDL-lowering drug to achieve an LDL-C level < 100 mg/dL is a therapeutic option.

Any person at high risk or moderately high risk who has lifestyle-related risk factors (eg, obesity, physical inactivity, elevated triglycerides, low HDL-C, or metabolic syndrome) is a candidate for TLC to modify these risk factors regardless of LDL-C level.

When LDL-lowering drug therapy is employed in high-risk or moderately high-risk persons, intensity of therapy should be sufficient to achieve at least a 30%–40% reduction in LDL-C levels.

Source: Implications of Recent Clinical Trials for the National Cholesterol Education Program Adult Treatment Panel III Guidelines. *Circulation.* 2004;110:227–239.

2011 EUROPEAN SOCIETY OF CARDIOLOGY/EUROPEAN ATHEROSCLEROSIS SOCIETY GUIDELINES FOR THE MANAGEMENT OF DYSLIPIDEMIA

ESC/EAS GUIDELINES

1. Screen with lipid profile:
   Men ≥ 40 years
   Women ≥ 50 years or post-menopausal with additional risk factors
   Evidence of atherosclerosis in any vascular bed
   Diabetes type 2
   Family history of premature CVD
2. Estimate total CV 10-year risk by *SCORE* (Systemic Coronary Risk Estimation), which has a large European cohort database or the *Framingham Risk Score.*

   If the 10-year risk is ≥ 5% at increased risk, recommend heart score modified to include HDL-C

2011 EUROPEAN SOCIETY OF CARDIOLOGY/EUROPEAN ATHEROSCLEROSIS SOCIETY GUIDELINES FOR THE MANAGEMENT OF DYSLIPIDEMIA (CONTINUED)

VERY HIGH RISK—LDL-C goal < 70 mg/dL

Documented CVD by invasive or noninvasive testing, previous MI, PCI, CABG, other arterial revascularization procedures, ischemic CVA or PAD

Type 2 diabetes; type 1 with end organ disease (microalbinuria)

Moderate to severe CKD GRF < 60mL/min/1.73 m²

Calculated 10-year risk SCORE ≥ 10%; FRS ≥ 20%.

HIGH RISK—LDL-C goal < 100 mg.dL

Markedly elevated lipids or BP

SCORE ≥ 5% and < 10% for the 10-year risk of fatal CVD; FRS ≥ 20%.

MODERATE RISK – LDL-C goal < 115 mg/dL

SCORE ≥ 1% and < 5% at 10 years; FRS 10–20%.

FH premature CAD

Obesity

Physical inactivity

Low HDL-C, high TG

LOW RISK

SCORE < 1 %; FRS ≤ 5%

3. Lipid analysis

LDL-C is the primary marker

TG , HDL-C, non HDL-C, Apo B (with diabetes and MetS), Lpa in selected high-risk patients with FH of premature disease. TC adds little to assessment.

4. Lifestyle management—same as ATP recommendations with additional use of phytosterols, soy protein, red yeast rice, polycosanol supplements

5. Secondary causes for hypercholesterolemia

hypothyroidism, nephrotic syndrome, pregnancy, Cushing syndrome, Anorexia nervosa, immunosuppressant agents, corticosteroids

6. Drug therapy

LDL-C

Statins—Initial agent in moderate, high, or very high risk.

Statin therapy in primary prevention patients should be limited to patients with moderate or high-risk patients.

Combined therapy: BAS + nicotinic acid, cholesterol absorption inhibitor + BAS + nicotinic acid

TG > 880 mg/dL—pancreatitis

Fibrates, nicotinic acid, n-3 fatty acids

HDL-C

Nicotinic acid, statin, nicotinic acid + statin

CKD stage 1–2

statin well tolerated; Stage > 3 more adverse events—use atorvastatin, fluvastatin, gemfibrozil

Source: ESC/EAS Guidelines. *Eur Heart J.* (2011) 32, 1769–1818
doi:10.1093/eurheartj/ehr158

CHOLESTEROL AND LIPID MANAGEMENT IN CHILDREN
Source: PEDIATRICS 2011

Children:
- Consider drug therapy if, after 6-month trial of lifestyle/diet management. Two determinations should be obtained at least 2 weeks apart.
- LDL ≥ 190 mg/dL for children aged 10 years or older or
- LDL > 160 mg/dL and positive family history of premature CHD; 1 high-level risk factor, ≥ 2 moderate-level risk factors are present
- Treatment goal in children and adolescense is to decrease LDL level to the 95th percentile (< 130 mf/dL)
- Do not start before age 10 years in boys and until after menarche in girls
- Statins (HMG-CoA reductase inhibitors) as first-line drug therapy

Source: Circulation. 2007;115:1948–1967. Pediatrics. 2011:128(5)

COLITIS, CLOSTRIDIUM DIFFICILE

Disease Management	Organization	Date	Population	Recommendations	Comments	Source

Colitis, *Clostridium difficile*	IDSA SHEA	2010	Adults	• Treatment of *C. difficile* infection (CDI)
				  ○ Discontinue antibiotics as soon as possible
				  ○ Avoid antiperistaltic agents
				  ○ Mild-moderate CDI: metronidazole 500 mg PO tid × 10–14 days
				  ○ Severe CDI: vancomycin 125 mg PO qid × 10–14 days
				  ○ Severe complicated CDI taking POs: vancomycin 500 mg PO qid +/− metronidazole 500 mg IV q8h
				  ○ Severe complicated CDI and NPO: 500 mg in 100 mL normal saline enema per rectum qid +/− metronidazole 500 mg IV q8h
				  ○ Administer vancomycin as a tapered regimen for recurrent CDI
					• Testing for *C. difficile* or its toxins should be performed only on diarrheal stool
					• Testing of stool on asymptomatic patients should be avoided
					• Enzyme immunoassay (EIA) testing for *C. difficile* toxin A and B is rapid but is less sensitive than the cell cytotoxin assay
					• Stool for *C. difficile* toxins by PCR is rapid and very sensitive and specific
						http://www.doh.state.fl.us/disease_ctrl/epi/HAI/SHEA_IDSA_Clinical_Practice_Cdiff_Guideline.pdf

CONSTIPATION

Disease Management	Organization	Date	Population	Recommendations	Comments	Source
Constipation, Idiopathic	NICE	2010	Children aged ≤ 18 years	1. Assess all children for fecal impaction. 2. Recommends polyethylene glycol (PEG) as first-line agent for oral disimpaction. 3. Add a stimulant laxative if PEG therapy is ineffective after 2 weeks. 4. Recommends sodium citrate enemas for disimpaction only if all oral medications have failed. 5. Recommends a maintenance regimen with PEG for several months after a regular bowel pattern has been established. 6. Recommends gradually tapering maintenance dose over several months as bowel pattern allows. 7. Recommends adequate fluid intake.	Minimal fluid intake for age: *Age* *Volume* 1–3 years 1300 mL 4–8 years 1700 mL 9–13 years 2200 mL 14–18 years 2500 mL	http://www.nice.org.uk/nicemedia/live/12993/48741/48741.pdf

CONTRACEPTION, EMERGENCY

Disease Management	Organization	Date	Population	Recommendations	Comments	Source
Contraception, Emergency	ACOG	2010	Women of childbearing age who had unprotected or inadequately protected sexual intercourse within the last 5 days and who do not desire pregnancy	• The levonorgestrel-only regimen is more effective and is associated with less nausea and vomiting compared with the combined estrogen–progestin regimen. • The two 0.75-mg doses of the levonorgestrel-only regimen are equally effective if taken 12 to 24 hours apart. • The single-dose 1.5-mg levonorgestrel-only regimen is as effective as the two-dose regimen. • Recommend an antiemetic agent 1 hour before the first dose of the combined estrogen–progestin regimen to reduce nausea • Treatment with emergency contraception should be initiated as soon as possible after unprotected or inadequately protected intercourse • Emergency contraception should be made available to patients who request it up to 5 days after unprotected intercourse.	• No clinician examination or pregnancy testing is necessary before provision or prescription of emergency contraception. • The copper intrauterine device (IUD) is appropriate for use as emergency contraception for women who desire long-acting contraception. • 0Information regarding effective long-term contraceptive methods should be made available whenever a woman requests emergency contraception.	http://www.guidelines.gov/content.aspx?id=15718&search=emergency+contraception

PERCENTAGE OF WOMEN EXPERIENCING AN UNINTENDED PREGNANCY DURING THE FIRST YEAR OF TYPICAL USE AND THE FIRST YEAR OF PERFECT USE OF CONTRACEPTION AND THE PERCENTAGE CONTINUING USE AT THE END OF THE FIRST YEAR—UNITED STATES

Method	Women Experiencing an Unintended Pregnancy Within the First Year of Use		Women Continuing Use at 1 Year[c]
	Typical Use[a]	Perfect Use[b]	
No method[d]	85%	85%	
Spermicides[e]	29%	18%	42%
Withdrawal	27%	4%	43%
Fertility awareness–based methods	25%		51%
Standard Days method[f]		5%	
TwoDay method[TM][f]		4%	
Ovulation method[f]		3%	
Sponge			
Parous women	32%	20%	46%
Nulliparous women	16%	9%	57%
Diaphragm[g]	16%	6%	57%
Condom[h]			
Female (Reality®)	21%	5%	49%
Male	15%	2%	53%
Combined pill and progestin-only pill	8%	0.3%	68%
Evra patch®	8%	0.3%	68%
NuvaRing®	8%	0.3%	68%
Depo-Provera®	3%	0.3%	56%
Intrauterine device			
ParaGard® (copper T)	0.8%	0.6%	78%
Mirena® (LNG-IUS)	0.2%	0.2%	80%

PERCENTAGE OF WOMEN EXPERIENCING AN UNINTENDED PREGNANCY DURING THE FIRST YEAR OF TYPICAL USE AND THE FIRST YEAR OF PERFECT USE OF CONTRACEPTION AND THE PERCENTAGE CONTINUING USE AT THE END OF THE FIRST YEAR—UNITED STATES (CONTINUED)

Method	Women Experiencing an Unintended Pregnancy Within the First Year of Use		Women Continuing Use at 1 Year[c]
	Typical Use[a]	Perfect Use[b]	
Implanon®	0.05%	0.05%	84%
Female sterilization	0.5%	0.5%	100%
Male sterilization	0.15%	0.10%	100%
Emergency contraceptive pills[i]	Not applicable	Not applicable	Not applicable
Lactational amenorrhea method[j]	Not applicable	Not applicable	Not applicable

Adapted from Trussell J. Contraceptive efficacy. In Hatcher RA, Trussell J, Nelson AL, Cates W, Stewart FH, Kowal D. *Contraceptive Technology*. 19th revised ed. New York, NY: Ardent Media; 2007.

[a]Among typical couples who initiate use of a method (not necessarily for the first time), the percentage who experience an unintended pregnancy during the first year if they do not stop use for any other reason. Estimates of the probability of pregnancy during the first year of typical use for spermicides, withdrawal, fertility awareness–based methods, the diaphragm, the male condom, the pill, and Depo-Provera are taken from the 1995 National Survey of Family Growth corrected for underreporting of abortion; see the text for the derivation of estimates for the other methods.

[b]Among couples who initiate use of a method (not necessarily for the first time) and who use it *perfectly* (both consistently and correctly), the percentage who experience an unintended pregnancy during the first year if they do not stop use for any other reason. See the text for the derivation of the estimate for each method.

[c]Among couples attempting to avoid pregnancy, the percentage who continue to use a method for 1 year.

[d]The percentages becoming pregnant in the typical use and perfect use columns are based on data from populations where contraception is not used and from women who cease using contraception to become pregnant. Of these, approximately 89% become pregnant within 1 year. This estimate was lowered slightly (to 85%) to represent the percentage who would become pregnant within 1 year among women now relying on reversible methods of contraception if they abandoned contraception altogether.

[e]Foams, creams, gels, vaginal suppositories, and vaginal film.

[f]The TwoDay and Ovulation methods are based on evaluation of cervical mucus. The Standard Days method avoids intercourse on cycle days 8–19.

[g]With spermicidal cream or jelly.

[h]Without spermicides.

PERCENTAGE OF WOMEN EXPERIENCING AN UNINTENDED PREGNANCY DURING THE FIRST YEAR OF TYPICAL USE AND THE FIRST YEAR OF PERFECT USE OF CONTRACEPTION AND THE PERCENTAGE CONTINUING USE AT THE END OF THE FIRST YEAR—UNITED STATES (CONTINUED)

Method	Women Experiencing an Unintended Pregnancy Within the First Year of Use			Women Continuing Use at 1 Year[c]
	Typical Use[a]	Perfect Use[b]		

[f]Treatment initiated within 72 hours after unprotected intercourse reduces the risk for pregnancy by at least 75%. The treatment schedule is 1 dose within 120 hours after unprotected intercourse and a second dose 12 hours after the first dose. Both doses of Plan B can be taken at the same time. Plan B (1 dose is 1 white pill) is the only dedicated product specifically marketed for emergency contraception. The Food and Drug Administration has in addition declared the following 22 brands of oral contraceptive to be safe and effective for emergency contraception: Ogestrel or Ovral (1 dose is 2 white pills); Levlen or Nordette (1 dose is 4 light-orange pills); Cryselle, Levora, Low-Ogestrel, Lo/Ovral, or Quasence (1 dose is 4 white pills); Tri-Levlen or Triphasil (1 dose is 4 yellow pills); Jolessa, Portia, Seasonale, or Trivora (1 dose is 4 pink pills); Seasonique (1 dose is 4 light blue-green pills); Empresse (1 dose is 4 orange pills); Alesse, Lessina, or Levlite (1 dose is 5 pink pills); Aviane (1 dose is 5 orange pills); and Lutera (1 dose is 5 white pills).

[g]Lactational amenorrhea method is a highly effective temporary method of contraception. However, to maintain effective protection against pregnancy, another method of contraception must be used as soon as menstruation resumes, the frequency or duration of breastfeeding is reduced, bottle feeds are introduced, or the baby reaches 6 months of age.

SUMMARY OF CHANGES IN CLASSIFICATIONS FROM WHO MEDICAL ELIGIBILITY CRITERIA FOR CONTRACEPTIVE USE, 4TH EDITION[ab]

Condition	COC/P/R	POP	DMPA	Implants	LNG-IUD	Cu-IUD	Clarification
Breastfeeding							The U.S. Department of Health and Human Services recommends that infants be exclusively breastfed during the first 4–6 months of life, preferably for a full 6 months. Ideally, breastfeeding should continue through the first year of life (1). {Not included in WHO MEC}
a. < 1 mo postpartum {WHO: < 6 wks post partum}	3[c] {4}	2[c] {3}	2[c] {3}	2[c] {3}			
b. 1 mo to < 6 mos {WHO: ≥ 6 wks to < 6 mos postpartum}	2[c] {3}						
Postpartum (in breastfeeding or nonbreastfeeding women), including post caesarean section					2 {1 if not breastfeeding and 3 if breastfeeding}		
a. < 10 min after delivery of the placenta {WHO: < 48 hrs, including insertion immediately after delivery of the placenta}							
b. 10 min after delivery of the placenta to < 4 wks {WHO: ≥ 48 hrs to < 4 wks}					2 {3}	2{3}	

SUMMARY OF CHANGES IN CLASSIFICATIONS FROM WHO MEDICAL ELIGIBILITY CRITERIA FOR CONTRACEPTIVE USE, 4TH EDITION[ab] (CONTINUED)

Condition	COC/P/R	POP	DMPA	Implants	LNG-IUD	Cu-IUD	Clarification
Deep venous thrombosis (DVT)/ pulmonary embolism (PE)							
a. History of DVT/PE, not on anticoagulant therapy							
i. Lower risk for recurrent DVT/PE (no risk factors)	3 {4}						
b. Acute DVT/PE		2 {3}	2 {3}	2 {3}	2 {3}	2 {1}	
c. DVT/PE and established on anticoagulant therapy for at least 3 mos						2 {1}	
i. Higher risk for recurrent DVT/PE (≥ 1 risk factors)							
• Known thrombophilia, including antiphospholipid syndrome							
• Active cancer (metastatic, on therapy, or within 6 mos after clinical remission), excluding nonmelanoma skin cancer							
• History of recurrent DVT/PE							

SUMMARY OF CHANGES IN CLASSIFICATIONS FROM WHO MEDICAL ELIGIBILITY CRITERIA FOR CONTRACEPTIVE USE, 4TH EDITION[a][b] (CONTINUED)

Condition	COC/P/R	POP	DMPA	Implants	LNG-IUD	Cu-IUD	Clarification
ii. Lower risk for recurrent DVT/ PE (no risk factors)	3* {4}					2 {1}	Women on anticoagulant therapy are at risk for gynecologic complications of therapy such as hemorrhagic ovarian cysts and severe menorrhagia. Hormonal contraceptive methods can be of benefit in preventing or treating these complications. When a contraceptive method is used as a therapy, rather than solely to prevent pregnancy, the risk/benefit ratio may be different and should be considered on a case-by-case basis. [Not included in WHO MEC]
Valvular heart disease a. Complicated (pulmonary hypertension, risk for atrial fibrillation, history of subacute bacterial endocarditis)						1 {2}	1 {2}
Ovarian cancer[d]						1 {Initiation = 3, Continuation = 2}	1 {Initiation = 3, Continuation = 2}

SUMMARY OF CHANGES IN CLASSIFICATIONS FROM WHO MEDICAL ELIGIBILITY CRITERIA FOR CONTRACEPTIVE USE, 4TH EDITION[a][b] (CONTINUED)

Condition	COC/P/R	POP[b]	DMPA	Implants	LNG-IUD	Cu-IUD	Clarification
Uterine fibroids						2 {1 if no uterine distortion and 4 if uterine distortion is present}	2 {1 if no uterine distortion and 4 if uterine distortion is present}

[a]For conditions for which classification changed for ≥ 1 methods or the condition description underwent a major modification, WHO conditions and recommendations appear in curly brackets.

[b]Abbreviations: WHO, World Health Organization; COC, combined oral contraceptive; F, combined hormonal contraceptive patch; R, combined hormonal vaginal ring; POP, progestin-only pill; DMPA, depot medroxyprogesterone acetate; LNG-IUD, levonorgestrel-releasing intrauterine device Cu-IUD, copper intrauterine device; DVT, deep venous thrombosis; PE, pulmonary embolism; VTE, venous thromboembolism.

[c]Consult the clarification column for this classification.

[d]Condition that exposes a women to increased risk as a result of unintended pregnancy.

SUMMARY OF RECOMMENDATIONS FOR MEDICAL CONDITIONS ADDED TO THE U.S. MEDICAL ELIGIBILITY CRITERIA FOR CONTRACEPTIVE USE[a]

Condition	COC/P/R	POP	DMPA	Implants	LNG-IUD	Cu-IUD	Clarification
History of bariatric surgery[†]							
a. Restrictive procedures: decrease storage capacity of the stomach (vertical banded gastroplasty, laparoscopic adjustable gastric band, laparoscopic sleeve gastrectomy)	1	1	1	1	1	1	
b. Malabsorptive procedures: decrease absorption of nutrients and calories by shortening the functional length of the small intestine (Roux-en-Y gastric bypass, biliopancreatic diversion)	COCs: 3 P/R: 1	3	1	1	1	1	
Peripartum cardiomyopathy[b]							
a. Normal or mildly impaired cardiac function (New York Heart Association Functional Class I or II: patients with no limitation of activities or patients with slight, mild limitation of activity) (2)							
i < 6 mos	4	1	1	1	2	2	
ii ≥ 6 mos	3	1	1	1	2	2	
b. Moderately or severely impaired cardiac function (New York Heart Association Functional Class III or IV: patients with marked limitation of activity or patients who should be at complete rest) (2)	4	2	2	2	2	2	

SUMMARY OF RECOMMENDATIONS FOR MEDICAL CONDITIONS ADDED TO THE U.S. MEDICAL ELIGIBILITY CRITERIA FOR CONTRACEPTIVE USE[a] (CONTINUED)

Condition	COC/P/R	POP	DMPA	Implants	LNG-IUD		Cu-IUD		Clarification
					Initiation	Continuation	Initiation	Continuation	
Rheumatoid arthritis									
a. On immunosuppressive therapy	2	1	2/3[c]	1	2	1	2	1	DMPA use among women on long-term corticosteroid therapy with a history of, or risk factors for, nontraumatic fracture is classified as Category 3. Otherwise, DMPA use for women with rheumatoid arthritis is classified as Category 2.
b. Not on immunosuppressive therapy	2	1	2	1	1		1		
Endometrial hyperplasia	1	1	1	1	1		1		

SUMMARY OF RECOMMENDATIONS FOR MEDICAL CONDITIONS ADDED TO THE U.S. MEDICAL ELIGIBILITY CRITERIA FOR CONTRACEPTIVE USE[a] (CONTINUED)

Condition	COC/P/R	POP	DMPA	Implants	LNG-IUD			Cu-IUD		Clarification
					Initiation	Continuation		Initiation	Continuation	
Inflammatory bowel disease (IBD) (ulcerative colitis, Crohn disease)	2/3[c]	2	2	1	1			1		For women with mild IBD, with no other risk factors for VTE, the benefits of COC/P/R use generally outweigh the risks (Category 2). However, for women with IBD with increased risk for VTE (eg, those with active or extensive disease, surgery, immobilization, corticosteroid use, vitamin deficiencies, fluid depletion), the risks for COC/P/R use generally outweigh the benefits (Category 3).
Solid organ transplantation†										
a. Complicated: graft failure (acute or chronic), rejection, cardiac allograft vasculopathy	4	2	2	2	3	2		3	2	

SUMMARY OF RECOMMENDATIONS FOR MEDICAL CONDITIONS ADDED TO THE U.S. MEDICAL ELIGIBILITY CRITERIA FOR CONTRACEPTIVE USE* (CONTINUED)							
Condition	COC/P/R	POP	DMPA	Implants	LNG-IUD	Cu-IUD	Clarification
b. Uncomplicated	2§	2	2	2	2	2	Women with Budd-Chiari syndrome should not use COC/P/R because of the increased risk for thrombosis.

*Abbreviations: COC, combined oral contraceptive; P, combined hormonal contraceptive patch; R, combined hormonal vaginal ring; POP, progestin-only pill; DMPA, depotmedroxyprogesterone acetate; LNG-IUD, levonorgestrel-releasing intrauterine device; Cu-IUD, copper intrauterine device; IIED, inflammatory bowel disease; VTE, venousthromboembolism.

†Condition that exposes a woman to increased risk as a result of unintended pregnancy.

‡Consult the clarification column for this classification.

SUMMARY OF ADDITIONAL CHANGES TO THE U.S. MEDICAL ELIGIBILITY CRITERIA FOR CONTRACEPTIVE USE	
Condition/Contraceptive Method	**Change**
Emergency contraceptive pills	History of bariatric surgery, rheumatoid arthritis, inflammatory bowel disease, and solid organ transplantation were added to Appendix D and given a Category 1.
Barrier methods	For 6 conditions—history of bariatric surgery, peripartum cardiomyopathy, rheumatoid arthritis, endometrial hyperplasia, inflammatory bowel disease, and solid organ transplantation—the barrier methods are classified as Category 1.
Sterilization	In general, no medical conditions would absolutely restrict a person's eligibility for sterilization. Recommendations from the World Health Organization (WHO) Medical Eligibility Criteria for Contraceptive Use about specific settings and surgical procedures for sterilization are not included here. The guidance has been replaced with general text on sterilization.
Other deleted items	Guidance for combined injectables, levonorgestrel implants, and norethisterone enanthate has been removed because these methods are not currently available in the United States. Guidance for "blood pressure measurement unavailable" and "history of hypertension, where blood pressure CANNOT be evaluated (including hypertension in pregnancy)" has been removed.
Unintended pregnancy and increased health risk	The following conditions have been added to the WHO list of conditions that expose a woman to increased risk as a result of unintended pregnancy: history of bariatric surgery within the past 2 years, peripartum cardiomyopathy, and receiving a solid organ transplant within 2 years.

CHRONIC OBSTRUCTIVE PULMONARY DISEASE (COPD), EXACERBATIONS

Disease Management	Organization	Date	Population	Recommendations	Comments	Source
Chronic Obstructive Pulmonary Disease (COPD), Exacerbations	NICE	2010	Adults	1. Recommends non-invasive positive pressure ventilation for moderate-severe hypercapnic respiratory failure. 2. Prednisolone 30 mg orally, or its equivalent IV, should be prescribed for 7–14 days. 3. Recommends antibiotics for COPD exacerbations associated with more purulent sputum. 4. Bronchodilators can be delivered by either nebulizers or meter-dosed inhalers depending on the patient's ability to use the device during a COPD exacerbation.	Initial empiric antibiotics should be an aminopenicillin, macrolide, or a tetracycline.	http://www.nice.org.uk/nicemedia/live/13029/49397/49397.pdf

Disease Management	Organization	Date	Population	Recommendations	Comments	Source

Chronic Obstructive Pulmonary Disease (COPD), Stable	NICE	2010	Adults	1. Recommends confirming all suspected COPD with postbronchodilator spirometry.
				2. Recommends spirometry in all persons aged >35 years who are current or ex-smokers and have a chronic cough to evaluate for early-stage COPD.
				3. Recommends smoking cessation counseling.
				4. Stepwise medication approach[a]:
				  a. Short-acting beta-agonist (SABA) as needed (prn)
				  b. If persistent symptoms, add:
				    i. $FEV_1 \geq 50\%$, add either a long-acting beta-agonist (LABA) or long-acting muscarinic agonist (LAMA)
				    ii. $FEV_1 < 50\%$, add either LABA + inhaled corticosteroid (ICS), or LAMA
				  c. If persistent symptoms, add:
				    i. LAMA to LABA + ICS
				5. Recommends pulmonary rehabilitation for symptomatic patients with moderate-severe COPD (FEV1 < 50%).
				6. Recommends calculating the BODE index (BMI, airflow obstruction, dyspnea, and exercise capacity on a 6-minute walk test) to calculate the risk of death in severe COPD.[b]
						http://www.nice.org.uk/nicemedia/live/13029/49397/49397.pdf

CHRONIC OBSTRUCTIVE PULMONARY DISEASE (COPD), STABLE

Disease Management	Organization	Date	Population	Recommendations	Comments	Source
Chronic Obstructive Pulmonary Disease (COPD), Stable (continued)	ACP	2011	Adults	• Spirometry should be obtained to diagnose airflow obstruction in patients presenting with respiratory symptoms • Bronchodilators should be prescribed for stable COPD patients with respiratory symptoms and a FEV_1 60%–80% of predicted. • Inhaled corticosteroids and long-acting anticholinergics or long-acting β-agonists should be prescribed for stable COPD patients with respiratory symptoms and a $FEV_1 < 60\%$ of predicted. • Pulmonary rehabilitation should be prescribed for symptomatic COPD patients with a $FEV_1 < 50\%$ of predicted. • Continuous oxygen therapy should be prescribed for COPD patients with resting hypoxemia ($PaO_2 \leq 55$ mm Hg or $SpO_2 \leq 88\%$	• No proven benefit for using spirometry to encourage smoking cessation • No role for periodic spirometry to monitor disease status • No role for spirometry for at-risk patients who are *asymptomatic*	http://www.annals.org/content/155/3/179.full.pdf-html

CHRONIC OBSTRUCTIVE PULMONARY DISEASE (COPD), STABLE

[a]SABA, short-acting beta-agonist: albuterol, fenoterol, levalbuterol, metaproterenol, pirbuterol, and terbutaline.
LABA, long-acting beta-agonists: arformoterol, formoterol, or salmeterol.
LAMA, long-acting muscarinic agonists: tiotropium.
ICS, inhaled corticosteroids: beclomethasone, budesonide, ciclesonide, flunisolide, fluticasone, mometasone, and triamcinolone.
[b]See http://www.nejm.org/doi/full/10.1056/NEJMoa021322#t=article

CORONARY ARTERY DISEASE: STENT THERAPY
USE OF TRIPLE ANTICOAGULATION TREATMENT
Source: AMERICAN COLLEGE OF CARDIOLOGY/AMERICAN HEART ASSOCIATION/EUROPEAN SOCIETY OF CARDIOLOGY

The prudent use of triple anticoagulation therapy with aspirin, clopidogrel, and warfarin in AF patients at high risk of thromboembolism and recent coronary stent placement remains a *matter of clinical judgment*, balancing the risk of thrombotic versus bleeding events.

Facts:

- Bare-metal stents are the stent of choice if TAT is required.
- Drug eluting stents should be reserved for high-risk clinical or anatomic situations (diabetic patients or if the coronary lesions are unusually long, totally occlusive, or in small blood vessels) if TAT is required.
- Dual antiplatelet therapy with clopidogrel (75 mg/day) and ASA (81 mg/day) is the most effective therapy to *prevent coronary stent thrombosis*.
- Warfarin anticoagulation is the most effective therapy to *prevent thromboembolism* in high-risk AF patients as defined by the $CHADS_2$ risk score (≥ 2) or the $CHA_2DS_2\text{-}VAS_c$ risk score (≥ 3).
- TAT is the most effective therapy to *prevent* both *coronary stent thrombosis* and the *occurrence* of embolic strokes in high-risk patients.
- However, the addition of DAPT to warfarin increases the bleeding risk by 3.7-fold.
- Therefore, awaiting a definitive clinical trial (WOEST Trial), risk stratification of patients to evaluate the *thromboembolic potential of AF* versus the *bleeding potential* should be performed.
- The HAS-BLED (see box below) bleeding risk score is the best measure of bleeding risk. A high risk of bleeding is defined by a score ≥ 3.

Hypertension (≥ 160 mm Hg), **A**bnormal kidney function (creatinine ≥ 2, chronic dialysis, transplant), **A**bnormal liver function (cirrhosis, bilirubin > 2×, AST > 3×), **S**troke, **B**leeding history or anemia, **L**abile INR (< 60% within range), **E**lderly (aged ≥ 65 years), **D**rugs/alcohol (use of ASA or clopidogrel) or alcohol (≥ 8 alcoholic drinks/week). *Each risk factor is assigned 1 point for a total of 9 points.*

- If DAPT or TAT is required, *prophylactic GI therapy* with an H_2 blocker (except cimetidine) or PPI agent should be maintained. If omeprazole (Prilosec) is considered, the risk-to-benefit ratio needs to be considered due to its possible interference with clopidogrel function.
- In patients with a high risk of bleeding, TAT should be reserved for AF patients with a high thromboembolic risk. If the bleeding risk is high but the AF thromboembolic risk is low, DAPT therapy is suggested.

TAT, triple anticoagulation therapy; AF, atrial fibrillation; ASA, aspirin; BMS, bare-metal stents; DES, drug-eluting stents; DAPT, dual antiplatelet therapy; AST, aspartate transaminase; INR, international normalized ratio; GI, gastrointestinal; H_2, histamine; PPI, proton pump inhibitor

Sources: Adapted from European Society of Cardiology Guidelines for the Management of Atrial Fibrillation. *Eur Heart J.* 2010;31:2369–2429. Managing the anticoagulated patient with atrial fibrillation at high risk of stroke who needs coronary intervention. *BMJ.* 2008;337a840. Coronary Stent Implantation in Patients Committed to Long-term Oral Anticoagulation. *Chest.* 2011;139(5):981–987. ACC/AHA/SCAI 2007 Focused Update of the 2005 Guidelines for PCI. *J Am Coll Cardiol.* 2008;51(2):172–208. ACC/AHA 2011 Guidelines for the Management of Patients With Unstable Angina/Non-ST-Elevation Myocardial Infarction. *J Am Coll Cardiol.* 2011; 57:1920–1959. ACCF/ACG/AHA 2010 Expert Consensus Document on the Concomitant Use of Protein Pump Inhibitors and Thienopyridines. *J Am Coll Cardiol.* 2010;56(24):2051–2066. Combined Antiplatelet and Anticoagulation Therapies. *J Am Coll Cardiol.* 2009;54(2):95–109.

CORONARY ARTERY DISEASE: STENT THERAPY
USE OF TRIPLE ANTICOAGULATION TREATMENT

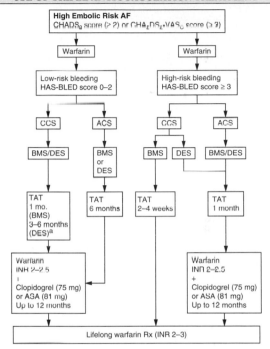

AF, atrial fibrillation; CCS, patient with chronic coronary syndrome (stable coronary artery disease); ACS, acute coronary syndrome; BMS, bare metal stent; DES, drug eluting stent; TAT, triple anticoagulation therapy; DES, drug eluting stent; ASA, aspirin; INR, international normalized ratio; Rx, therapy [warfarin (INR 2–2.5) + aspirin (81 mg daily) + clopidogrel (75 mg daily)].

a DES stents if sirolimus, everolimus or tacrolimus require 3-month dual platelet therapy (aspirin plus clopidogrel). If DES stent is paclitaxel, 6-month dual therapy is required.

Sources: Adopted from European Society of Cardiology Guidelines for the Management of Atrial Fibrillation. *Euro Heart J*. 2010;31:2369–2429. Managing the anticoagulated patient with atrial fibrillation at high risk of stroke who needs coronary intervention. *BMJ*. 2008;337a840. Coronary Stent Implantation in Patients Committed to Long-term Oral Anticoagulation. *CHEST*. 2011;139(5):981–987. ACC/AHA/SCAI 2007 Focused Update of the 2005 Guidelines for PCI. *J Am Coll Cardiol*. 2008;51(2):172–208. ACC/AHA 2011 Guidelines for the Management of Patients With Unstable Angina/Non-ST-Elevation Myocardial Infarction. *J Am Coll Cardiol*. 2011; 57:1920–1959. ACCF/ACG/AHA 2010 Expert Consensus Document on the Concomitant Use of Protein Pump Inhibitors and Thienopyridines. *J Am Coll Cardiol*. 2010;56(24):2051–2066. Combined Antiplatelet and Anticoagulation Therapies. *J Am Coll Cardiol*. 2009;54(2):95–109.

CORONARY ARTERY DISEASE: THERAPY FOR UNSTABLE ANGINA/ NON-ST-ELEVATION MI
ACCF/AHA 2011
CLASS 1 RECOMMENDATIONS

1. Aspirin (ASA) 325 mg should be administered promptly to all patients unless contraindicated.

2. Clopidogrel 300–600 mg bolus or prasugrel 60 mg should be administered to all ASA-allergic patients.

3. Risk stratification to *initial invasive* or *conservative therapy* is required. Early invasive therapy is indicated with refractory angina, hemodynamic or electrical instability. Most procedures are performed within 2–24 hours depending on the stability of the patient. TIMI and GRACE scores are often employed to select invasive versus conservative therapy.

4. Dual antiplatelet (ASA + clopidogrel) therapy is indicated *upstream* (before the heart catheterization) in the invasive group and in the conservative group.

5. If a history of GI bleeding is noted, a PPI agent or H2 blocker should be added to the dual antiplatelet therapy.

6. In the conservative group, if recurrent ischemia, heart failure, or serious arrhythmias occur, coronary arteriogram is indicated.

7. Nasal oxygen is indicated if arterial saturation is < 90%, if respiratory distress is present, or other high-risk features for hypoxemia.

8. Sublingual and intravenous NTG are indicated for clinical angina.

9. Oral beta-blockers should be administered within the first 24 hours unless contraindicated. Intravenous beta-blocker if chest pain is ongoing.

10. ACE inhibitor should be administered within 24 hours in patients with clinical HF with decreased ejection fraction (> 40%), if not contraindicated.

11. Consider percutaneous coronary intervention (PCI) of the *culprit coronary vessel* (the vessel causing the acute ischemia) with staged PCIs for other significant but less critical lesions. Consider CABG for significant left main lesion, double or triple vessel disease with decreased ejection fraction. The SYNTAX score may have predictive value in selecting PCI versus CABG.

12. Myocardial perfusion imaging (MPI) is indicated prior to discharge if conservative therapy chosen.

13. Dual anti-platelet (ASA 81 mg and clopidogrel 75 mg or prasugrel 10 mg) is indicated for at least 12 months. ASA should be continued lifelong.

14. If warfarin is indicated post-coronary stent, see Anticoagulation with Stent section.

15. Post-discharge medications include: ASA, clopidogrel 75 mg, beta-blocker dose to control heart rate, statin agent and possible ACE inhibitor if decreased ejection fraction or clinical heart failure, diabetes or hypertension is present.

Source: ACC/AHA 2007 Guidelines J Am Coll Cardiol. 2007;50(7):652–726. ACCF/AHA 2011 Guidelines J Am Coll Cardiol. 2011;57(19(:1920–1959. ESC 2011. ECS Guidelines European Heart J http://eurheartj.oxfordjournals.org/at OCLC, Accessed 11/21/2011. SYNTAX Score J Am Coll Cardiol. 2011;57(24):2389–2397. ACCF/SCAI/STS/AATS/AHA/ASNC/HFSA/SCCT 2012, J Am Coll Cardiol 59(9): 857–876.

				DELIRIUM		

Disease Management	Organization	Date	Population	Recommendations	Comments	Source

Delirium	NICE	2010	Adults aged ≥ 18 years in the hospital or in long-term care facilities	1. Perform a short Confusion Assessment Method (CAM) screen to confirm the diagnosis of delirium.
				2. Recommended approach to the management of delirium:
				  a. Treat the underlying cause
				  b. Provide frequent reorientation and reassurance to patients and their families
				  c. Provide cognitively stimulating activities
				  d. Ensure adequate hydration
				  e. Prevent constipation
				  f. Early mobilization
				  g. Treat pain if present
				  h. Provide hearing aids or corrective lenses if sensory impairment is present
				  i. Promote good sleep hygiene
				  j. Consider short-term antipsychotic use (< 1 week) for patients who are distressed or considered at risk to themselves or others
					Recommended antipsychotics are haloperidol or olanzapine given at the lowest effective dose.	http://www.nice.org.uk/ nicemedia/live/ 13060/49909/49909.pdf

					DEMENTIA	

Disease Management	Organization	Date	Population	Recommendations	Comments	Source
Dementia	ACP AAFP	2008 2008	Adults with dementia	1. Recommend a trial of therapy with a cholinesterase inhibitor or memantine based on individual assessment of relative risks versus benefits. 2. The choice of medication is based on tolerability, side effect profile, ease of use, and medication cost. 3. The evidence is insufficient to compare the relative efficacy of different medications for dementia. 4. Evidence is insufficient to determine the optimal duration of therapy.	1. A beneficial effect of cholinesterase inhibitors or memantine is generally observed within 3 months. 2. Good-quality data in mild-moderate Alzheimer and vascular dementia showed that cholinesterase inhibitors provide a modest improvement in global assessment, but no clinically important cognitive improvement. Subsets of patients may have significant cognitive improvement. 3. Five high-quality studies evaluated memantine use in moderate-severe Alzheimer and vascular dementia and showed statistically significant improvement in global assessment, but no clinically important cognitive improvement.	http://www.annals.org/content/148/5/370.full.pdf

DEMENTIA, ALZHEIMER'S DISEASE						
Disease Management	Organization	Date	Population	Recommendations	Comments	Source
Dementia, Alzheimer's Disease	NICE	2011	Adults	• Donepezil, galantamine, and rivastigmine are recommended as options for mild-moderate Alzheimer's disease. • Memantine is recommended as an option for managing moderate Alzheimer's disease in patients who can't tolerate acetylcholinesterase inhibitors	• Common adverse effects of acetylcholinesterase inhibitors include diarrhea, nausea, vomiting, muscle cramps, and insomnia • Common adverse effects of memantine are dizziness, headache, constipation, somnolence, and hypertension	http://www.nice.org.uk/nicemedia/live/13419/53619_pdf

	DEPRESSION					

Disease Management	Organization	Date	Population	Recommendations	Comments	Source
Depression	USPSTF	2009	Children and adolescents	1. Adequate evidence showed that SSRIs, psychotherapy, and combined therapy will decrease symptoms of major depressive disorder in adolescents aged 12–18 years. 2. Insufficient evidence to support screening and treatment of depression in children aged 7–11 years.	1. Good evidence showed that SSRIs may increase absolute risk of suicidality in adolescents by 1%–2%. Therefore, SSRIs should be used only if close clinical monitoring is possible. 2. Fluoxetine and citalopram yielded statistically significant higher response rates than did other SSRIs.	http://www.uspreventiveservicestaskforce.org/uspstf09/depression/chdeprrs.pdf

DIABETES MELLITUS (DM), TYPE 1					
Disease Management	Organization	Date	Population	Recommendations	Comments	Source

Diabetes Mellitus (DM), Type 1	ADA	2012	Adults and children	1. Recommends intensive insulin therapy with ≥ 3 injections daily using both basal and prandial insulin or an insulin pump.
				 2. Self-monitoring blood glucose ≥ 3 times daily in all patients using multiple insulin injections or an insulin pump.
				 3. Recommends assessment of psychological and social situation as part of diabetic evaluation.
				 4. Recommends glucose (15–20 g) for all conscious patients with hypoglycemia.
				 5. Advise all patients not to smoke.
				 6. Recommends beginning these screening tests after 5 years with type 1 DM
				   a. Urine albumin/creatinine ratio and serum creatinine annually
				   b. Dilated funduscopic exam annually
				   c. Monofilament screening for diabetic neuropathy annually
				   d. Comprehensive foot exam at least annually
				 7. Recommends screening at diagnosis for other autoimmune conditions:
				   a. Tissue transglutaminase IgA antibodies
				   b. Thyroperoxidase and thyroglobulin antibodies
				   c. TSH
					1. Glycemic control recommendations for **toddlers (aged 0–6 years):**
					   a. Before meals, CPG 100–180 mg/dL
					   b. Bedtime CPG, 110–200 mg/dL
					   c. HgbA1c < 8.5%
					 2. Glycemic control recommendations for **school-aged (aged 6–12 years):**
					   a. Before meals, CPG 90–180 mg/dL
					   b. Bedtime CPG, 100–180 mg/dL
					   c. HgbA1c < 8%
						http://care.diabetesjournals.org/content/34/Supplement_1/S11.full.pdf+html

DIABETES MELLITUS (DM), TYPE 1					
Disease Management	Organization	Date	Population	Recommendations	Comments	Source
Diabetes Mellitus (DM), Type 1 (continued)				7. Fasting lipid panel at age 10 years or at puberty (consider as early as age 2 years for a strong family history of hyperlipidemia). 　a. Repeat annually if results abnormal or every 5 years if results acceptable 8. Consider statin therapy if aged ≥ 10 years and LDL > 160 mg/dL despite good glycemic control and lifestyle modification. 9. Aspirin 75–162 mg/day if: 　a. Primary prevention of CVD if 10-year risk of coronary artery disease (CAD) > 10% 　b. Secondary prevention of CVD	3. Glycemic control recommendations for **adolescents (aged 13–19 years):** 　a. Before meals, CPG 90–130 mg/dL 　b. Bedtime CPG, 90–150 mg/dL 　c. HgbA1c < 7.5%	

DIABETES MELLITUS (DM), TYPE 2

Disease Management	Organization	Date	Population	Recommendations	Comments	Source
Diabetes Mellitus (DM), Type 2	AACE	2010	Nonpregnant adults	1. Endorsed the use of HgbA1c ≥ 6.5% as a means of diagnosing type 2 DM. 2. HgbA1c is not recommended for diagnosing type 1 DM or gestational diabetes.		http://www.aace.com/pub/pdf/guidelines/AACEpositionA1cfeb2010.pdf
	NICE	2009	Adults	1. Consider adding a dipeptidyl peptidase-4) DPP-4 inhibitor* or pioglitazone to metformin as a second-line agent if glycemic control is inadequate and a significant risk of hypoglycemia or sulfonylurea contraindications exist. 2. Consider adding a DPP-4 inhibitor* or pioglitazone to a sulfonylurea as a second-line agent if glycemic control is inadequate and a metformin contraindication exists. 3. Consider a glucagon-like peptide-1 (GLP-1) mimetic (eg, exenatide) as a third-line agent when glycemic control is inadequate (HgbA1c ≥ 7.5% with metformin and a sulfonylurea. 4. Consider adding insulin when glycemic control is inadequate (HgbA1c ≥ 7.5%) with oral agents alone.	1. Avoid pioglitazone in people with heart failure or who have a higher risk of fracture. 2. Avoid metformin if the glomerular filtration rate (GFR) is < 45 mL/min/1.73 m².	http://www.nice.org.uz/nicemedia/live/12165/44318/44318.pdf

Disease Management	Organization	Date	Population	Recommendations	Comments	Source
DIABETES MELLITUS (DM), TYPE 2						

Diabetes Mellitus (DM, Type 2 (continued)	ADA	2012	Adults and children	1. Self-monitoring blood glucose ≥ 3 times daily in all patients using multiple insulin injections or an insulin pump
				2. Recommends HgbA1c every 3 months if therapy has changed or if blood glucose control is inadequate
				3. Provide diabetes self-management education, including education about hypoglycemia management and adjustments during illness
				4. Provide family planning for women of reproductive age
				5. Provide medical nutrition therapy
				6. Weight loss is recommended for all overweight or obese diabetic patients
				7. Keep saturated fat intake < 7% of total calories
				8. Reduction of protein intake to 0.8–1 gm/kg/d for early stages of CKD and 0.8 gm/kg/d for later stages of CKD
				9. Recommends at least 150 min/week of moderate physical activity
					1. Glycemic control recommendations:
					  a. Preprandial capillary blood gas (CPG) 70–130 mg/dL
					  b. Postprandial CPG < 180 mg/dL (1–2 hour post-meals)
					  c. HgbA1c < 7%
					2. Consider bariatric surgery if BMI > 35 kg/m^2 and if diabetes is difficult to control with lifestyle modification and medications.
					3. Angiotensin-converting enzyme inhibitors (ACEIs) or angiotensin receptor blockers (ARBs) are first-line antihypertensives.
						http://care.diabetesjournals.org/content/35/Supplement_1/S11.full.pdf+html

DIABETES MELLITUS (DM), TYPE 2					
Disease Management	Organization	Date	Population	Recommendations	Comments	Source
Diabetes Mellitus (DM), Type 2 (continued)				10. The glucose range for critically ill patients is 140–180 mg/dL (7.8–10 mmol/L)	4. Second-line antihypertensives are a thiazide diuretic if GFR $\geq$ 30 mL/min/1.73m^2 or a loop diuretic if GFR < 30 mL/min/1.73m^2.	
				11. The glucose range for non-critically ill patients in the hospital is < 140 mg/dL premeal (< 7.8 mmol/L) and random blood glucose < 180 mg/dL (< 10 mmol/L)	5. Clopidogrel 75 mg/day is an alternative for persons ASA intolerant.	
				12. Recommends the following: a. Immunizations: annual influenza vaccination if aged ≥ 6 months, pneumococcal polysaccharide vaccine if aged ≥ 2 years, and 1 x revaccination if aged ≥ 65 years, and hepatitis B vaccination per CDC recommendations b. Target blood pressure (BP) < 130/80 mm Hg	6. Nephrology referral indicated if GFR < 60 mL/min/1.73m^2, or if heavy proteinuria or structural kidney disease present 7. Consider a serum TSH in women aged > 50 years.	

					DIABETES MELLITUS (DM), TYPE 2	
Disease Management	Organization	Date	Population	Recommendations	Comments	Source

Diabetes Mellitus (DM), Type 2 (continued)				c. Statin therapy if:
				  i. Overt cardiovascular disease (CVD) present
				  ii. Aged > 40 years and ≥ 1 cardiovascular (CV) risk factor*
				  iii. Low-density lipoprotein (LDL) > 100 mg/dL despite lifestyle modification
				d. Aspirin 75–162 mg/day if:
				  i. Primary prevention of CVD if 10-year risk of coronary artery disease (CAD) > 10%
				  ii. Secondary prevention of CVD
				e. Annual check of urine albumin/creatinine ratio and serum creatinine
				f. Annual serum creatinine and fasting lipid profile
				g. Annual dilated funduscopic exam
				h. Annual monofilament screening for diabetic neuropathy
				i. At minimum, annual comprehensive foot exam
					8. Consider assessing patients for the following comorbidities that are increased with DM:
					a. Hearing impairment
					b. Obstructive sleep apnea
					c. Fatty liver disease
					d. Low testosterone in men
					e. Periodontal disease
					f. Cognitive impairment	

					DIABETES MELLITUS (DM), TYPE 2	
Disease Management	Organization	Date	Population	Recommendations	Comments	Source
Diabetes Mellitus (DM), Type 2 (continued)	ACP	2012	Adults older than 18 years	• Oral pharmacologic therapy should be added for treatment of type 2 DM when lifestyle modifications, including diet, exercise, and weight loss, have failed to adequately control hyperglycemia • Recommends metformin as the initial pharmacologic agent to treat most patients with type 2 DM • Recommend adding another oral agent to metformin if patients have persistent hyperglycemia despite metformin and lifestyle modifications	• All dual-regimens were more effective than monotherapy and decreased the HbA1c levels by an average of 1% more • Most monotherapy regimens had similar efficacy and reduced HbA1c levels by an average of 1% • Studies suggest that metformin decreases all-cause mortality slightly more than sulfonylureas with a much lower rate of hypoglycemia	http://www.annals.org/content/156/3/1-36.full.pdf+html
		2011	Hospitalized adults older than 18 years	• Avoid intensive insulin therapy in hospitalized patients (even if in SICU/MICU) • Recommends a target blood glucose level of 140–200 mg/dL if insulin therapy is used in SICU/MICU patients	• Intensive insulin therapy (targeting blood glucose levels of 80–110 mg/dL) in SICU/MICU patients does not improve mortality, but has a five-fold increased risk of hypoglycemia	http://www.annals.org/content/154/4/260.full.pdf+html

^aSitagliptin or vildagliptin.
^bCardiovascular risk factors: hypertension, smoking, positive family history, men aged ≥45 years and women aged ≥55 years, or hyperlipidemia.

BLOOD-GLUCOSE-LOWERING THERAPY: NICE, 2009

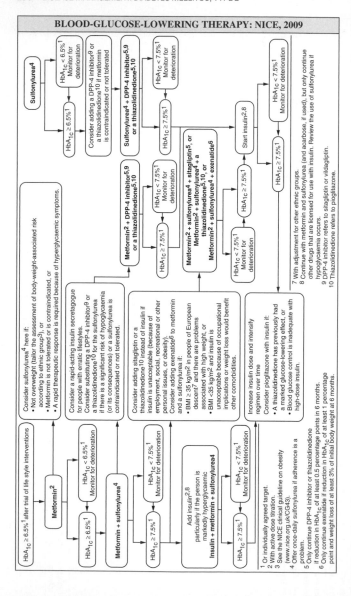

	DIABETIC FOOT PROBLEMS, INPATIENT MANAGEMENT				
Disease Management	Organization	Date	Population	Recommendations	Comments	Source

Diabetic Foot Problems, Inpatient Management	NICE	2011	Hospitalized adults older than 18 years with diabetic foot problems	• Every hospital should have a multidisciplinary foot care team to assess and treat any diabetic patient with foot problems
				• Every patient with a diabetic foot problem should undergo an assessment for:
				  ○ Need for debridement, pressure off-loading
				  ○ Vascular inflow
				  ○ Infection of the foot
				  ○ Glycemic control
				  ○ Neuropathy
				• If osteomyelitis is suspected, obtain an x-ray and if x-ray is normal obtain an MRI
				• Provide off-loading for diabetic foot ulcers
				• For mild diabetic foot infections, treat with empiric antibiotics that provide good gram-positive organisms coverage
				• For moderate-severe diabetic foot infections, treat with empiric antibiotics that provide coverage of gram-positive, gram-negative, and anaerobic bacteria
					• The diabetic foot care team should include:
					  ○ Diabetologist
					  ○ Surgeon with expertise managing DM foot problems
					  ○ DM nurse specialist
					  ○ Podiatrist
					  ○ Tissue viability nurse
						http://www.nice.org.uk/nicemedia/live/13416/53556/53556.pdf

ERECTILE DYSFUNCTION (ED)

Disease Management	Organization	Date	Population	Recommendations	Comments	Source

Erectile Dysfunction (ED)	EAU	2009	Adult men	1. Recommends a medical and psychosexual history on all patients
				2. Recommends a focused physical exam to assess CV status, neurologic status, prostate disease, penile abnormalities, and signs of hypogonadism
				3. Recommends checking a fasting glucose, lipid profile, and total testosterone levels
				4. Recommends psychosexual therapy for psychogenic ED
				5. Recommends testosterone therapy for androgen deficiency if no contraindications present[a]
				6. Selective phosphodiesterase 5 (PDE5) inhibitors are first-line therapy for idiopathic ED
					1. Selective PDE5 inhibitors:
					  a. Sildenafil
					  b. Tadalafil
					  c. Vardenafil
					2. Avoid nitrates and use alpha-blockers with caution when prescribing a selective PDE5 inhibitor
						http://www.uroweb.org/gls/EU/2010%20Male%20Sex%20Dysfunction.pdf

[a]Prostate CA , breast CA, or signs of prostatism.

GLAUCOMA, CHRONIC OPEN ANGLE

Disease Management	Organization	Date	Population	Recommendations	Comments	Source

Glaucoma, Chronic Open Angle	NICE	2009	Adults	1. All persons with known or suspected chronic open angle glaucoma (COAG) or ocular hypertension (OHT) should undergo the following:
				  a. Intraocular pressure monitoring using tonometry
				  b. Central corneal thickness measurement
				  c. Peripheral anterior chamber depth assessments using gonioscopy
				  d. Visual field testing
				  e. Optic nerve assessment using slit-lamp exam
				2. Recommends monitoring patients with OHT at least annually for COAG (every 6 months for high-risk patients).
				3. Recommends monitoring patients with COAG every 6–12 months based on disease progression.
				4. Recommends prostaglandin analogue therapy for early-moderate COAG patients at risk of visual loss.
				5. Consider surgery with pharmacologic augmentation for advanced COAG.
				6. Recommends beta-blocker drops for mild OHT until age 60 years.
				7. Recommends prostaglandin analogue drops for any degree of OHT.
				8. Recommends additional medication therapy for uncontrolled OHT despite single-agent therapy.
					1. Alternative pharmacologic treatments for OHT or suspected COAG in patients whose intraocular pressures remain elevated on monotherapy include:
					  a. Prostaglandin analogues
					  b. Beta-blockers
					  c. Carbonic anhydrase inhibitors
					  d. Sympathomimetics
						http://www.guidelines.gov/content.aspx?id=14444

	HEADACHE, MIGRAINE PROPHYLAXIS					
Disease Management	Organization	Date	Population	Recommendations	Comments	Source

Headache, Migraine Prophylaxis	AAN	2012	Adults	• The following medications have **established efficacy** for migraine prophylaxis:
				  ○ Divalproex sodium
				  ○ Sodium valproate
				  ○ Topiramate
				  ○ Metoprolol
				  ○ Propranolol
				  ○ Timolol
				• Frovatriptan is effective for menstrual migraine prophylaxis
				• The following medications are **probably effective** for migraine prophylaxis:
				  ○ Amitriptyline
				  ○ Venlafaxine
				  ○ Atenolol
				  ○ Nadolol
					• Lamotrigine and clomipramine is ineffective for migraine prevention	http://www.neurology.org/content/78/17/1337.full.pdf+html

HEADACHE DIAGNOSIS ALGORITHM: ICSI, 2011

Patient presents with complaint of a headache A

Detailed History
- Characteristics of the headache
- Assess functional impairment
- Past medical history
- Family history of migraines
- Current medications and previous medications for headache (Rx and over-the-counter)
- Social history
- Review of systems-to rule out systemic illness

All algorithm boxes with an "A" and those that refer to other algorithm boxes link to annotation content.

Causes for concern:
- Subacute and/or progressive headache over months
- New or different headache
- "Worst headache ever"
- Any headache of maximum severity at onset
- Onset after the age of 50 years old
- Symptoms of systemic illness
- Seizures
- Any neurological signs

Critical first steps:
- Detailed history
- Focused physical examination
- Focused neurological examination A

Causes for concern? A → Yes → Consider secondary headache disorder A

No ↓

Headaches other than primary headache out of guideline ← No ← Meets criteria for primary headache disorder? A

Specialty consultation indicated? A → Yes → Refer to headache specialist

No ↓

Perform diagnostic testing if indicated A

Diagnosis of primary headache confirmed? → Yes

No ↓

Findings consistent with secondary headache? A → No / Yes → Determine secondary headache type out of guideline

Yes ↓

Evaluate type of primary headache. Initiate patient education and lifestyle management A

- Migraine (See Migraine algorithm)
- Tension-type (See Tension-Type Headache algorithm)
- Cluster (see Cluster Headache algorithm)
- Chronic daily headache A
- Other headache A

Sinus Headache

Migraine-associated symptoms are often misdiagnosed as "sinus headache" by patients and providers. Most headaches characterized as "sinus headaches" are migraines.

The International Classifications of Headache Disorders (ICHD-II) defines sinus headache by purulent nasal discharge, pathologic sinus finding by imaging, simultaneous onset of headache and sinusitis, and headache localized to specific facial and cranial areas of the sinuses.

A = Annotation

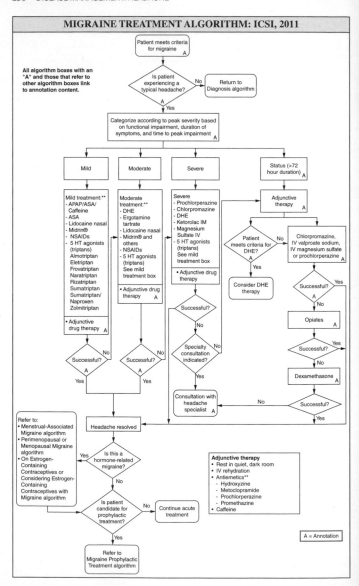

MIGRAINE TREATMENT ALGORITHM: ICSI, 2011

Patient meets criteria for migraine
A

All algorithm boxes with an "A" and those that refer to other algorithm boxes link to annotation content.

Is patient experiencing a typical headache?
A — Yes / No → Return to Diagnosis algorithm

Categorize according to peak severity based on functional impairment, duration of symptoms, and time to peak impairment A

Mild / **Moderate** / **Severe** / **Status (>72 hour duration)** A

Mild treatment:**
- APAP/ASA/Caffeine
- ASA
- Lidocaine nasal
- Midrin®
- NSAIDs
- 5 HT agonists (triptans)
  Almotriptan
  Eletriptan
  Frovatriptan
  Naratriptan
  Rizatriptan
  Sumatriptan
  Sumatriptan/Naproxen
  Zolmitriptan
• Adjunctive drug therapy A

Moderate treatment:**
- DHE
- Ergotamine tartrate
- Lidocaine nasal
- Midrin® and others
- NSAIDs
- 5 HT agonists (triptans)
  See mild treatment box
• Adjunctive drug therapy A

Severe
- Prochlorperazine
- Chlorpromazine
- DHE
- Ketorolac IM
- Magnesium Sulfate IV
- 5 HT agonists (triptans)
  See mild treatment box
• Adjunctive drug therapy

Adjunctive therapy A

Patient meets criteria for DHE? A — No / Yes → Consider DHE therapy

Chlorpromazine, IV valproate sodium, IV magnesium sulfate or prochlorperazine A

Successful? A — Yes / No

Opiates A

Successful? — Yes / No

Dexamethasone A

Successful? — Yes / No

Successful? A — Yes / No

Successful? A — Yes / No

Successful? — Yes / No

Specialty consultation indicated? — No / Yes

Consultation with headache specialist A

Refer to:
• Menstrual-Associated Migraine algorithm
• Perimenopausal or Menopausal Migraine algorithm
• On Estrogen-Containing Contraceptives or Considering Estrogen-Containing Contraceptives with Migraine algorithm

Headache resolved

Is this a hormone-related migraine? — Yes / No

Is patient candidate for prophylactic treatment? — No → Continue acute treatment / Yes

Refer to Migraine Prophylactic Treatment algorithm

Adjunctive therapy
• Rest in quiet, dark room
• IV rehydration
• Antiemetics**
  - Hydroxyzine
  - Metoclopramide
  - Prochlorperazine
  - Promethazine
• Caffeine

A = Annotation

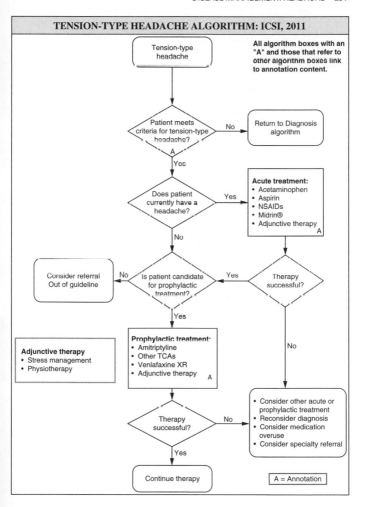

TENSION-TYPE HEADACHE ALGORITHM: ICSI, 2011

Tension-type headache

All algorithm boxes with an "A" and those that refer to other algorithm boxes link to annotation content.

Patient meets criteria for tension-type headache? — No → Return to Diagnosis algorithm

A / Yes

Does patient currently have a headache? — Yes →

Acute treatment:
- Acetaminophen
- Aspirin
- NSAIDs
- Midrin®
- Adjunctive therapy A

No

Consider referral Out of guideline ← No — Is patient candidate for prophylactic treatment? ← Yes — Therapy successful?

Yes

No

Adjunctive therapy
- Stress management
- Physiotherapy

Prophylactic treatment:
- Amitriptyline
- Other TCAs
- Venlafaxine XR
- Adjunctive therapy A

Therapy successful? — No →

- Consider other acute or prophylactic treatment
- Reconsider diagnosis
- Consider medication overuse
- Consider specialty referral

Yes

Continue therapy

A = Annotation

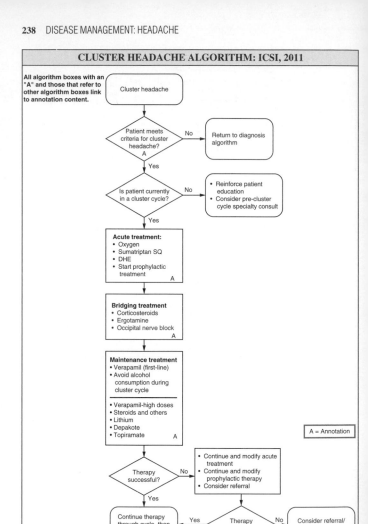

CLUSTER HEADACHE ALGORITHM: ICSI, 2011

All algorithm boxes with an "A" and those that refer to other algorithm boxes link to annotation content.

Cluster headache

Patient meets criteria for cluster headache? — No → Return to diagnosis algorithm

Yes

Is patient currently in a cluster cycle? — No → • Reinforce patient education • Consider pre-cluster cycle specialty consult

Yes

Acute treatment:
• Oxygen
• Sumatriptan SQ
• DHE
• Start prophylactic treatment
A

Bridging treatment
• Corticosteroids
• Ergotamine
• Occipital nerve block
A

Maintenance treatment
• Verapamil (first-line)
• Avoid alcohol consumption during cluster cycle

• Verapamil-high doses
• Steroids and others
• Lithium
• Depakote
• Topiramate
A

A = Annotation

Therapy successful? — No → • Continue and modify acute treatment • Continue and modify prophylactic therapy • Consider referral

Yes

Continue therapy through cycle, then taper ← Yes — Therapy successful? — No → Consider referral/ Out of guideline

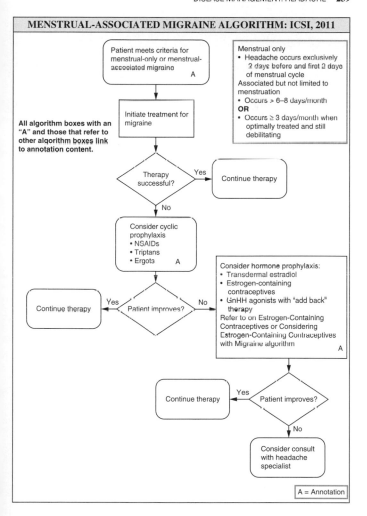

MENSTRUAL-ASSOCIATED MIGRAINE ALGORITHM: ICSI, 2011

Patient meets criteria for menstrual-only or menstrual-associated migraine   A

Menstrual only
• Headache occurs exclusively 2 days before and first 2 days of menstrual cycle
Associated but not limited to menstruation
• Occurs > 6–8 days/month
OR
• Occurs ≥ 3 days/month when optimally treated and still debilitating

All algorithm boxes with an "A" and those that refer to other algorithm boxes link to annotation content.

Initiate treatment for migraine

Therapy successful? → Yes → Continue therapy

No

Consider cyclic prophylaxis
• NSAIDs
• Triptans
• Ergots   A

Patient improves? → Yes → Continue therapy

No →

Consider hormone prophylaxis:
• Transdermal estradiol
• Estrogen-containing contraceptives
• GnRH agonists with "add back" therapy
Refer to on Estrogen-Containing Contraceptives or Considering Estrogen-Containing Contraceptives with Migraine algorithm   A

Patient improves? → Yes → Continue therapy

No

Consider consult with headache specialist

A = Annotation

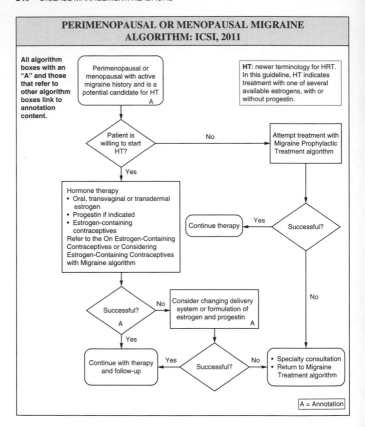

PERIMENOPAUSAL OR MENOPAUSAL MIGRAINE ALGORITHM: ICSI, 2011

All algorithm boxes with an "A" and those that refer to other algorithm boxes link to annotation content.

Perimenopausal or menopausal with active migraine history and is a potential candidate for HT
A

HT: newer terminology for HRT. In this guideline, HT indicates treatment with one of several available estrogens, with or without progestin.

Patient is willing to start HT? — No → Attempt treatment with Migraine Prophylactic Treatment algorithm

Yes

Hormone therapy
- Oral, transvaginal or transdermal estrogen
- Progestin if indicated
- Estrogen-containing contraceptives
Refer to the On Estrogen-Containing Contraceptives or Considering Estrogen-Containing Contraceptives with Migraine algorithm

Successful? — Yes → Continue therapy

No

Successful?
A
— No → Consider changing delivery system or formulation of estrogen and progestin
A

Yes

Continue with therapy and follow-up ← Yes — Successful? — No → • Specialty consultation
• Return to Migraine Treatment algorithm

A = Annotation

ON ESTROGEN-CONTAINING CONTRACEPTIVES OR CONSIDERING ESTROGEN-CONTAINING CONTRACEPTIVES WITH MIGRAINE ALGORITHM: ICSI, 2011

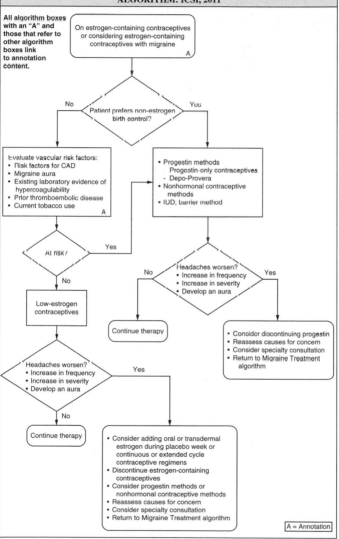

All algorithm boxes with an "A" and those that refer to other algorithm boxes link to annotation content.

On estrogen-containing contraceptives or considering estrogen-containing contraceptives with migraine
A

Patient prefers non-estrogen birth control?

No / Yes

Evaluate vascular risk factors:
- Risk factors for CAD
- Migraine aura
- Existing laboratory evidence of hypercoagulability
- Prior thromboembolic disease
- Current tobacco use
A

- Progestin methods
  Progestin-only contraceptives
  - Depo-Provera
- Nonhormonal contraceptive methods
- IUD; barrier method

At risk?

Yes / No

Low-estrogen contraceptives

Headaches worsen?
- Increase in frequency
- Increase in severity
- Develop an aura

No / Yes

Continue therapy

- Consider discontinuing progestin
- Reassess causes for concern
- Consider specialty consultation
- Return to Migraine Treatment algorithm

Headaches worsen?
- Increase in frequency
- Increase in severity
- Develop an aura

No / Yes

Continue therapy

- Consider adding oral or transdermal estrogen during placebo week or continuous or extended cycle contraceptive regimens
- Discontinue estrogen-containing contraceptives
- Consider progestin methods or nonhormonal contraceptive methods
- Reassess causes for concern
- Consider specialty consultation
- Return to Migraine Treatment algorithm

A = Annotation

MIGRAINE PROPHYLACTIC TREATMENT ALGORITHM: ICSI, 2011

All algorithm boxes with an "A" and those that refer to other algorithm boxes link to annotation content.

Patient meets criteria for migraine headache

Prophylactic treatment
Assess factors that may trigger migraine
Treatment:
• Medication
  - Beta-blocker
  - Tricyclic antidepressants
  - Ca++ channel blockers
  - Antiepileptic drugs
    • Divalproex
    • Topiramate
    • Gabapentin
• Reinforce education and lifestyle management
• Consider other therapies (biofeedback, relaxation)
• Screen for depression and generalized anxiety

A

Successful?* ──Yes──▶ Continue treatment for 6–12 months, then reassess   A

Successful?
Success as determined by:
• Headaches decrease by 50% or more
• An acceptable side effect profile

No

Try different first-line medication or different drug of same class   A

Successful? * ──Yes──▶ Continue treatment for 6–12 months, then reassess

No

Try combination of beta-blockers and tricyclics   A

Successful? * ──Yes──▶ Continue treatment for 6–12 months, then reassess

No

Third-line prophylaxis treatment or consultation with headache specialist   A

A = Annotation

HEARING LOSS, SUDDEN

Disease Management	Organization	Date	Population	Recommendations	Comments	Source
Hearing Loss, Sudden	AAO-HNS	2012	Adults 18 years and older	• Distinguish hearing loss into sensorineural or conductive hearing loss • Counsel patients with incomplete recovery of hearing about the benefits of hearing aids • Evaluate patients with idiopathic sudden sensorineural hearing loss (ISSNHL) for retrocochlear pathology by obtaining an MRI of the internal auditory canal, auditory brainstem responses, and an audiology exam • Consider treatment of ISSNHL with incomplete hearing recovery with systemic or intratympanic steroids or hyperbaric oxygen therapy • In patients with ISSNHL, recommend against antivirals, thrombolytics, vasodilators, or antioxidants for treatment and against CT scanning of the head or routine lab testing.		http://oto.sagepub.com/content/146/3_suppl/S1.full.pdf+html

HEART FAILURE
Source: ADAPTED FROM ACC/AHA, 2005

Stage A	Stage B	Stage C	Stage D
At high risk for HF but without structural heart disease or symptoms of HF	Structural heart disease but without signs or symptoms of HF	Structural heart disease with prior or current symptoms of HF	Refractory HF requiring specialized interventions

Structural heart disease → Development of symptoms of HF → Refractory symptoms of HF at rest

Therapy	**Therapy**	**Therapy**	**Therapy**

• Treat hypertension
• Encourage smoking cessation
• Treat lipid disorders
• Encourage regular exercise
• Discourage alcohol intake, illicit drug use
• Control metabolic syndrome
• ACE inhibition or ARB in appropriate patients[a]
	• All measures under stage A
	• ACE inhibitors or ARB in appropriate patients[b]
	• Beta-blockers in appropriate patients[b]
	• Devices in selected patients
	  - Implantable defibrillators
		• All measures under stage A, B
		• Dietary salt restriction
		• Drugs for routine use[c]:
		  Diuretics
		  ACE inhibitors
		  Beta-blockers
		• Drugs in selected patients
		  - Aldosterone agonist
		  - ARBs
		  - Digitalis
		  - Hydralazine/nitrates
		• Devices in selected patients
		  - Biventricular pacing
		  - Implantable defibrillators
			• Appropriate measures under stages A, B, and C
			• Decision re: appropriate level of care
			• Options
			  - Hospice (end-of-life care)
			  - Extraordinary measures
			  - Heart transplant
			  - Chronic inotropes
			  - Permanent mechanical support
			  - Experimental surgery or drugs

Stage A: Patients with hypertension, atherosclerotic disease, diabetes mellitus, metabolic syndrome, *or* those using cardiotoxins or having a family history of cardiomyopathy

Stage B: Patients with previous MI, LV remodeling including LVH and low EF, or asymptomatic valvular disease

Stage C: Patients with known structural heart disease; shortness of breath and fatigue, reduced exercise tolerance

Stage D: Patients who have marked symptoms at rest despite maximal medical therapy (eg, those who are recurrently hospitalized or cannot be safely discharged from the hospital without specialized interventions)

[a]History of atherosclerotic vascular disease, diabetes mellitus, or hypertension and associated cardiovascular risk factors.

[b]Recent or remote MI, regardless of ejection fraction; or reduced ejection fraction regardless of MI Hx. Use ARB in patients post-MI who cannot tolerate ACE inhibitors.

[c]Evidence suggests that isosorbide dinitrate plus hydralazine reduces mortality in blacks with advanced heart failure. (*NEJM.* 2004;351:2049)

Comments: Exercise training in patients with HF seems to be safe and beneficial overall in improving exercise capacity, quality of life, muscle structure, and physiologic responses to exercise. (*Circulation.* 2003;107:1210–1225)

HF, heart failure; LV, left ventricle

Source: Adapted from the American College of Cardiology, American Heart Association, Inc. *J Am Coll Cardiol.* 2005;46:1–82 and *Circulation.* 2005;112:154–235.
2009 ACCF/AHA Guidelines. *J Am Coll Cardiol.* 2009;53(150):1334–1378.

HEART FAILURE
SOURCE: ADOPTED FROM ACCF/AHA, 2009, 2011

CLINICAL ASSESSMENT IN HEART FAILURE
CLASS 1 RECOMMENDATION

1. Identify prior cardiac or noncardiac disease that may lead to HF.

2. Obtain history to include diet or medicine nonadherence; current or past use of alcohol, illicit drugs, and chemotherapy; or recent viral illness.

3. Identify the patient's present activity level and desired post-treatment level.

4. Assess the patient's volume status, orthostatic BP changes, height and weight, and body mass index.

5. Initial blood work to include at least CBC, chemistry panel, lipid profile, troponin I level, NT-proBNP, and TSH level.

6. 12-lead ECG should be obtained.

7. 2D echocardiogram is indicated to determine the systolic function, diastolic function, valvular function, and pulmonary artery pressure.

8. Coronary arteriography to be performed in patients with angina or significant ischemia with HF unless the patient is not eligible for surgery.

9. Initiate diuretic therapy and salt restriction if volume overloaded. Diuretics do not improve long-term survival but improve symptoms and short-term survival. Once euvolemic and symptoms have resolved, carefully start to wean dosage as a outpatient to lowest dose possible to prevent electrolyte disorders and activation of the renin angiotensin system.

10. ACE inhibitor or ARB agent should be considered early in the initial course to decrease afterload unless contraindicated if decreased ejection fraction noted (systolic dysfunction). Both agents improve long-term survival but are seldom employed together due to marginal benefit. Titrate dosage to that employed in clinical studies as BP allows.

11. Specific beta-blockers (carvedilol, sustained release metoprolol succinate, bisoprolol) should be added to improve long-term survival. These specific beta-blocker improve survival the most in systolic heart failure. Titrate dosage to heart rate 65–70 bpm.

12. Start aldosterone antagonist in patients with moderate or severe symptoms and reduced ejection fraction. Creatinine should be less than 2.5 mg/dL in men and less than 2 mg/dL in women, and the potassium should be less than 5 mEq/L.

13. The combination of hydralazine and nitrates should be employed to improve outcome in African Americans with moderate to severe HF with decreased ejection fraction in addition to optimal therapy. If ACE inhibitor or ARB agent is contraindicated, hydralazine and nitrates may be used as alternative therapy.

14. Discontinue anti-inflammatory agents, diltiazem, and verapamil.

15. Remember exercise training is beneficial in heart failure patients with decreased ejection fraction (systolic dysfunction) or preserved ejection fraction (diastolic dysfunction) once therapy is optimized.

16. Intracardiac cardiac defibrillator is indicated for secondary survival benefit in patients who survive cardiac arrest, ventricular fibrillation, or hemodynamically significant ventricular tachycardia.

17. Intracardiac cardiac defibrillator is indicated for primary survival benefit in patients with ischemic or nonischemic cardiomyopathy with EF equal or less than 35% with NYHA class II or III. The patient should be stable on optimal chronic medical HF therapy and at least 40 days post MI.

HEART FAILURE
SOURCE: ADOPTED FROM ACCF/AHA, 2009, 2011
(CONTINUED)

CLINICAL ASSESSMENT IN HEART FAILURE
CLASS 1 RECOMMENDATION

18. Biventricular heart pacemaker should be considered in refractory HF with ejection fraction equal or less than 35% with NYHA class III or ambulatory class IV. The rhythm should be sinus and the QRS duration should be equal or greater than 120 msec.

19. Long-term warfarin therapy in patients with marked decreased ejection fraction while in sinus rhythm in the absence of valve disease or endocardial clot offers no significant difference is frequency of ischemic stroke, intracerebral hemorrhage, or death.

20. In HF patients with preserved systolic function (diastolic dysfunction), randomized data on therapy are lacking. The goal is to control blood volume (diuretic), control systolic blood pressure (beta-blocker, ACE inhibitor, ARB agent, or diuretic), slow heart rate (beta-blocker), and treat coronary artery ischemia. Whether beta-blockers, ACE inhibitors, ARB agents, or aldosterone antagonists improve survival independently is yet to be proven.

21. Comprehensive written discharge instruction should be given to all patients. Diet, weight monitoring, medicine, and salt adherence should be emphasized. Activity should be discussed along with education of symptoms of worsening HF.

22. Post-discharge appointment with physician and health care team with attention o information on discharge medications.

Source: Adopted from theACCF/AHA 2009 Guidelines. *J Am Coll Cardiol* 2009;53(15):1333–1378; *N Engl J Med*. 2012;WARCET Trial; ACCF/AHA/AMA-PCPI 2011 *J Am Coll Cardiol* 2012;59(20):1812–1832.

HEMOCHROMATOSIS						
Disease Management	Organization	Date	Population	Recommendations	Comments	Source

Hemochromatosis	AASLD	2011	Adults	• Patients with abnormal iron studies should be evaluated for hemochromatosis
				  ○ Transferrin saturation ≥ 45%
				  ○ Elevated ferritin
				• Serum HFE mutation analysis should be performed in patients with possible hemochromatosis
				• All patients with unexplained liver disease should be evaluated for hemochromatosis
				• Liver biopsy is recommended to stage the degree of liver disease in C282Y homozygotes or compound heterozygotes if liver enzymes are elevated or ferritin > 1,000 mcg/L
				  ○ Treatment of hemochromatosis:
				  ○ Therapeutic phlebotomy weekly until the ferritin is 50–100 mcg/L
				  ○ Avoid vitamin C and iron supplements
				  ○ Iron chelation with deferoxamine mesylate or deferasirox is recommended in iron-overloaded patients with dyserythropoietic syndromes or chronic hemolytic anemia
						http://www.aasld.org/practiceguidelines/Practice%20Guideline%20Archive/Diagnosis%20and%20Management%20of%20Hemochromatosis.pdf

	HEPATITIS B VIRUS (HBV)				
Disease Management	Organization	Date	Population	Recommendations	Comments	Source
Hepatitis B Virus (HBV)	NIH AASLD	2009 2009	Adults and children with HBV infection	1. Recommend HBV immunoglobulin and HBV vaccine to all infants born to HBsAg-positive women. 2. Recommend antiviral therapy for adults and alanine transaminase (ALT) > 2× normal, moderate-severe hepatitis on biopsy, compensated cirrhosis or advanced fibrosis and HBV DNA > 20,000 IU/mL; or for reactivation of chronic HBV after chemotherapy or immunosuppression. 3. Recommend antiviral therapy in children for ALT > 2× normal and HBV DNA >20,000 IU/mL for at least 6 months. 4. Optimal monitoring practices have not been defined.	1. The most important predictors of cirrhosis or hepatocellular carcinoma (HCC) in chronic HBV infection are persistently elevated HBV DNA and serum ALT levels, HBV genotype C infection, male gender, older age, and coinfection with hepatitis C virus or human immunodeficiency virus (HIV). a. Persons at risk for HCC should be screened by ultrasound every 6–12 months 2. No randomized controlled trials have demonstrated a decrease in overall mortality, liver-specific mortality, or the rate of HCC with anti-HBV therapies. 3. Consider lamivudine or interferon-alpha for initial anti-HBV therapy.	http://www.guidelines.gov/content.aspx?id=14240 http://www.guidelines.gov/content.aspx?id=15475

Disease Management	Organization	Date	Population	Recommendations	Comments	Source
HEPATITIS C VIRUS (HCV)						

Hepatitis C Virus (HCV)	AASLD	2009	Adults with HCV infection	1. Recommends education on methods to avoid transmission to others.
				2. Recommends antiviral treatment for:
				  a. Bridging fibrosis or compensated cirrhosis
				  b. Consideration of acute HCV infection
				3. Test quantitative HCV RNA before treatment and at 12 weeks of therapy.
				4. Patients who lack antibodies for hepatitis A and B viruses should receive vaccination.
				5. Recommend abstaining from alcohol consumption.
				6. Insufficient evidence to recommend herbal therapy.
					1. Optimal therapy is the combination of peginterferon-alfa and ribavirin
					  a. Duration of therapy is 48 weeks for HCV genotypes 1 and 4
					  b. Duration of therapy is 24 weeks for HCV genotypes 2 and 3
						http://www.guidelines.gov/content.aspx?id=14708

Disease Management	Organization	Date	Population	Recommendations	Comments	Source
Hoarseness	AAO-HNS	2009	Persons with hoarseness	1. Recommends against the routine use of antibiotics to treat hoarseness. 2. Recommends voice therapy for all patients with hoarseness and a decreased voice quality of life. 3. All patients with chronic hoarseness > 3 months should undergo laryngoscopy. 4. Recommends against routine use of antireflux medications unless the patient exhibits signs or symptoms of gastroesophageal reflux disease. 5. Recommends against the routine use of corticosteroids to treat hoarseness. 6. Recommends against screening neck imaging (CT or MRI scanning) for chronic hoarseness prior to laryngoscopy. 7. Consider surgery for possible laryngeal CA, benign laryngeal soft tissue lesions, or glottis insufficiency. 8. Consider botulinum toxin injections for spasmodic dysphonia.	Nearly one-third of Americans will have hoarseness at some point in their lives.	http://www.guidelines.gov/content.aspx?id=15203

HOARSENESS

HUMAN IMMUNODEFICIENCY VIRUS (HIV)

Disease Management	Organization	Date	Population	Recommendations	Comments	Source

Human Immunodeficiency Virus (HIV)	IDSA	2009	HIV-infected adults and children	1. Recommends education to avoid high-risk behaviors to minimize risk of HIV transmission.
				2. Assess for the presence of depression, substance abuse, or domestic violence.
				3. Baseline labs: CD4 count; quantitative HIV RNA by PCR (viral load); HIV genotyping; CBC; chemistry panel; G6PD testing; fasting lipid profile; HLA B5701 test (if abacavir is used); urinalysis; PPD; *Toxoplasma* antibodies; HBsAg, HBsAb, and HCV antibodies; VDRL; urine NAAT for gonorrhea; and urine NAAT for chlamydia (except in men aged <25 years); Pap smear in women[a]
				4. Monitoring labs:
				  a. CD4 counts and HIV viral load every 3–4 months.
				  b. Frequency of repeat sexually transmitted disease (STD) screening is undefined.
				  c. Annual PPD test.
				  d. Persons starting antiretroviral medications should have a repeat fasting glucose and lipid panel 4–6 weeks after initiation of therapy.
					1. Homosexual men and women with abnormal cervical Pap smear results and persons with a history of genital warts should undergo anogenital human papilloma virus (HPV) screening and anal Pap testing.
					2. Serum testosterone level should be considered in men complaining of fatigue, ED, or decreased libido.
					3. Chest x-ray should be obtained in persons with pulmonary symptoms or who have a positive PPD test result.
						http://www.guidelines.gov/content.aspx?id=15440

HUMAN IMMUNODEFICIENCY VIRUS (HIV)

Disease Management	Organization	Date	Population	Recommendations	Comments	Source
Human Immunodeficiency Virus (HIV) (continued)				5. Vaccination for pneumococcal infection, influenza, varicella, hepatitis A, and hepatitis B virus according to standard immunization charts. 6. All HIV-infected women of childbearing age should be counseled regarding contraception. 7. Pap smear in women every 6 months. 8. Consider annual mammography in all women aged ≥ 40 years. 9. Hormone replacement therapy is not recommended. 10. All women aged ≥ 65 years should have a dual-energy x-ray absorptiometry (DXA) test of spine/hips.		

ªPCR, polymerase chain reaction; CBCD, complete blood count with differential; RNA, ribonucleic acid; G6PD, glucose-6-phosphate dehydrogenase; HLA, human leukocyte antigen; PPD, purified protein derivative; HB, hepatitis B; VDRL, Venereal Disease Research Laboratory; NAAT, nucleic acid amplification test

HUMAN IMMUNODEFICIENCY VIRUS, ANTIRETROVIRAL THERAPY (ART)

Disease Management	Organization	Date	Population	Recommendations	Comments	Source

Human Immunodeficiency Virus (HIV), Antiretroviral Therapy (ART)	HHS	2010	HIV-infected children	1. ART is recommended for all children with symptomatic HIV disease.
				2. Recommends ART for:
				  a. Infants aged < 12 months
				  b. Asymptomatic children with HIV RNA ≥ 100,000 copies/mL
				  c. Children aged 1–5 years with CD4 < 25%
				  d. Children aged ≥ 5 years with CD4 < 350 cells/mm^3
				  e. Children aged ≥ 1 year with acquired immunodeficiency syndrome (AIDS) or symptomatic HIV infection
				3. HIV genotype testing is recommended:
				  a. Prior to initiation of therapy in all treatment-naïve children
				  b. Prior to changing therapy for treatment failure
				4. Recommends evaluating all children 4–8 weeks after initiation of ART for possible side effects and to evaluate response to therapy.
				  a. Reevaluate children every 3–4 months thereafter.
					Specific ART recommendations are beyond the scope of this book	http://www.guidelines.gov/content.aspx?id=23916

	HUMAN IMMUNOVIRUS-1 (HIV-1), ANTIRETROVIRAL USE				
Disease Management	Organization	Date	Population	Recommendations	Comments	Source

Human Immunovirus-1 (HIV-1), Antiretroviral Use	HHS	2011	Adults and adolescents	• Non-nucleoside reverse transcriptase inhibitor-based (NNRTI) regimens
				  ○ Rilpivirine is an alternative NNRTI option for initial therapy in treatment-naïve patients
				  ○ All nevirapine-based regimens are acceptable options for treatment-naïve patients
				• Protease inhibitor–based regimens
				  ○ Ritonavir-boosted darunavir + abacavir/lamivudine is an alternative regimen
				  ○ Unboosted fosamprenavir is NOT an acceptable option
				• Raltegravir-based regimens
				  ○ Ralteravir + abacavir/lamivudine is an alternative regimen
				• Dual-nucleoside reverse transcriptase inhibitor (NRTI) options
				  ○ Zidovudine + lamivudine is an acceptable regimen
				  ○ Didanosine + lamivudine is NOT an acceptable option
				• Management of a treatment-experienced patient is complex and should be managed by an HIV specialist
					• This guideline focuses on what antiretroviral regimen to start
					• Baseline evaluation should include:
					  ○ CD4 T-cell count
					  ○ HIV RNA viral load
					  ○ CBC, chemistry panel, liver panel, urinalysis
					  ○ Fasting glucose and lipid panel
					  ○ HIV-1 genotypic resistance testing
					  ○ STD screening
					  ○ Psychosocial assessment
					  ○ Substance abuse screening
					• Antiretroviral therapy should be started in patients with:
					  ○ AIDS-defining illness
					  ○ $CD_4 < 350$ cells/mm^3
					  ○ Consider for CD_4 350–500 cells/mm^3
					  ○ Pregnant women to prevent perinatal transmission
					  ○ HIV-associated nephropathy
						http://aidsinfo.nih.gov/contentfiles/lvguidelines/adultandadolescentgl.pdf

HUMAN IMMUNODEFICIENCY VIRUS (HIV), PREGNANCY

Disease Management	Organization	Date	Population	Recommendations	Comments	Source

Human Immunodeficiency Virus (HIV), Pregnancy	CDC	2010	HIV-infected pregnant women	1. Recommend combination antiretroviral (ART) regimens during the antepartum period.
				2. Women who were taking ART prior to conception should have their regimen reviewed (ie, teratogenic potential of drugs), but continue combination ART throughout the pregnancy.
				3. Initial prenatal labs should include a CD4 count, HIV viral load, and hepatitis C virus (HCV) antibody.
				  a. If HIV RNA is detectable (> 500–1000 copies/mL), perform HIV genotypic resistance testing to help guide antepartum therapy.
				4. Women who do not require ART for their own health should initiate combination ART between 14–28 gestational weeks and continue until delivery.
				  a. Zidovudine should be a component of the regimen when feasible.
				  b. Recommend against single-dose intrapartum/newborn nevirapine in addition to antepartum ART.
					1. Avoid Methergine for postpartum hemorrhage in women receiving a protease inhibitor or efavirenz.
					2. If women do not receive antepartum/intrapartum ART prophylaxis, infants should receive zidovudine for 6 weeks.
					3. Infants born to HIV-infected women should have an HIV viral load checked at 14 days, at 1–2 months, and at 4–6 months.
						http://www.guidelines.gov/content.aspx?id= 6305

| | HUMAN IMMUNODEFICIENCY VIRUS (HIV), PREGNANCY | | | | | |

Disease Management	Organization	Date	Population	Recommendations	Comments	Source
Human Immunodeficiency Virus (HIV), Pregnancy (continued)				5. Antepartum monitoring: a. Monitor CD4 count every 3 months. b. HIV viral load should be assessed 2–4 weeks after initiating or changing ART, monthly until undetectable, and then at 34–36 weeks. c. Recommend a first-trimester ultrasound to confirm dating. d. Screen for gestational diabetes at 24–28 weeks. 6. Scheduled cesarean delivery is recommended for HIV-infected women who have HIV RNA levels > 1000 copies/mL and intact membranes near term. 7. Intrapartum IV zidovudine is recommended for all HIV-infected pregnant women. 8. Avoid artificial rupture of membranes. 9. Avoid routine use of fetal scalp electrodes. 10. Breast-feeding is not recommended.		

HYPERTENSION: INITIATING TREATMENT
Source: THE 7TH REPORT OF THE JOINT NATIONAL COMMITTEE ON
PREVENTION, DETECTION, EVALUATION, AND TREATMENT OF HIGH
BLOOD PRESSURE, 2003

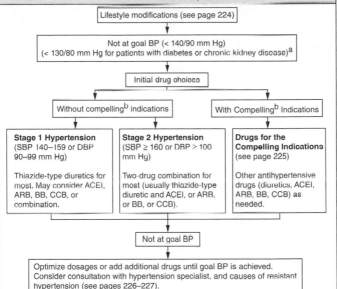

ACEI, ACE inhibitor; ARB, angiotensin receptor blocker; BB, beta-blocker; CCB, calcium channel blocker.

[a]AHA also recommends BP < 130/80 mm Hg for patients with known CHD, carotid artery disease, peripheral arterial disease, abdominal aortic aneurysm, or 10 year Framingham risk score ≥ 10%; and BP < 120/80 for patients with left ventricular dysfunction. (*Circulation.* 2007;115:2761–2788)

[b]Compelling indications: CHF, high CHD risk, diabetes, chronic kidney disease, recurrent stroke prevention, post-MI.

Source: JNC VII, 2003. (*Hypertension.* 2003;42:1206–1252)

Note: Similar recommendations from the Canadian Hypertension Education Program (http://www.hypertension.ca), and the joint European Society of Hypertension and European Society of Cardiology Task Force [*J Hypertension.* 2007;25(9):1751–1762].

Cochrane review (2007): Available evidence does not support use of BB as first-line drugs in treatment of hypertension. BB were inferior to CCB, renin-angiotensin system inhibitors, and thiazide diuretics (although most trials used atenolol). [*Cochrane Database of Systematic Reviews* 2007, Issue 1 (CD002003), http://www.cochrane.org]

LIFESTYLE MODIFICATIONS FOR TREATMENT OF HYPERTENSION[a,b]

Modification	Recommendation	Approximate SBP Reduction (Range)
Weight reduction	Maintain normal body weight (BMI 18.5–24.9 kg/m^2).	5–20 mm Hg per 10-kg weight loss
Adopt DASH eating plan	Consume diet rich in fruits, vegetables, and low-fat dairy products with a reduced content of saturated and total fat.	8–14 mm Hg
Dietary sodium reduction	Reduce dietary sodium intake to less than 100 mmol/day (2.4 g sodium or 6 g sodium chloride).	2–8 mm Hg
Physical activity	Engage in regular aerobic physical activity such as brisk walking (at least 30 min/day, most days of the week).	4–9 mm Hg
Moderation of alcohol consumption	Limit consumption to no more than 2 drinks (1 oz or 30 mL ethanol; eg, 24 oz beer, 10 oz wine, or 3 oz 80-proof whiskey) per day in most men and to no more than 1 drink per day in women and lighter-weight persons.	2–4 mm Hg

[a]For overall cardiovascular risk reduction, stop smoking.
[b]The effects of implementing these modifications are dose- and time dependent and could be greater for some individuals.
DASH = Dietary Approaches to Stop Hypertension
DASH diet found to be effective in lowering SBP in adolescents.
Source: J Pediatr. 2008;152(4):494–501, ACCF/AHA *J Am Coll Cardiol.* 2011:57(20):2037–2110, *J Am Coll Cardiology.* 201:57(20):2037–2110.

RECOMMENDED MEDICATIONS FOR COMPELLING INDICATIONS

Compelling Indication[a]	Diuretic	BB	ACEI	ARB	CCB	AldoANT
Heart failure	X	X	X	X		X
Post-MI		X	X			X
High coronary disease risk	X	X	X		X	
Diabetes	X	X	X	X	X	
Chronic kidney disease[b]			X	X		
Recurrent stroke prevention	X		X			

ACEI, ACE inhibitor; ARB, angiotensin receptor blocker;
AldoANT, aldosterone antagonist; BB, beta-blocker; CCB, calcium channel blocker
[a]Compelling indications for antihypertensive drugs are based on benefits from outcome
studies or existing clinical guidelines; the compelling indication is managed in parallel with the BP.
[b]ALLHAT: Patients with hypertension and reduced GFR. no difference in renal outcomes
(development of ESRD and/or decrement in GFR of > 50% from baseline) comparing amlodipine,
lisinopril, and chlorthalidone. (*Arch Intern Med*. 2005 Apr 25;165(8):936–946) Data do *not* support
preference for CCB, alpha-blockers, or ACEI compared with thiazide diuretics in patients with
metabolic syndrome [*Arch Intern Med*. 2008;168(2):207–217; *J Am Coll Cardiol*. 2011;57(20):
2037–2110; 2012 CHEP Recommendations www.hypertension.ca].

REFRACTORY HYPERTENSION
Source: **AMERICAN COLLEGE OF CARDIOLOGY/AMERICAN HEART ASSOCIATION/EUROPEAN SOCIETY OF CARDIOLOGY**

Definition:

Failure to reach BP goal (< 140/90 mm Hg, or 130/80 mm Hg in patients with diabetes, heart disease, or chronic kidney disease) using three different antihypertensive drug classes.

Incidence: 20%–30% of HTN patients

Common Causes:

1. Nonadherence to drugs/diet
2. Suboptimal therapy/BP measurement (fluid retention, inadequate dosage)
3. Diet/drug interactions (caffeine, cocaine, alcohol, nicotine, NSAIDs, steroids, BCP, erythropoietin, natural licorice, herbs)
4. Common secondary causes:
   Obstructive sleep apnea
   Diabetes
   Chronic kidney disease
   Renal artery stenosis
   Obesity
   Endocrine disorders (primary hyperaldosteronism, hyperthyroidism, hyperparathyroidism, Cushing syndrome), pheochromocytoma

Therapy:

- Exclude nonadherence and incorrect BP measurement
- Review drug and diet history
- Screen for secondary causes:

History of sleep disorders/daytime sleepiness/tachycardias/BPs in both arms

Routine labs: sodium, potassium, creatinine, CBC, ECG, urinalysis, blood glucose, cholesterol

Additional evaluation: aldosterone:renin ratio/renal ultrasound with Doppler flow study/serum or urine catecholamine levels/morning cortisol level

REFRACTORY HYPERTENSION (CONTINUED)
Source: AMERICAN COLLEGE OF CARDIOLOGY/AMERICAN HEART ASSOCIATION/EUROPEAN SOCIETY OF CARDIOLOGY

- Lifestyle therapy:

Weight loss (10-kg weight loss results in a 5–20 mm Hg decrease in SBP); diet consult for low sodium (2.3 g daily), high fiber, and high potassium (DASH diet results in an 8–14 mm Hg decrease in SBP); exercise aerobic training results in a 4–9 mm Hg decrease in SBP; and restriction of excess alcohol (1 oz in men and 0.5 oz in women) results in a 2–4 mm Hg decrease in SBP

- Pharmacologic therapy:

Consider volume overload

- Switch from HCTZ to chlorthalidone (especially if GFR < 40 mL/min)
- Switch to loop diuretic if GFR < 30 mL/min (eg, furosemide 40 mg bid)
- Use CCB (amlodipine or nifedipine) + ACE inhibitor or ARB

Consider catecholamine excess

- Switch to vasodilating beta-blocker (carvedilol, labetalol, nebivolol)

Consider aldosterone excess (even with normal serum K + level)

- Spironolactone or eplerenone

Finally, consider hydralazine or minoxidil

    If already on beta-blocker, clonidine adds little BP benefit

---

- Nonpharmacologic therapy: still under investigation

Carotid baroreceptor stimulation (*Hypertension.* 2010;55:1–8)

    May lower BP 33/22 mm Hg

Renal artery nerve ablation (*N Engl J Med.* 2009;361:932–934)

    May lower BP 32/12 mm Hg with no change in GFR

BP, blood pressure; HTN, hypertension; NSAIDs, nonsteroidal anti-inflammatory drugs; BCP, birth control pill; CBC, complete blood count; ECG, electrocardiogram; SBP, systolic blood pressure; DASH diet, Dietary Approaches to Stop Hypertension diet, HCTZ, hydrochlorothiazide; GFR, glomerular filtration rate; bid, twice a day; CCB, calcium channel blocker; ACE, angiotensin-converting enzyme; ARB, angiotensin receptor blocker.
Sources: AHA Scientific Statement 2008. *Circulation.* 117:e510–e526. JNC VII. *Arch Intern Med.* 2003;289:2560–2572. European 2007 Guidelines. 2007;28:1462–1536.

HYPERTENSION: CHILDREN AND ADOLESCENTS

Indications for Antihypertensive Drug Therapy in Children and Adolescents

- Symptomatic hypertension
- Secondary hypertension
- Hypertensive target organ damage
- Diabetes (types 1 and 2)
- Persistent hypertension despite nonpharmacologic measures (weight management counseling if overweight; physical activity; diet management)

Sources: Pediatrics. 2011;128 (5): December and *Circulation.* 2006:2710–2738

2012 JOINT NATIONAL COMMITTEE JNC 8

• Projected release data late 2012

• A new nine-step systemic review and development process in issuing guidelines is demonstrated below:

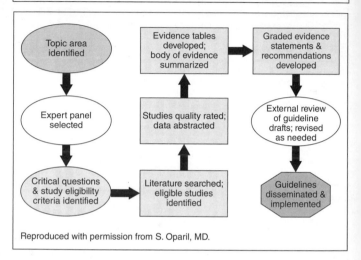

Reproduced with permission from S. Oparil, MD.

Three major areas emphasized in JNC 8:
- ✓ Threshold for drug initiation
- ✓ Target BP goal
- ✓ Most appropriate drug selection in specific populations

• Current target BP goals are based on expert opinion not randomized controlled trials and whether JNC 8 will adjust is awaiting guideline release

HYPOGONADISM, MALE					
Disease Management	**Organization**	**Date**	**Population**	**Recommendations**	**Comments**	**Source**

Disease Management	Organization	Date	Population	Recommendations	Comments	Source
Hypogonadism, Male	EAU	2012	Adults	• Testosterone testing should be done in: ○ Pituitary masses ○ ESRD ○ Moderate-severe COPD ○ Infertility ○ Osteoporosis ○ HIV infection ○ DM 2 • Signs and symptoms of hypogonadism • Indications for testosterone treatment are patients with low testosterone and: ○ Hypogonadism ○ Delayed puberty ○ Klinefelter syndrome ○ Sexual dysfunction ○ Low bone mass ○ Hypopituitarism • Contraindications to testosterone use: ○ Prostate CA ○ PSA > 4 ng/mL ○ Male breast CA ○ Severe sleep apnea ○ Male infertility ○ Hematocrit > 50% ○ Symptomatic BPH • Monitor response to therapy. PSA and hematocrit 3, 6, and 12 months after starting therapy	• Caused by androgen deficiency • Primary hypogonadism ○ Klinefelter syndrome ○ Cryptorchidism ○ Congenital anorchia ○ Testicular CA ○ Orchitis ○ Chemotherapy • Secondary hypogonadism ○ Kallmann syndrome ○ Pituitary tumor ○ Renal failure ○ Hemochromatosis ○ Hypothyroidism ○ Anabolic steroid abuse ○ Morbid obesity ○ Radiotherapy ○ Idiopathic hypogonadotrophic hypogonadism ○ Androgen insensitivity syndrome	http://www.uroweb.org/gls/pdf/16_Male-Hypogonadism_LR%20II.pdf

INFERTILITY, MALE

Disease Management	Organization	Date	Population	Recommendations	Comments	Source
Infertility, Male	EAU	2012	Adults	• Assessment of male infertility includes: 　○ Semen analysis 　○ Check FSH, LH, and testosterone levels 　○ Screen for gonorrhea and chlamydia 　○ Substance abuse screening • Refer patients with abnormal screens to a specialist in male infertility for potential treatments that may include clomiphene citrate, tamoxifen, hCG, dopamine agonists or surgical treatments depending on the underlying etiology	• Infertility is defined as the inability of a sexually active couple not using contraception to conceive in 1 year	http://www.uroweb.org/gls/pdf/15_Male_Infertility_LR%20II.pdf

Disease Management	Organization	Date	Population	Recommendations	Comments	Source
INFLUENZA						
Influenza	IDSA	2009	Adults and children	1. Antiviral treatment is recommended for: a. Lab-confirmed cases of influenza within 48 hours of symptom onset. b. Strongly suspected influenza within 48 hours of symptom onset. c. Hospitalized patients with severe, complicated, or progressive influenza or lab-confirmed influenza-like illness with high likelihood of complications even if >48 hours from symptom onset. 2. Antiviral options include oseltamivir and zanamivir. a. Oseltamivir for influenza A or B: 75 mg by mouth (PO) twice daily (bid) (adults); 30 mg PO bid (≤15 kg); 45 mg PO bid (16–23 kg); 60 mg PO bid (24–40 kg); 75 mg PO bid (>40 kg or aged ≥ 13 years) × 5 days. Avoid in children aged < 1 year. b. Zanamivir for influenza A or B: 2 puffs bid × 5 days (children aged ≥7 years and adults) Avoid in asthmatic patients	1. Consider an influenza nasal swab for diagnosis during influenza season in: a. Persons with acute onset of fever and respiratory illness b. Persons with fever and acute exacerbation of chronic lung disease c. Infants and children with fever of unclear etiology d. Severely ill persons with fever or hypothermia 2. Rapid influenza antigen tests have a 70%–90% sensitivity in children and a 40%–60% sensitivity in adults. 3. Direct or indirect fluorescent antibody staining are useful screening tests. 4. Influenza PCR may be used as a confirmatory test.	http://www.guidelines.gov/content.aspx?id=14173

KIDNEY DISEASE, CHRONIC

Disease Management	Organization	Date	Population	Recommendations	Comments	Source

Kidney Disease, Chronic	NICE	2008	Adults	1. Recommends the modification of diet in renal disease (MDRD) equation to estimate GFR.
				  a. Advise patients not to eat any meat in the 12 hours before a blood test for GFR estimation.
				2. Frequency of GFR testing by chronic kidney disease (CKD) stage:
				  i. Stages 1–2: annually
				  ii. Stage 3: every 6 months
				  iii. Stage 4: every 3 months
				  iv. Stage 5: every 6 weeks
				2. Recommends urine albumin to creatinine ratio (ACR) to detect low levels of proteinuria.
				  a. Levels ≥ 30 mg/mmol are significant
				3. Recommends checking for urinary tract malignancy for persistent hematuria.
				4. Recommends a renal ultrasound in CKD and if patient is/has:
				  a. A GFR decline > 5 mL/min/1.73m² in 1 year or > 10 mL/min/1.73m² in 5 years
				  b. Persistent hematuria
				  c. Symptoms of urinary tract obstruction
				  d. Aged > 20 years and has a family history of polycystic kidney disease
				  e. Stage 4–5 CKD
				  f. Being considered for a renal biopsy
						http://www.nice.org.uk/nicemedia/live/12069/42117/42117.pdf

Disease Management	Organization	Date	Population	Recommendations	Comments	Source
KIDNEY DISEASE, CHRONIC						

Kidney Disease, Chronic (continued)				5. Recommends nephrology referral for:
				  a. Stage 4–5 CKD
				  b. ACR ≥ 70 mg/mmol
				  c. Proteinuria ≥ 1 g/24 h
				  d. Poorly controlled HTN
				  e. Suspected renal artery stenosis
				  f. Rapidly progressive renal impairment
				6. Recommends a check of serum calcium, phosphate, intact parathyroid hormone (iPTH), 25-OH vitamin D, and hemoglobin levels for all stage 4–5 CKD.		

KIDNEY DISEASE, CHRONIC-MINERAL AND BONE DISORDERS (CKD-MBDS)

Disease Management	Organization	Date	Population	Recommendations	Comments	Source

Kidney Disease, Chronic-Mineral and Bone Disorders (CKD-MBDs)	NKF	2009	Adults and children	1. Recommends monitoring serum calcium, phosphorus, iPTH, and alkaline phosphatase levels for:
				  a. Stage 3 CKD (adults)
				  b. Stage 2 CKD (children)
				2. Measure 25-OH vitamin D levels beginning in stage 3 CKD.
				3. Recommends treating all vitamin D deficiency with vitamin D supplementation.
				4. In stages 3–5 CKD, consider a bone biopsy before bisphosphonate therapy if a dynamic bone disease is a possibility.
				5. In stages 3–5 CKD, aim to normalize calcium and phosphorus levels.
				6. In Stage 5 CKD, maintain a PTH level of 130–600 pg/mL.
					1. Options for oral phosphate binders:
					  a. Calcium acetate
					  b. Calcium carbonate
					  c. Calcium citrate
					  d. Sevelamer-HCl
					  e. Sevelamer carbonate
					  f. Lanthanum carbonate
						http://www.kdigo.org/guidelines/mbd/index.html

Disease Management	Organization	Date	Population	Recommendations	Comments	Source
KIDNEY STONES						

Kidney Stones	EAU	2010	Adults and children with kidney stone disease	1. Recommended imaging study for patients with acute flank pain is a non-contrast CT urogram.
				2. Recommended evaluation for renal colic:
				  a. Urinalysis
				  b. Serum CBC, creatinine, uric acid, calcium, and albumin
				  c. Stone analysis by x-ray crystallography or infrared spectroscopy
				3. Recommends 24-hour urine analysis for complicated calcium stone disease: calcium; oxalate; citrate; creatinine; urate; magnesium; phosphate; sodium; and phosphate.
				4. Recommends a thiazide diuretic for patients with hypercalciuria.
				5. Recommends treatment with analkaline citrate for hypocitraturia, type 1 renal tubular acidosis (RTA), hypercalciuria, and hyperoxaluria.
				6. Recommends that adults with a history of urinary stones drink sufficient water to maintain a urine output ≥ 2 L/day.
				7. Consider use of an alpha receptor blocker to facilitate spontaneous passage of ureteral stones < 10 mm.
				8. Consider active ureteral stone removal for persistent obstruction, failure of spontaneous passage, or the presence of severe, unremitting colic.
				  a. Options include shockwave lithotripsy or ureteroscopy
					1. Patients at high risk for recurrent stone formation:
					  a. ≥ 3 stones in 3 years
					  b. Infection stones
					  c. Urate stones
					  d. Children and adolescents with stones
					  e. Cystinuria
					  f. Primary hyperoxaluria
					  g. Type 1 RTA
					  h. Cystic fibrosis
					  i. Hyperparathyroidism
					  j. Crohn disease
					  k. Malabsorption syndromes
					  l. Nephrocalcinosis
					  m. Family history of kidney stone disease
						http://www.uroweb.org/gls/pdf/18_Urolithiasis.pdf

BACK PAIN, LOW

Disease Management	Organization	Date	Population	Recommendations	Comments	Source

Back Pain, Low	NICE	2009	Adults	1. Educate patients and promote self-management of low back pain.
				 2. Recommends offering one of the following treatment options:
				   a. Structure exercise program
				   b. Manual therapy[a]
				   c. Acupuncture
				 3. Consider a psychology referral for patients with a high disability and/or who experience significant psychological distress from their low back pain.
				 4. Recommends against routine lumbar spine x-rays.
				 5. Recommends an MRI scan of lumbar spine only if spinal fusion is under consideration.
				 6. Consider a referral for surgery in patients with refractory, severe nonspecific low back pain who have completed the programs above and would consider spinal fusion.
					1. Analgesic ladder for low back pain
					   a. Recommend scheduled acetaminophen
					   b. Add nonsteroidal anti-inflammatory drugs (NSAIDs) and/or weak opioids
					   c. Consider adding a tricyclic antidepressant
					   d. Consider a strong opioid for short-term use for people in severe pain.
					   e. Refer for specialist assessment for people who may require prolonged use of strong opioids
						http://www.nice.org.uk/nicemedia/live/11887/44343/44343.pdf

	ICSI	2010	Adults	See table.		http://www.icsi.org/low_back_pain/adult_low_back_pain__8.html

[a]Manual therapy includes spinal manipulation, spinal mobilization, and massage.

EVALUATION AND MANAGEMENT OF ACUTE LOW BACK PAIN
Source: ICSI, November 2010

Acute low back pain (LBP) or sciatica/radiculopathy

Emergent or urgent evaluation?
- Bowel or bladder incontinence
- Related to trauma
- Sudden bilateral leg weakness
- Saddle numbness
- Fever ≥ 100.4°F for > 48 hours
- Unrelenting night pain or pain at rest
- Progressive pain with distal leg numbness or leg weakness
- Progressive neurological deficit

Definitions
- Acute low back pain (LBP) has a duration ≤ 6 weeks and does NOT radiate past the knee
- Acute sciatica/radiculopathy has a duration 6 weeks and pain radiates past the knee

Refer to ER for evaluation ◄— Yes

Red Flags for metastases?
- ≥ 50 years
- History of cancer
- Unexplained weight loss
- Unrelenting back pain despite 4–6 weeks of conservative LBP therapy

Red Flags for spine infection?
- IV drug use
- Immunosuppression
- History of tuberculosis
- Unrelenting back pain with fever ≥ 38°C
- Urinary tract infection

Red Flags for spine fracture?
- Onset after trauma
- Osteoporosis
- Chronic steroid use

Red Flags for cord or nerve root compression?
- New onset urinary incontinence or urinary retention
- Saddle anesthesia
- Acute sciatica
- Acute radiculopathy
- New onset numbness and weakness in the legs

No

Any of the following present?
- Back pain lasting longer than 6 weeks
- Unexplained weight loss (greater than 10 lb in 6 months)
- Over age 50
- History of cancer
- Moderate to severe new onset back pain or leg pain

No → Patient should be seen within 7 days

Yes

Patient should be seen in 2–7 days

Treatment of Acute LBP
- Light duty activities
- Regular walking
- Avoid heavy lifting
- Acetaminophen and NSAIDS
- Opioids can be used to control refractory pain for the short term
- Muscle relaxants may be beneficial as needed for the first several days
- Apply ice packs or heat to affected area
- Identify and manage stressors

Evaluation and Management
- Lumbar x-rays if fracture or metastases suspected
- Blood work if cancer or infection suspected
- MRI lumbar spine if a spine infection or cord compression is suspected
- Specialty referral dependent upon etiology
- Early referral to physical therapy for any disabling back or leg pain is present

Elements of Back Pain Evaluation
- Screen for mood disorders
- Assess functional limitations
- Palpate for spine tenderness
- Assess posture, gait, rang of motion
- Strength testing
- Reflex testing
- Sensory testing
- Straight leg raise
- Lumbar x-rays if fracture or metastases suspected
- Blood work if cancer or infection suspected

Treatment of Persistent Pain
- Physical therapy
- Graded exercise program
- Practice good body mechanics to avoid exacerbations of back pain
- Consider a referral to a spine specialist
- Consider lumbar x-rays
- Consider an epidural steroid injection for radiculopathy

					MENOPAUSE		

Disease Management	Organization	Date	Population	Recommendations	Comments	Source
Menopause	AACE	2011	Menopausal women	• Indications for menopausal hormone therapy: 　○ Severe menopausal symptoms 　○ Severe vulvovaginal atrophy 　○ Consider transdermal or topical estrogens which may reduce the risk of VTE 　○ Treatment of osteoporosis • Cautions with menopausal hormone therapy: 　○ Avoid unopposed estrogen use in women with an intact uterus 　○ Use hormonal therapy in the lowest effective dose for the shortest duration possible 　○ Custom compounded bioidentical hormone therapy is NOT recommended 　○ Not appropriate for prevention or treatment of dementia 　○ Avoid if at high risk for VTE 　○ Not recommended for prevention or treatment of cardiovascular disease • Contraindications of menopausal hormone therapy: 　○ History of breast CA 　○ Suspected estrogen-sensitive malignancy 　○ Undiagnosed vaginal bleeding 　○ Endometrial hyperplasia 　○ History of VTE 　○ Untreated hypertension 　○ Active liver disease 　○ Porphyria cutanea tarda	• Use of hormone therapy should always occur after a thorough discussion of the risks, benefits, and alternatives of this treatment with the patient	https://www.aace.com/files/menopause.pdf

METABOLIC SYNDROME: IDENTIFICATION & MANAGEMENT *Source*: NCEP, ATP III, 2005	
Clinical Identification	
Risk Factor	**Defining Level**[a]
Abdominal obesity (waist circumference)[b]	
Men	> 102 cm (> 40 in)
Women	> 88 cm (> 35 in)
Triglycerides	≥ 150 mg/dL
HDL cholesterol	
Men	< 40 mg/dL
Women	< 50 mg/dL
Blood pressure	≥ 135 / ≥ 85 mm Hg
Fasting glucose	> 100 mg/dL

Management

- First-line therapy: Lifestyle modification leading to weight reduction and increased physical activity
- Goal: ↓ Body weight by ~ 7%–10% over 6–12 months
- At least 30 minutes of daily moderate-intensity physical activity
- Low intake of saturated fats, trans fats, and cholesterol
- Reduced consumption of simple sugars
- Increased intake of fruits, vegetables, and whole grains
- Avoid extremes in intake of either carbohydrates or fats
- Smoking cessation
- Drug therapy for HTN, elevated LDL cholesterol, and diabetes
- Consider combination therapy with fibrates or nicotinic acid plus a statin
- Low-dose ASA for patients at intermediate and high risk
- Bariatric surgery for BMI > 35 mg/kg^2
- If one component is identified, a systematic search for the others is indicated, together with an active approach to managing all risk factors. (*Eur Heart J.* 2007;28:2375–2414)
- Metabolic syndrome is associated with the presence of subclinical ischemic brain lesions independent of other risk factors. (*Stroke.* 2008;39:1607–1609)
- In patients with atherosclerosis, the presence of metabolic syndrome is associated with an increased risk of cardiovascular event and all-cause mortality, independent of the presence of diabetes. (*Eur Heart J.* 2008;29:213–223)

HDL, high-density lipoprotein; LDL, low-density lipoprotein; ASA, aspirin; BMI, body mass index; HTN, hypertension

[a]NCEP ATP III definition (*Circulation.* 2005;112:2735–2752)—Requires any 3 of the listed components.
[b]Waist circumference can identify persons at greater cardiometabolic risk than are identified by BMI alone. However, further studies are needed to establish waist circumference cutpoints that assess risk not adequately captured by BMI. (*Am J Clin Nutr.* 2007;85:1197–1202)
Note: The World Health Organization (WHO) and International Diabetes Federation (IDF, http://www. idf.org) define metabolic syndrome slightly differently. One study found a 5-fold difference in the prevalence of metabolic syndrome depending on which of seven diagnostic criteria were used [*Metabolism.* 2008;57(3):355–361]. There is no official definition of metabolic syndrome in children, but a constellation of conditions confers significant increased risk of coronary heart disease. (*Circulation.* 2007;115:1948–1967).

TREATMENT OF METHICILLIN-RESISTANT *STAPHYLOCOCCUS AUREUS* INFECTIONS (MRSA) IN ADULTS AND CHILDREN

Source: IDSA 2011 Clinical Practice Guideline: *Clin Infect Dis.* 2011;52:1–38

Infection	Primary Therapy	Alternative Therapy	Comments

Abscess associated with extensive involvement; cellulitis; systemic illness; immunosuppression; extremes of age; involvement of face, hands, or genitalia; septic phlebitis; trauma; infected ulcer or burn; or poor response to incision and drainage	1. Incision and drainage
	2. Antibiotics
	  a. Outpatient
	    i. Clindamycin
	    ii. Trimethoprim-sulfamethoxazole (TMP-SMX)
	  b. Inpatient
	    i. Vancomycin
	    ii. Linezolid
	    iii. Daptomycin
		1. Outpatient antibiotics
		  a. Tetracycline
		  b. Linezolid
		2. Inpatient antibiotics
		  a. Telavancin
		  b. Clindamycin
			1. Tetracyclines should not be used in children aged <8 years.
			2. Vancomycin is recommended for hospitalized children.
			3. Clindamycin and linezolid are alternative choices for children.

Recurrent skin and soft tissue infections (SSTIs)	1. Cover draining wounds.
	2. Maintain good hygiene.
	3. Avoid reusing or sharing personal toiletries.
	4. Use oral antibiotics only for active infections.
		1. Decolonization only if recurrent SSTI despite good hygiene
		  a. Mupirocin per nares bid × 5–10 days
		  b. Chlorhexidine or dilute bleach baths twice weekly (biw) × 1–2 weeks
			Screening cultures prior to decolonization or surveillance cultures after decolonization is not recommended.

Uncomplicated MRSA bacteremia[a]	Vancomycin × 2 weeks	Daptomycin × 2 weeks	Echocardiography is recommended for all MRSA bacteremia.

TREATMENT OF METHICILLIN-RESISTANT *STAPHYLOCOCCUS AUREUS* INFECTIONS (MRSA) IN ADULTS AND CHILDREN (CONTINUED)

Infection	Primary Therapy	Alternative Therapy	Comments
MRSA native valve endocarditis	Vancomycin × 6 weeks	Daptomycin × 6 weeks	1. Synergistic gentamicin or rifampin is not indicated for native valve endocarditis. 2. Vancomycin is the drug of choice for children.
MRSA prosthetic valve endocarditis	1. Vancomycin plus rifampin × 6 weeks 2. Gentamicin 1 mg/kg IV q8h × 2 weeks		Recommend early evaluation for valve replacement surgery.
MRSA pneumonia	1. Vancomycin 2. Linezolid	Clindamycin	1. Duration of therapy is 7–21 days 2. Vancomycin for children
MRSA osteomyelitis	1. Surgical débridement 2. Vancomycin 3. Daptomycin 4. Duration of therapy is at least 8 weeks	1. Linezolid 2. TMP-SMX plus rifampin 3. Clindamycin	
MRSA septic arthritis	1. Drain or débride the joint space 2. Vancomycin	Daptomycin	Duration of therapy is 3–4 weeks
MRSA meningitis	1. Vancomycin × 2 weeks	1. Linezolid 2. TMP-SMX	Consider adding rifampin

*No endocarditis, no implanted prostheses, defervescence within 72 hours, sterile blood cultures within 72 hours, no evidence of metastatic sites of infection.

					FEBRILE NEUTROPENIA	

Disease management	Organization	Population	Recommendations	Comments	Source
Febrile Neutropenia (FN)	Infectious Disease Society of America 2011	Patients with single temperature >38.3°C or ≥ 38.0°C for >1hr in the setting of neutropenia (absolute neutrophil count including granulocytes and bands <500/mm³)	• Two sets of blood cultures/urine C+S/ chemistries. CXR/ancillary studies based on clinical evaluation. Begin antibiotics as rapidly as possible • Stratify into **LOW RISK**ᵃ (absence of comorbidity, no cardiovascular compromise, expected duration of neutropenia <7days, compliant) vs. **HIGH RISK**ᵃ (ANC <100 comorbidity, cardiovascular compromise, unreliable, expected duration of neutropenia >7days) • High risk patients must be admitted to hospital with rapid initiation of single agent antibiotic (cefepine, imipenem, ceftazidine) or combination therapy (extended spectrum beta lactam plus either aminoglycide or fluoroquinolone) depending on clinical features. Add antifungal agent if continued fever and negative cultures after 4–7 days. • Selected low risk patients can be treated with oral cipro 500 mg BID and augmentin 875 mg BID with < 5% requiring hospitalization for worsening symptoms. Close communication with patient is essential.	• Prophylactic granulocyte colony stimulating factor (GCSF) should be used in patients on chemotherapy with an expected rate of febrile neutropenia (FN) of ≥ 20%. Secondary use of GCSF after FN (shortens hospital stay by 1 day but no impact on survival) • Vancomycin should not be given empirically unless history of methicillin resistant staph aureus (MRSA), catheter tunnel infection, presence of pneumonia or soft tissue infection • Three other unique organisms requiring antibiotic adjustment: • Vancomycin resistant enterococci (VRE) – Use line linezolid or daptomycin • Extended spectrum beta lactamase (ESBL) producing gram negative bacteria – Use carbapenem • Carbapenemase producing organism (*klebsiella*) – Use polymixin-colistin or tigecycline	*Clin Infect Dis.* 2011; Feb; 52:e56–93

FEBRILE NEUTROPENIA					
Disease management	Organization	Population	Recommendations	Comments	Source
Febrile Neutropenia (FN) (continued)			• Continue broad spectrum antibiotics in both low and high risk groups until ANC >500. Adjust antibiotics based on positive cultures and switch to oral to complete a 10–14 day course of antibiotics.	• If central venous catheter (CVC) line infection suspected, draw blood cultures from CVC and peripheral vein. If CVC culture grows out >120 minutes before peripheral blood cultures then CVC is source of infection. • CVC must be removed if infected with staph aureus, pseudomonas and other gram negative bacteria, fungi or mycobacterial infection as well as tunnel or port pocket infection. If coag negative staph, retain CVC and treat with an antibiotic ×4–6 weeks with 85% success. • In afebrile patients with ANC<100 treat with oral fluoroquinolone to lower risk of severe infection • With ANC<100 risk of serious infection is 10% per day	

[a]Multinational Association for Supportive Care in Cancer (MASCC)
• Symptoms → no or mild = 5, moderate = 3, severe = 0
• No hypotension – 5
• No COPD – 4
• No previous fungal infection – 4
• No dehydration requiring parenteral fluids – 3
• Outpatient status – 3
• Age < 60 – 2
• High risk = < 21; Low risk = > 21

MANAGEMENT OF OBESITY IN MATURE ADOLESCENTS AND ADULTS

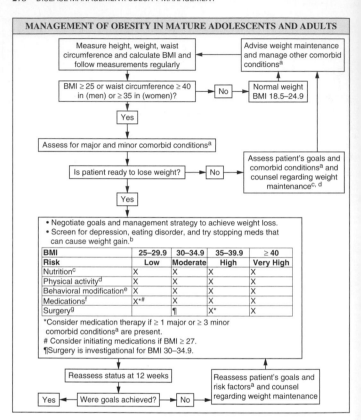

Measure height, weight, waist circumference and calculate BMI and follow measurements regularly

Advise weight maintenance and manage other comorbid conditions[a]

BMI ≥ 25 or waist circumference ≥ 40 in (men) or ≥ 35 in (women)? → No → Normal weight BMI 18.5–24.9

Yes

Assess for major and minor comorbid conditions[a]

Is patient ready to lose weight? → No → Assess patient's goals[a] and comorbid conditions[a] and counsel regarding weight maintenance[c, d]

Yes

- Negotiate goals and management strategy to achieve weight loss.
- Screen for depression, eating disorder, and try stopping meds that can cause weight gain.[b]

| BMI | 25–29.9 | 30–34.9 | 35–39.9 | ≥ 40 |
Risk	Low	Moderate	High	Very High
Nutrition[c]	X	X	X	X
Physical activity[d]	X	X	X	X
Behavioral modification[e]	X	X	X	X
Medications[f]	X*#	X	X	X
Surgery[g]		¶	X*	X

*Consider medication therapy if ≥ 1 major or ≥ 3 minor comorbid conditions[a] are present.
Consider initiating medications if BMI ≥ 27.
¶Surgery is investigational for BMI 30–34.9.

Reassess status at 12 weeks

Yes ← Were goals achieved? → No → Reassess patient's goals and risk factors[a] and counsel regarding weight maintenance

[a]**Minor comorbid conditions:** cigarette smoking; hypertension; LDL cholesterol >130 mg/dL; HDL cholesterol < 40 mg/dL (men) or < 50 mg/dL (women); glucose intolerance; family history of premature CAD; age ≥ 65 years (men) or ≥ 55 years (women)
Major comorbid conditions: waist circumference ≥ 40 inches (men) or ≥ 35 inches (women); CAD; peripheral vascular disease; abdominal aortic aneurysm; symptomatic carotid artery disease; type 2 diabetes; and obstructive sleep apnea.
[b]Sulfonylureas; thiazolidinediones; olanzapine, clozapine, resperidone, quetiapine; lithium; paroxetine, citalopram, sertraline; carbamazepine; pregabalin; corticosteroids; megestrol acetate; cyproheptadine; tricyclic antidepressants; monoamine oxidase inhibitors; mirtazapine; valproic acid; and gabapentin.
[c]Encourage a healthy, balanced diet with daily intake of ≥ 5 servings of fruits/vegetables; 35 g fiber; < 30% calories from fat; eliminate take out, fast food, soda, and desserts; dietician consultation for a calorie reduction between 500 and 1000 kcal/kg/day to achieve a 1–2 lb weight reduction per week.
[d]Recommend 30–60 minutes of moderate activity at least 5 days a week.

MANAGEMENT OF OBESITY IN MATURE ADOLESCENTS AND ADULTS (CONTINUED)

[e]Identify behaviors that may contribute to weight gain (stress, emotional eating, boredom) and use cognitive behavioral counseling, stimulus control, relapse prevention, and goal setting to decrease caloric intake and increase physical activity.

[f]Medications that are FDA approved for weight loss: phentermine; orlistat; phendimetrazine; diethylpropion; and benzphetamine can be used for up to 3 months as an adjunct for weight loss.

[g]Bariatric surgery is indicated for patients at high risk for complications. They should be motivated, psychologically stable, have no surgical contraindications, and must accept the operative risk involved.

Source: Adapted from the ICSI Guideline on the Prevention and Management of Obesity available at http://www.icsi.org/obesity/obesity_3398.html

	OSTEOARTHRITIS (OA)				
Disease Management	Organization	Date	Population	Recommendations	Comments	Source

Osteoarthritis (OA)	ACR	2012	Adults	• Nonpharmacologic recommendations for the management of hand OA
				  ○ Evaluate ability to perform ADLs
				  ○ Instruct in joint protection techniques
				  ○ Provide assistive devices to help perform ADLs
				  ○ Instruct in use of thermal modalities
				  ○ Provide splints for trapeziometacarpal joint OA
				• Nonpharmacologic recommendations for the management of knee or hip OA
				  ○ Participate in aquatic exercise
				  ○ Lose weight
				  ○ Start aerobic exercise program
				  ○ Instruct in use of thermal modalities
				  ○ Consider for knee OA:
				    - Medially directed patellar taping
				    - Wedged insoles for either medial- or lateral compartment OA
				• Pharmacologic options for OA
				  ○ Topical capsaicin
				  ○ Topical or PO NSAIDS
				  ○ Acetaminophen
				  ○ Tramadol
				  ○ Intraarticular steroids is an option for refractory knee or hip OA
					• The following should NOT be used for OA:
					  ○ Chondroitin sulfate
					  ○ Glucosamine
					  ○ Opiates (if possible)
						http://www.rheumatology.org/practice/clinical/guidelines/PDFs/ACR_OA_Guidelines_FINAL.pdf

Disease Management	Organization	Date	Population	Recommendations	Comments	Source

Osteoporosis	ICSI	2011	Adults at risk for osteoporosis or have confirmed osteoporosis	• Evaluate all patients with a low-impact fracture for osteoporosis
				• Advise smoking cessation and alcohol moderation (≤2 drinks per day)
				• Advise 1,500 mg elemental calcium daily for established osteoporosis, glucocorticoid therapy, or age >65 years
				• Assess for vitamin D deficiency with a 25-hydroxy vitamin D level
				   ○ Treat vitamin D deficiency if present
				• Treatment of osteoporosis
				   ○ Bisphosphonate therapy
				   ○ Consider estrogen therapy in menopausal women under 50 years of age
				   ○ Consider parathyroid hormone in women with very high risk for fracture
				• Fall prevention program
				   ○ Home safety evaluation
				   ○ Avoid medications that can cause sedation, orthostatic hypotension, or affect balance
				   ○ Assistive walking devices as necessary
					• All patients should have serial heights and observed for kyphosis
					• Obtain a lateral vertebral assessment with DEXA scan or x-ray if height loss exceeds 4 cm
					• DEXA bone mineral densitometry should be repeated no more than every 12–24 months
						http://www.icsi.org/osteoporosis/diagnosis_and_treatment_of_osteoporosis_3.html

Disease Management	Organization	Date	Population	Recommendations	Comments	Source
OSTEOPOROSIS						
Osteoporosis (continued)	NAMS AACE	2010 2010	Postmenopausal women	1. Recommend maintaining a healthy weight, eating a balanced diet, avoiding excessive alcohol intake, avoiding cigarette smoking, and utilizing measures to avoid falls. 2. Recommend supplemental calcium 1200 mg/day and vitamin D_3 800–1000 international units (IU)/day. 3. Recommend an annual check of height and weight, and assess for chronic back pain. 4. DXA of the hip, femoral neck, and lumbar spine should be measured in women aged ≥ 65 years or postmenopausal women with a risk factor for osteoporosis.[a] 5. Recommend repeat DXA testing every 1–2 years for women taking therapy for osteoporosis and every 2–5 years for untreated postmenopausal women.	1. Options for osteoporosis drug therapy: a. Bisphosphonates i. First-line therapy ii. Options include alendronate, risedronate, or zoledronic acid b. Denosumab i. Consider for women at high fracture risk c. Raloxifene i. Second-line agent in younger women with osteoporosis d. Teriparatide is an option for high fracture risk when bisphosphonates have failed. i. Therapy should not exceed 24 months.	http://www.guidelines.gov/content.aspx?id=15500 http://www.aace.com/pub/pdf/guidelines/OsteoGuidelines2010.pdf

OSTEOPOROSIS

Disease Management	Organization	Date	Population	Recommendations	Comments	Source
Osteoporosis (continued)				6. Recommend against measurement of biochemical markers of bone turnover. 7. Recommend drug therapy for osteoporosis for: a. Osteoporotic vertebral or hip fracture b. DXA with T score ≤ −2.5 c. DXA with T score ≤ −1 to −2.4 and a 10-year risk of major osteoporotic fracture of ≥ 20% or hip fracture ≥ 3% based on FRAX calculator, available at http://www.shef.ac.uk/FRAX/ 8. Consider the use of hip protectors in women at high risk of falling.	e. Calcitonin i. Third-line therapy for osteoporosis ii. May be used for bone pain from acute vertebral compression fractures. 2. Vitamin D therapy should maintain a 25-OH vitamin D level between 30–60 ng/mL.	

ªPrevious fracture after menopause, weight < 127 lb, BMI < 21 kg/m², parent with a history of hip fracture, current smoker, rheumatoid arthritis, or excessive alcohol intake.

OSTEOPOROSIS, GLUCOCORTICOID-INDUCED

Disease Management	Organization	Date	Population	Recommendations	Comments	Source

Osteoporosis, Glucocorticoid-Induced	ACR	2010	Glucocorticoid-induced osteoporosis	1. All patients receiving glucocorticoid therapy should receive education and assess risk factors for osteoporosis.
				2. FRAX calculator should be used to place patients at low risk, medium risk, or high risk for major osteoporotic fracture.
				3. If glucocorticoid treatment is expected to last ≥3 months, recommend:
				  a. Weight-bearing activities
				  b. Smoking cessation
				  c. Avoid >2 alcoholic drinks/day
				  d. Calcium 1200–1500 mg/day
				  e. Vitamin D 800–1000 IU/day
				  f. Fall risk assessment
				  g. Baseline DXA test and then every 2 years
				  h. Annual 25-OH vitamin D
				  i. Baseline and annual height measurement
				  j. Assessment of prevalent fragility fractures
				  k. X-rays of spine
				  l. Assessment of degree of osteoporosis medication compliance, if applicable
					1. Clinical factors that may increase the risk of osteoporotic fracture estimated by FRAX calculator:
					  a. BMI < 21 kg/m^2
					  b. Parental history of hip fracture
					  c. Current smoking
					  d. ≥ 3 alcoholic drinks/day
					  e. Higher glucocorticoid doses or cumulative dose
					  f. IV pulse glucocorticoid use
					  g. Declining central bone mineral density measurement
						http://www.rheumatology.org/practice/clinical/guidelines/ACR_2010_GIOP_Recomm_Clinicians_Guide.pdf

OSTEOPOROSIS, GLUCOCORTICOID-INDUCED					
Disease Management	Organization	Date	Population	Recommendations	Comments	Source
Osteoporosis, Glucocorticoid-Induced (continued)				4. For postmenopausal women or men aged > 50 years: a. Low-risk group i. Bisphosphonae if equivalent of prednisone ≥ 7.5 mg/day b. Medium-risk group i. Bisphosphonate if equivalent of prednisolone ≥ 5 mg/day c. High-risk group i. Bisphosphonate for any dose of glucocorticoid 5. For premenopausal women or men aged < 50 years with a prevalent fragility (osteoporotic) fracture and glucocorticoid use ≥ 3 months: a. For prednisone ≥ 5 mg/day, use alendronate or risedronate b. For prednisone ≥ 7.5 mg/day, use zoledronic acid c. Consider teriparatide for bisphosphonate failures	2. Bisphosphonates recommended: a. Low- to medium-risk patients i. Alendronate ii. Risedronate iii. Zoledronic acid b. High-risk patients i. Same + teriparatide	

Disease Management	Organization	Date	Population	Recommendations	Comments	Source
OTITIS MEDIA, ACUTE						
Otitis Media, Acute	ICSI	2008	Children aged 3 months–18 years	1. Diagnosis should be made with pneumatic otoscopy.	1. Amoxicillin is first-line therapy for low-risk children:	http://www.icsi.org/ otitis_media/ diagnosis_and_ treatment_of_otitis_ media_in_ children_2304.html
				2. Children at low risk[a] should use a wait-and-see approach for 48–72 hours with oral analgesics.	a. 40 mg/kg/day if no antibiotics used in last 3 months	
				3. Recommends symptomatic relief with acetaminophen or ibuprofen and warm compresses to the ear.	b. 80 mg/kg/day if child is not low risk	
				4. Educate caregivers about prevention of otitis media: encourage breast-feeding, feed child upright if bottle fed, avoid passive smoke exposure, limit exposure to groups of children, careful handwashing prior to handling child, avoid pacifier use > 10 months, ensure immunizations are up to date.	2. Alternative antibiotics: a. Amoxicillin-clavulanate b. Cefuroxime axetil c. Ceftriaxone d. Cefprozil e. Loracarbef f. Cefdinir g. Cefixime h. Cefpodoxime i. Clarithromycin j. Azithromycin k. Erythromycin	
				5. Amoxicillin is the first-line antibiotic for low-risk children.		
				6. Alternative medication if failure to respond to initial treatment; penicillin allergy: presence of a resistant organism found on culture.		

OTITIS MEDIA, ACUTE					

Disease Management	Organization	Date	Population	Recommendations	Comments	Source
Otitis Media, Acute (continued)				7. Consider prophylactic antibiotics for recurrent acute otitis media: a. ≥ 5 episodes in 6 months or ≥ 4 episodes in a year 8. Recommends referral to an ENT specialist for a complication of otitis media: mastoiditis, facial nerve palsy, lateral sinus thrombosis, meningitis, brain abscess, or labyrinthitis. 9. Recommends against routine recheck at 10–14 days in children feeling well. 10. Management of otitis media with effusion: a. Educate that effusion will resolve on its own b. Recommends against antihistamines or decongestants c. Recommends a trial of antibiotics for 10–14 days prior to referral for tympanostomy tubes		

ªChildren older than age 2 years without severe disease (temperature > 39°C and moderate-severe otalgia), otherwise healthy, do not attend daycare and have had no prior ear infections within the last month.

PALLIATIVE & END-OF-LIFE CARE: PAIN MANAGEMENT	
Principles of Analgesic Use	
By the mouth	The oral route is the preferred route for analgesics, including morphine.
By the clock	Persistent pain requires around-the-clock treatment to prevent further pain. As-needed (prn) dosing is irrational and inhumane; it requires patients to experience pain before becoming eligible for relief. Relief is accomplished with long-acting delayed-release preparations (fentanyl patch, slow-release morphine, or oxycodone).
By the WHO ladder	If a maximum dose of medication fails to adequately relieve pain, move up the ladder, not laterally to a different drug in the same efficiency group. Severe pain requires immediate use of an opioid recommended for controlling severe pain, without progressing sequentially through Steps 1 and 2. When using a long-acting opioid, the dose for breakthrough pain should be 10% of the 24-hour opioid dose (ie, if a patient is on 100 mg/day of an extended-release morphine preparation, their breakthrough dose is 10 mg of morphine or equivalent every 1–2 hours until pain relief is achieved.
Individualize treatment	The right dose of an analgesic is the dose that relieves pain with acceptable side effects for a specific patient.
Monitor	Monitoring is required to ensure the benefits of treatment are maximized while adverse effects are minimized.
Use adjuvant drugs	For example, a nonsteroidal anti-inflammatory drug (NSAID) is often helpful in controlling bone pain. Nonopioid analgesics, such as NSAIDs or acetaminophen, can be used at any step of the ladder. Adjuvant medications also can be used at any step to enhance pain relief or counteract the adverse effects of medications. Neuropathic pain should be treated with gabapentin, nortriptyline, or pregabalin. Moderate to high-dose dexamethasone is effective as an adjunct to opioids in a pain crisis situation.

Source: Reprinted with permission from the American Academy of Hospice and Palliative Medicine. *Pocket Guide to Hospice/Palliative Medicine.*

ABNORMAL PAP SMEAR ALGORITHM

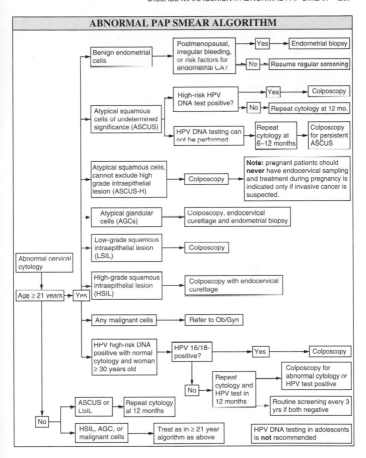

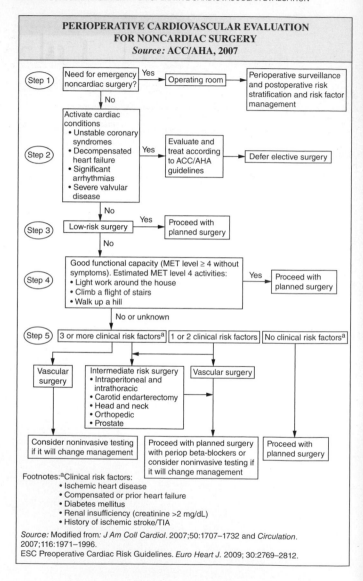

PERIOPERATIVE CARDIOVASCULAR EVALUATION FOR NONCARDIAC SURGERY
Source: ACC/AHA, 2007

(Step 1) Need for emergency noncardiac surgery? → Yes → Operating room → Perioperative surveillance and postoperative risk stratification and risk factor management

No ↓

(Step 2) Activate cardiac conditions
- Unstable coronary syndromes
- Decompensated heart failure
- Significant arrhythmias
- Severe valvular disease

→ Yes → Evaluate and treat according to ACC/AHA guidelines → Defer elective surgery

No ↓

(Step 3) Low-risk surgery → Yes → Proceed with planned surgery

No ↓

(Step 4) Good functional capacity (MET level ≥ 4 without symptoms). Estimated MET level 4 activities:
- Light work around the house
- Climb a flight of stairs
- Walk up a hill

→ Yes → Proceed with planned surgery

No or unknown ↓

(Step 5) 3 or more clinical risk factors[a] | 1 or 2 clinical risk factors | No clinical risk factors[a]

Vascular surgery

Intermediate risk surgery
- Intraperitoneal and intrathoracic
- Carotid endarterectomy
- Head and neck
- Orthopedic
- Prostate

Vascular surgery

Consider noninvasive testing if it will change management

Proceed with planned surgery with periop beta-blockers or consider noninvasive testing if it will change management

Proceed with planned surgery

Footnotes:[a]Clinical risk factors:
- Ischemic heart disease
- Compensated or prior heart failure
- Diabetes mellitus
- Renal insufficiency (creatinine >2 mg/dL)
- History of ischemic stroke/TIA

Source: Modified from: *J Am Coll Cardiol.* 2007;50:1707–1732 and *Circulation.* 2007;116:1971–1996.
ESC Preoperative Cardiac Risk Guidelines. *Euro Heart J.* 2009; 30:2769–2812.

PERIOPERATIVE CARDIOVASCULAR EVALUATION
Source: ACCF/AHA/ESC, 2009

Perioperative Beta-Blocker Therapy:

- Perioperative beta-blocker recommendations have become more limited.
- Chronic beta-blocker should be continued to prevent rebound HTN, arrhythmias, or myocardial infarction.
- Beta-blockers titrated to heart rate and blood pressure are *probably recommended* for patients undergoing vascular surgery who have CAD or findings of ischemia on preoperative testing.
- Beta-blockers titrated to heart rate and blood pressure are *probably recommended* for patients undergoing intermediate surgery who have CAD or ≥ 1 clinical risk factors.
- Beta-blockers should optimally be started 30 days before surgery, but at least 1 week prior to surgery to allow titrating dose to optimal heart rate and blood pressure.
- Initiation of high-dose beta-blockers should NOT be administered for *potential* benefit due to the observed increased risk of overall death, stroke, and risk of hemodynamic instability. (POISE Trial. *Lancet.* 2008;371:1839–1847)
- A long-acting beta-blocker should be used without intrinsic sympathomimetic activity.
- Beta-blocker therapy should be continued at least 2 months in the postoperative period if there is no other indication for long-term use.

Sources: ACC/AHA 2007 Guidelines. *J Am Coll Cardiol.* 2007;50:1707–1732. 2009 Focused Update on Perioperative Beta Blockade. *J Am Coll Cardiol.* 2009;54(22):2102–2128. European Guidelines. *Eur Heart J.* 2009;30:2769–2812.

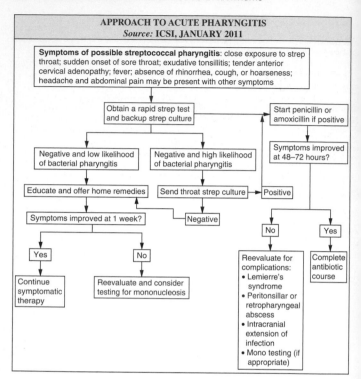

APPROACH TO ACUTE PHARYNGITIS
Source: **ICSI, JANUARY 2011**

Symptoms of possible streptococcal pharyngitis: close exposure to strep throat; sudden onset of sore throat; exudative tonsillitis; tender anterior cervical adenopathy; fever; absence of rhinorrhea, cough, or hoarseness; headache and abdominal pain may be present with other symptoms

Obtain a rapid strep test and backup strep culture

Start penicillin or amoxicillin if positive

Symptoms improved at 48–72 hours?

Negative and low likelihood of bacterial pharyngitis

Negative and high likelihood of bacterial pharyngitis

Educate and offer home remedies

Send throat strep culture → Positive

Negative

Symptoms improved at 1 week?

No

Yes

Yes

No

Reevaluate for complications:
• Lemierre's syndrome
• Peritonsillar or retropharyngeal abscess
• Intracranial extension of infection
• Mono testing (if appropriate)

Complete antibiotic course

Continue symptomatic therapy

Reevaluate and consider testing for mononucleosis

PNEUMONIA, COMMUNITY-ACQUIRED: EVALUATION
Source: IDSA, ATS, 2007

Diagnostic Testing	Admission Decision

• CXR or other chest imaging required for diagnosis
• Sputum Gram stain and culture
  • Outpatients: optional
  • Inpatients: if unusual or antibiotic resistance suspected
	• Severity of illness (eg, CURB-65) and prognostic indices (eg, PSI) support decision
	• One must still recognize social and individual factors

CURB-65
(*Thorax.* 2003;58:337–382)

Clinical Factor	Points
Confusion	1
BUN > 19 mg/dL	1
Respiratory rate ≥ 30 breaths/min	1
Systolic BP < 90 mm Hg or Diastolic BP ≤ 60 mm Hg	1
Aged > 65 years	1
Total points	

• CURB-65 ≥ 2 suggest need for hospitalization

Score	In-hospital mortality
0	0.7%
1	3.2%
2	3.0%
3	17%
4	42%
5	57%

Pneumonia Severity Index
(*N Engl J Med.* 1997;336:243–250)

Demographic Factor	Points
Demographic factor	
Men age	Age in years
Women age	Age in years –10
Nursing home resident	+10
Coexisting illnesses	
Neoplastic disease	+30
Liver disease	+20
Congestive heart failure	+10
Cerebrovascular disease	+10
Renal disease	+10
Physical exam findings	
Altered mental status	+20
Respiratory rate 30 breaths/min	+20
Systolic BP < 90 mm Hg	+20
Temperature < 35°C (95°F)	+15
Temperature > 40°C (104°F)	+15
Pulse > 125 beats/min	+10
Laboratory and radiographic findings	
Arterial blood pH < 7.35	+30
BUN > 30 mg/dL	+20
Sodium level < 130 mmol/L	+20
Glucose level > 250 mg/dL	+10
Hematocrit < 30%	+10
PaO_2 < 60 mm Hg or O_2 sat. < 90%	+10
Pleural effusion	+10

Add up total points to estimate mortality risk

Class	Points	Overall Mortality
I	< 51	0.1%
II	51–70	0.6%
III	71–90	0.9%
IV	91–130	9.5%
V	> 130	26.7%

CXR, chest x-ray; CURB-65, confusion, urea nitrogen, respiratory rate, blood pressure, 65 years of age and older; PSI, pneumonia severity index; BP, blood pressure; BUN, blood urea nitrogen
Sources: IDSA and ATS Consensus Guidelines, 2007. (*Clin Infect Diseases.* 2007;44:S27–S72)
Pneumonia Severity Index. (*N Engl J Med.* 1997;336:243)

PNEUMONIA, COMMUNITY-ACQUIRED: SUSPECTED PATHOGENS
Source: IDSA, ATS, 2007

Condition and Risk Factors	Commonly Encountered Pathogens
Alcoholism	*Streptococcus pneumoniae, oral anaerobes, Klebsiella pneumoniae, Acinetobacter* species, *Mycobacterium tuberculosis*
COPD and/or smoking	*Haemophilus influenzae, Pseudomonas aeruginosa, Legionella* species, *S. pneumoniae, Moraxella catarrhalis, Chlamydia pneumoniae*
Aspiration	Gram-negative enteric pathogens, oral anaerobes
Lung abscess	CA-MRSA, oral anaerobes, endemic fungal pneumonia, *M. tuberculosis*, and atypical mycobacteria
Exposure to bat or bird droppings	*Histoplasma capsulatum*
Exposure to birds	*Chlamydophila psittaci* (if poultry: avian influenza)
Exposure to rabbits	*Francisella tularensis*
Exposure to farm animals or parturient cats	*Coxiella burnetii* (Q fever)
HIV infection (early)	*S. pneumoniae, H. influenzae*, and *M. tuberculosis*
HIV infection (late)	The pathogens listed for early infection plus *Pneumocystis jiroveci, Cryptococcus, Histoplasma, Aspergillus*, atypical mycobacteria (especially *Mycobacterium kansasii*), *P. aeruginosa, H. influenzae*
Hotel or cruise ship stay in previous 2 weeks	*Legionella* species
Travel to or residence in southwestern United States	*Coccidioides* species, *Hantavirus*
Travel to or residence in Southeast and East Asia	*Burkholderia pseudomallei*, avian influenza, SARS
Influenza active in community	Influenza, *S. pneumoniae, S. aureus, H. influenzae*
Cough ≥ 2 weeks with whoop or posttussive vomiting	*Bordetella pertussis*
Structural lung disease (eg, bronchiectasis)	*P. aeruginosa, Burkholderia cepacia*, and *S. aureus*
Injection drug use	*S. aureus*, anaerobes, *M. tuberculosis*, and *S. pneumoniae*
Endobronchial obstruction	Anaerobes, *S. pneumoniae, H. influenzae, S. aureus*
In context of bioterrorism	*Bacillus anthracis* (anthrax), *Yersinia pestis* (plague), *Francisella tularensis* (tularemia)

CA-MRSA, community-acquired methicillin-resistant *S. aureus*; COPD, chronic obstructive pulmonary disease; SARS, severe acute respiratory syndrome

ROUTINE PRENATAL CARE

Preconception Visit

1. Measure height, weight, blood pressure, and total and HDL cholesterol.
2. Determine rubella, rubeola, and varicella immunity status.
3. Assess all patients for pregnancy risk: substance abuse, domestic violence, sexual abuse, psychiatric disorders, risk factors for preterm labor, exposure to chemicals or infectious agents, hereditary disorders, gestational diabetes, or chronic medical problems.
4. Educate patients about proper nutrition; offer weight reduction strategies for obese patients.
5. Immunize if not current on the following: Tdap, MMR, varicella, or hepatitis B vaccine.
6. Initiate folic acid 400–800 mcg/day; 4 mg/day for a history of a child affected by a neural tube defect.

Initial Prenatal Visit

1. Medical, surgical, social, family, and obstetrical history and do complete exam.
2. Pap smear, urine NAAT for gonorrhea and *Chlamydia*, and assess for history of genital herpes.
3. Consider a varicella antibody test if patient unsure about prior varicella infection.
4. Urinalysis for proteinuria and glucosuria, and urine culture for asymptomatic bacteriuria.
5. Order prenatal labs to include a complete blood count, blood type, antibody screen, rubella titer, VDRL, hepatitis B surface antigen, and an HIV test.
6. Order an obstetrical ultrasound for dating if any of the following: beyond 16 weeks gestational age, unsure last menstrual period, size/dates discrepancy on exam, or for inability to hear fetal heart tones by 12 gestational weeks.
7. Discuss fetal aneuploidy screening and counseling regardless of maternal age.
8. Prenatal testing offered for: sickle cell anemia (African descent), thalassemia (African, Mediterranean, Middle Eastern, Southeast Asians), Canavan disease and Tay-Sachs (Jewish patients), cystic fibrosis (Caucasians and Ashkenazi Jews) and Fragile X syndrome (family history of nonspecified mental retardation).
9. Place a tuberculosis skin test for all medium-to-high risk patients.[a]
10. Consider a 1-hour 50-g glucose tolerance test for certain high-risk groups.[b]
11. Obtain an operative report in all women who have had a prior cesarean section
12. Psychosocial risk assessment for mood disorders, substance abuse, or domestic violence.

Frequency of Visits for Uncomplicated Pregnancies

1. Every 4 weeks until 28 gestational weeks; q2 weeks from 28 to 36 weeks; weekly > 36 weeks

Routine Checks at Follow-up Prenatal Visits

1. Assess weight, blood pressure, and urine for glucose and protein.
2. Exam: edema, fundal height, and fetal heart tones at all visits; fetal presentation starting at 36 weeks.
3. Ask about regular uterine contractions, leakage of fluid, vaginal bleeding, or decreased fetal movement.
4. Discuss labor precautions.

Antepartum Lab Testing

1. All women should be offered either first trimester, second trimester, or combined testing to screen for fetal aneuploidy; invasive diagnostic testing for fetal aneuploidy should be available to all women regardless of maternal age.
   a. First trimester
   b. Second trimester screening options: amniocentesis at 14 weeks; a Quad Marker Screen at 16–18 weeks; and/or a screening ultrasound with nuchal translucency assessment
2. Consider serial transvaginal sonography of the cervix every 2–3 weeks to assess cervical length for patients at high risk for preterm delivery starting at 16 weeks.

ROUTINE PRENATAL CARE (CONTINUED)

3. No role for routine bacterial vaginosis screening.
4. 1-hour 50-g glucose tolerance test in all women between 24 and 28 weeks.
5. Rectovaginal swab for group B streptococcal (GBS) testing between 35 and 37 weeks.
6. Recommend weekly amniotic fluid assessments and twice weekly nonstress testing starting at 41 weeks.

Prenatal Counseling

1. Cessation of smoking, drinking alcohol, or use of any illicit drugs.
2. Avoid cat litter boxes, hot tubs, certain foods (ie, raw fish or unpasteurized cheese)
3. Proper nutrition and expected weight gain: National Academy of Sciences advises weight gain 28–40 lb (pre-pregnancy BMI < 20), 25–35 lb (BMI 20–26), 15–25 lb (BMI 26–29) and 15–20 lb (BMI ≥ 30).
4. Inquire about domestic violence and depression at initial visit, at 28 weeks, and at postpartum visit.
5. Recommend regular mild-moderate exercise 3 or more times a week.
6. Avoid high-altitude activities, scuba diving, and contact sports during pregnancy.
7. Benefits of breast-feeding versus bottle feeding.
8. Discuss postpartum contraceptive options (including tubal sterilization) during third trimester.
9. Discuss analgesia and anesthesia options and offer prenatal classes at 24 weeks.
10. Discuss repeat c-section versus vaginal birth after cesarean (if applicable).
11. Discuss the option of circumcision if a boy is delivered.
12. Avoid air travel and long train or car trips beyond 36 weeks.

Prenatal Interventions

1. Suppressive antiviral medications starting at 36 weeks for women with a history of genital herpes.
2. Cesarean delivery is indicated for women who are HIV-positive or have active genital herpes and are in labor.
3. For patients who report a history of abuse, offer interventions and resources to increase their safety during and after pregnancy.
4. For patients with severe depression, consider treatment with an SSRI (avoid paroxetine if possible).
5. Rh immune globulin 300 mcg IM for all Rh-negative women with negative antibody screens between 26 and 28 weeks.
6. Refer for nutrition counseling at 10–12 weeks for BMI < 20 kg/m² or at any time during pregnancy for inadequate weight gain.
7. Start prenatal vitamins with iron and folic acid 400–800 mcg/day and 1200 mg elemental calcium/day starting at 4 weeks preconception (or as early as possible during pregnancy) and continued until 6 weeks postpartum.
8. Give inactivated influenza vaccine IM to all pregnant women during influenza season.
9. Consider progesterone therapy IM weekly or intravaginally daily to women at high risk for preterm birth.
10. Recommend an external cephalic version at 37 weeks for all noncephalic presentations.
11. Offer labor induction to women at 41 weeks by good dates.
12. Treat all women with confirmed syphilis with penicillin G during pregnancy.
13. Treat all women with gonorrhea with ceftriaxone; follow treatment with a test of cure.
14. Treat all women with *Chlamydia* with azithromycin; follow treatment with a test of cure.
15. Treat all GBS-positive women with penicillin G when in labor or with spontaneous rupture of membranes.

ROUTINE PRENATAL CARE (CONTINUED)

Postpartum Interventions

1. Treat all infants born to HBV-positive women with hepatitis B immunoglobulin (HBIG) and initiate HBV vaccine series within 12 hours of life.
2. All women with a positive tuberculosis skin test and no evidence of active disease should receive a postpartum chest x-ray; treat with isoniazid 300 mg PO daily for 9 months if chest x-ray is negative.
3. Administer a Tdap booster if tetanus status is unknown or the last Td vaccine has been over 10 years.
4. Administer an MMR vaccine to all rubella nonimmune women.
5. Offer HPV vaccine to all women ≤ 26 weeks who have not been immunized.
6. Initiate contraception.
7. Repeat Pap smear at 6-week postpartum check.

---

[a]Post-gastrectomy, gastric bypass, immunosuppressed (HIV-positive, diabetes, renal failure, chronic steroid/immunosuppressive therapy, head/neck or hematologic malignancies), silicosis, organ transplant recipients, malabsorptive syndromes, alcoholics, intravenous drug users, close contacts of persons with active pulmonary tuberculosis, medically underserved, low socioeconomic class, residents/ employees of long-term care facilities and jails, healthcare workers, and immigrants from endemic areas.

[b]Overweight (BMI ≥ 25 kg/m² and an additional risk factor: physical inactivity; first-degree relative with DM; high-risk ethnicity (eg, African American, Latino, Native American, Asian American, Pacific Islander); history of GDM; prior baby with birthweight > 9 lb; unexplained stillbirth or malformed infant, HTN on therapy or with BP ≥ 140/90 mmHg; HDL cholesterol level < 35 mg/dL (0.90 mmol/L) and/or a triglyceride level > 250 mg/dL (2.82 mmol/L); polycystic ovary syndrome; history of impaired glucose tolerance or HgbA1c ≥ 5.7%; acanthosis nigicans; cardiovascular disease; or ≥ 2+ glucosuria.

Adapted from ACOG ICSI Guideline on Routine Prenatal Care, July 2010 available at http://www.icsi.org/prenatal_care_4/prenatal_care__routine__full_version__2.html and VA/DoD Clinical Practice Guideline for Management of Pregnancy, 2009 at http://www.guidelines.gov/content.aspx?id=15678

PERINATAL & POSTNATAL GUIDELINES *Source:* AAP, AAFP	
Breast-feeding	Strongly recommends education and counseling to promote breast-feeding
Hemoglobinopathies	Strongly recommends ordering screening tests for hemoglobinopathies in neonates
Hyperbilirubinemia	Perform ongoing systematic assessments during the neonatal period for the risk of an infant developing severe hyperbilirubinemia
Phenylketonuria	Strongly recommends ordering screening tests for phenylketonuria in neonates
Thyroid function abnormalities	Strongly recommends ordering screening tests for thyroid function abnormalities in neonates
Source: Pediatrics. 2004;114:297–316. *Pediatrics.* 2005;115:496–506. (http://www.aafp.org/online/en/home/clinical/exam.html)	

PRETERM LABOR, TOCOLYSIS					
Disease Management	Organization	Date	Population	Recommendations	Comments	Source
Preterm Labor, Tocolysis	RCOG	2011	Pregnant women in preterm labor	• There is no clear evidence that tocolysis improves perinatal outcomes and therefore it is reasonable not to use them • Nifedipine and atosiban have comparable effectiveness in delaying birth up to seven days • Avoid the use of multiple tocolytic drugs simultaneously • Maintenance tocolytic therapy following threatened preterm labor is not recommended	• Tocolysis may be considered for women with suspected preterm labor who require *in utero* transfer or to complete a course of corticosteroids.	http://www.rcog.org.uk/files/rcog-corp/GTG1b26072011.pdf

Disease Management, Plaque-Type	Organization	Date	Population	Recommendations	Comments	Sources
PSORIASIS						

Psoriasis, Plaque-Type	AAD	2009	Adults	Topical Therapies
				1. Topical therapies are most effective for mild-moderate disease.
				2. Topical corticosteroids daily—bid
				  a. Cornerstone of therapy
				  b. Limit class 1 topical steroids to 4 weeks maximum
				3. Topical agents that have proven efficacy when combined with topical corticosteroids
				  a. Topical vitamin D analogues
				  b. Topical tazarotene
				  c. Topical salicylic acid
				4. Emollients applied 1–3 times daily are a helpful adjunct.
					1. Approximately, 2% of population has psoriasis.
					2. 80% of patients with psoriasis have mild-moderate disease.
					3. Topical steroid toxicity
					  a. Local: skin atrophy, telangiectasia, striae, purpura, or contact dermatitis
					  b. Hypothalamic-pituitary-adrenal axis may be suppressed with prolonged use of medium-high potency steroids
						http://www.aad.org/research/documents/JAADarticle-Section3PsoriasisGuidelines.pdf

	AAD	2009	Adults	Systemic Therapies
				1. Indicated for severe, recalcitrant, or disabling psoriasis
				2. Methotrexate (MTX)
				  a. Dose: 7.5–30 mg PO weekly
				  b. Monitor CBC and liver panel monthly
				3. Cyclosporine
				  a. Initial dose: 2.5–3 mg/kg divided bid
				  b. Monitor for nephrotoxicity, HTN, and hypertrichosis
				4. Acitretin
				  a. Dose: 10–50 mg PO daily
				  b. Monitor: liver panel
					1. MTX contraindications: pregnancy; breast-feeding; alcoholism; chronic liver disease; immunodeficiency syndromes; cytopenias; hypersensitivity reaction
					2. Cyclosporine contraindications: CA; renal impairment; uncontrolled HTN
					3. Acitretin contraindications: pregnancy; chronic liver or renal disease
						http://www.aad.org/research/documents/JAADarticle-Section4PsoriasisGuidelines.pdf

	PSORIASIS					

Disease Management	Organization	Date	Population	Recommendations	Comments	Source
Psoriasis and Psoriatic Arthritis	AAD	2010	Adults	• Treatment options for patients with limited plaque-type psoriasis 　○ First-line therapy 　　- Topical corticosteroids 　　- Topical calcipotriene/calcitriol 　　- Topical calcipotriene/steroid 　　- Topical tazarotene 　　- Topical calcineurin inhibitors (flexural surfaces and face) 　　- Targeted phototherapy 　○ Second-line therapy 　　- Systemic agents • Treatment of extensive plaque-type psoriasis 　○ First-line therapy 　　- UVB phototherapy +/- acitretin 　　- Topical PUVA 　○ Second-line therapy 　　- Acitretin + biologic 　　- Cyclosporine + biologic 　　- Cyclosporine + methotrexate 　　- Methotrexate + biologic 　　- UVB + biologic • Treatment of palmoplantar psoriasis 　○ First-line therapy 　• Topical corticosteroids 　• Topical calcipotriene/calcitriol 　• Topical calcipotriene/steroid 　• Topical tazarotene	• Use of potent topical corticosteroids should be limited to 4 weeks duration	http://www.guideline.gov/content.aspx?id=15650

				PSORIASIS		
Disease Management	Organization	Date	Population	Recommendations	Comments	Source

Psoriasis and Psoriatic Arthritis (continued)				○ Second-line therapy
				  - Acitretin
				  - Targeted UVB
				  - Topical PUVA
				○ Third-line therapy
				  - Adalimumab
				  - Alefacept
				  - Cyclosporine
				  - Etanercept
				  - Infliximab
				  - Methotrexate
				  - Ustekinumab
				• Treatment of erythrodermic psoriasis
				○ Acitretin
				○ Adalimumab
				○ Cyclosporine
				○ Infliximab
				○ Methotrexate
				○ Ustekinumab
				• Treatment of psoriatic arthritis
				○ First-line therapy
				  - Adalimumab
				  - Etanercept
				  - Golimumab
				  - Infliximab
				  - Methotrexate
				  - TNF blocker + methotrexate
				○ Second-line therapy
				  - Ustekinumab and methotrexate		

RESPIRATORY TRACT INFECTIONS, LOWER

Disease Management	Organization	Date	Population	Recommendations	Comments	Source

Respiratory Tract Infections, Lower	ESCMID	2011	Adults	• For Streptococcus pneumonia:
				  ○ Erythromycin MIC > 0.5 mg/L predicts clinical failure
				  ○ Penicillin MIC ≤ 8 mg/L predicts IV penicillin susceptibility
				• The role of community-acquired MRSA in CAP is poorly defined in Europe
				• A CRP < 2 mg/dL at presentation with symptoms > 24h makes pneumonia highly unlikely; a CRP > 10 mg/dL makes pneumonia likely
				• Indications for antibiotics in LRTIs:
				  ○ Suspected pneumonia
				  ○ Acute exacerbation of COPD with increased dyspnea, sputum volume, and sputum purulence
				• Evaluation of patients admitted for CAP
				  ○ Two sets of blood cultures
				  ○ Pleural fluid analysis is indicated when a significant parapneumonic effusion exists
				  ○ Sputum Gram stain and culture should be obtained if a purulent sputum sample can be obtained
				  ○ Consider testing for urine pneumococcal antigen
				  ○ Antibiotic duration for CAP should not exceed 8 days
					• Consider aspiration pneumonia in patients with a pneumonia and dysphagia
					• Empiric antibiotics of choice for LRTI in outpatient setting are amoxicillin or tetracycline
						http://www.escmic.org/fileadmin/src/media/PDFs/4ESCMID_Library/2Medical_Guidelines/ESCMID_Guidelines/Woodhead_et_al_CMI_Sep_2011_LRTI_GL_fulltext.pdf

RHEUMATOID ARTHRITIS (RA), BIOLOGIC DISEASE-MODIFYING) ANTIRHEUMATIC DRUGS (DMARDS)

Disease Management	Organization	Date	Population	Recommendations	Comments	Source
Rheumatoid Arthritis (RA), Biologic Disease-Modifying Antirheumatic Drugs (DMARDs)	ACR	2008	Adults	1. Anti-(tumor necrosis factor) TNF-α agents a. A tuberculosis (Tb) skin test or IGRA must be checked before initiating these medications b. Any patient with latent Tb needs at least 1 month treatment prior to the initiation of a TNF-α or biologic agent. c. Recommended for all patients with high disease activity and presence of poor prognostic features of any duration of disease. 2. Recommended for patients with disease ≥ 6 months who have failed nonbiologic DMARD therapy and have moderate-high disease activity, especially if poor prognostic features are present 3. Abatacept has same indications as anti-TNF-α agents. 4. Rituximab has same indications as anti-TNF-α agents. 5. Recommends withholding all biologic DMARDs 1 week before or after surgery.	1. Anti-TNF-α agents, abatacept, and rituximab all contraindicated in: a. Serious bacterial, fungal, and viral infections, or with latent Tb b. Acute viral hepatitis or Child's B or Child's C cirrhosis c. Instances of a lymphoproliferative disorder treated ≤ 5 years ago; decompensated congestive heart failure (CHF); or any demyelinating disorder	http://www.rheumatology.org/practice/clinical/guidelines/Singh%20bet%20al-ACR%20RA%20GL-May%202012%20AC&R.PDF#toolbar=1

RHEUMATOID ARTHRITIS (RA), NONBIOLOGIC DISEASE-MODIFYING ANTIRHEUMATIC DRUGS (DMARDS)

Disease Management	Organization	Date	Population	Recommendations	Comments	Source
Rheumatoid Arthritis (RA), Nonbiologic Disease-Modifying Antirheumatic Drugs (DMARDs) (continued)	ACR	2012	Adults	1. Target low disease activity or remission. 2. MTX or leflunomide monotherapy may be used for patients with any disease severity or duration. 3. Hydroxychloroquine or minocycline monotherapy recommended if low disease activity and duration ≤ 24 months. 4. Sulfasalazine recommended for all disease durations and without poor prognostic features.[a] 5. MTX plus either hydroxychloroquine or leflunomide recommended for moderate-high disease activity regardless of disease duration. 6. MTX plus sulfasalazine recommended for high disease activity and poor prognostic features.	1. Contraindications to DMARD therapy: a. Serious bacteria, fungal, or viral infections b. Only DMARDs safe with latent Tb are hydroxychloroquine, minocycline, and sulfasalazine. c. Avoid MTX for interstitial pneumonitis and for creatinine clearance < 30 mL/min. d. Avoid MTX and leflunomide for cytopenias, hepatitis, pregnancy, and breast-feeding (also minocycline). e. Avoid all DMARDs in Child's B or Child's C cirrhosis.	http://www.rheumatology.org/practice/clinical/guidelines/Sir_gh%20et%20al-ACR%20RA%20GL-May%2020 20.2%20AC&R. PDF#toolbar=1

[a] Functional limitation, presence of rheumatoid nodules, secondary Sjögren syndrome, RA vasculitis, Felty syndrome, and RA lung disease.

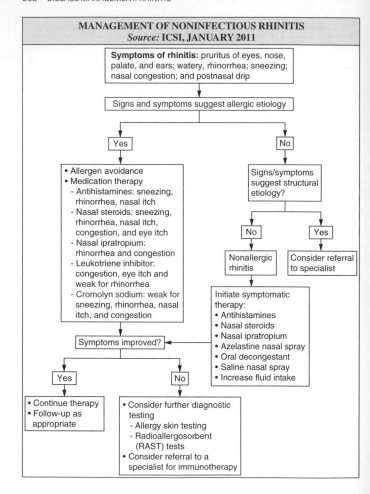

MANAGEMENT OF NONINFECTIOUS RHINITIS
Source: **ICSI, JANUARY 2011**

Symptoms of rhinitis: pruritus of eyes, nose, palate, and ears; watery, rhinorrhea; sneezing; nasal congestion; and postnasal drip

Signs and symptoms suggest allergic etiology

Yes

No

- Allergen avoidance
- Medication therapy
  - Antihistamines: sneezing, rhinorrhea, nasal itch
  - Nasal steroids: sneezing, rhinorrhea, nasal itch, congestion, and eye itch
  - Nasal ipratropium: rhinorrhea and congestion
  - Leukotriene inhibitor: congestion, eye itch and weak for rhinorrhea
  - Cromolyn sodium: weak for sneezing, rhinorrhea, nasal itch, and congestion

Signs/symptoms suggest structural etiology?

No

Yes

Nonallergic rhinitis

Consider referral to specialist

Initiate symptomatic therapy:
- Antihistamines
- Nasal steroids
- Nasal ipratropium
- Azelastine nasal spray
- Oral decongestant
- Saline nasal spray
- Increase fluid intake

Symptoms improved?

Yes

No

- Continue therapy
- Follow-up as appropriate

- Consider further diagnostic testing
  - Allergy skin testing
  - Radioallergosorbent (RAST) tests
- Consider referral to a specialist for immunotherapy

SEIZURES, FEBRILE

Disease Management	Organization	Date	Population	Recommendations	Comments	Source

Seizures, Febrile	AAP	2011	Children 6 months to 5 years old	• A lumbar puncture should be performed in any child who presents with a fever and seizure and has meningeal signs or whose history is concerning for meningitis
				• Lumbar puncture is an option in children 6–12 months of age who present with a fever and seizure and are not up to date with their *Haemophilus influenzae* or *S. pneumoniae* vaccinations
				• Lumbar puncture is an option in a child presenting with a fever and a seizure who has been pretreated with antibiotics
				• Studies that should not be performed for a simple febrile seizure:
				  ○ An EEG
				  ○ Routine labs including a basic metabolic panel, calcium, phosphorus, magnesium, glucose or CBC
				  ○ Neuroimaging
					• A febrile seizure is a seizure accompanied by fever (T ≥ 100.4°F) without CNS infection in a child aged 6 months to 5 years.	http://pediatrics.aappublications.org/content/127/2/389.full.pdf+html

SEXUALLY TRANSMITTED DISEASES TREATMENT GUIDELINES
ADAPTED FROM CDC GUIDELINES, *MMWR.* 2010;59(RR-12):1–116.

Infection	Recommended Treatment	Alternative Treatment
Chancroid	• Azithromycin 1 g PO × 1 • Ceftriaxone 250 mg IM × 1	• Ciprofloxacin 500 mg PO bid for 3 days • Erythromycin base 500 mg PO tid for 7 days
First episode of genital HSV	• Acyclovir 400 mg PO tid × 7–10 days[a] • Famciclovir 250 mg PO tid × 7–10 days[a] • Valacyclovir 1 g PO bid × 7–10 days[a]	• Acyclovir 200 mg PO five times a day for 7–10 days[a]
Suppressive therapy for genital HSV	• Acyclovir 400 mg PO bid • Famciclovir 250 mg PO bid	• Valacyclovir 1 g PO daily
Episodic therapy for recurrent genital HSV	• Acyclovir 400 mg PO tid × 5 days • Famciclovir 125 mg PO bid × 5 days • Valacyclovir 500 mg PO bid × 3 days	• Acyclovir 800 mg PO bid × 5 days • Acyclovir 800 mg PO tid × 2 days • Famciclovir 1000 mg PO bid × 1 day • Famciclovir 500 mg PO × 1 then 250 mg bid × 2 days • Valacyclovir 1 g PO daily × 5 days
Suppressive therapy for HIV-positive patients	• Acyclovir 400–800 mg PO bid-tid • Famciclovir 500 mg PO bid • Valacyclovir 500 mg PO bid	
Episodic therapy for recurrent genital HSV in HIV-positive patients	• Acyclovir 400 mg PO tid × 5–10 days • Famciclovir 500 mg PO bid × 5–10 days • Valacyclovir 1 g PO bid × 5–10 days	
Granuloma inguinale (Donovanosis)	• Doxycycline 100 mg PO bid × ≥ 3 weeks and until all lesions have completely healed	• Azithromycin 1 g PO weekly × ≥ 3 weeks • Ciprofloxacin 750 mg PO bid × ≥ 3 weeks • Erythromycin base 500 mg PO qid × ≥ 3 weeks • TMP-SMX one double-strength (160 mg/800 mg) tablet PO bid × ≥ 3 weeks • Continue all of these treatments until all lesions have completely healed
Lymphogranuloma venereum	• Doxycycline 100 mg PO bid for × 21 days	• Erythromycin base 500 mg PO qid × 21 days

SEXUALLY TRANSMITTED DISEASES TREATMENT GUIDELINES (CONTINUED) ADAPTED FROM CDC GUIDELINES, *MMWR*. 2010;59(RR-12):1–116.		
Infection	Recommended Treatment	Alternative Treatment
Syphilis in adults	• Benzathine penicillin G 2.4 million units IM × 1	
Syphilis in infants and children	• Benzathine penicillin G 50,000 units/kg IM, up to the adult dose of 2.4 million units × 1	
Early latent syphilis in adults	• Benzathine penicillin G 2.4 million units IM × 1	
Early latent syphilis in children	• Benzathine penicillin G 50,000 units/kg IM, up to the adult dose of 2.4 million units × 1	
Late latent syphilis or latent syphilis of unknown duration in adults	• Benzathine penicillin G 2.4 million units IM weekly × 3 doses	
Late latent syphilis or latent syphilis of unknown duration in children	• Benzathine penicillin G 50,000 units/kg, up to the adult dose of 2.4 million units, IM weekly × 3 doses	
Tertiary syphilis	• Benzathine penicillin G 2.4 million units IM weekly × 3 doses	
Neurosyphilis	• Aqueous crystalline penicillin G 3–4 million units IV q4h × 10–14 days	• Procaine penicillin 2.4 million units IM daily × 10–14 days **PLUS** • Probenecid 500 mg PO qid × 10–14 days
Syphilis, pregnant women	• Pregnant women should be treated with the penicillin regimen appropriate for their stage of infection	
Congenital syphilis	• Aqueous crystalline penicillin G 50,000 units/kg/dose IV q12h × 7 days; then q8h × 3 more days	• Procaine penicillin G 50,000 units/kg/dose IM daily × 10 days • Benzathine penicillin G 50,000 units/kg/dose IM × 1
Older children with syphilis	• Aqueous crystalline penicillin G 50,000 units/kg IV q4–6h × 10 days	
Nongonococcal urethritis	• Azithromycin 1 g PO × 1 • Doxycycline 100 mg PO bid × 7 days	• Erythromycin base 500 mg PO qid × 7 days • Erythromycin ethylsuccinate 800 mg PO qid × 7 days • Levofloxacin 500 mg PO daily × 7 days • Ofloxacin 300 mg PO bid × 7 days

SEXUALLY TRANSMITTED DISEASES TREATMENT GUIDELINES (CONTINUED)
ADAPTED FROM CDC GUIDELINES, *MMWR.* 2010;59(RR-12):1–116.

Infection	Recommended Treatment	Alternative Treatment
Recurrent or persistent urethritis	• Metronidazole 2 g PO × 1 • Tinidazole 2 g PO × 1 • Azithromycin 1 g PO × 1	
Cervicitis[b]	• Azithromycin 1 g PO × 1 • Doxycycline 100 mg PO bid × 7 days	
Chlamydia infections in adolescents, adults[b]	• Azithromycin 1 g PO × 1 • Doxycycline 100 mg PO bid × 7 days	• Erythromycin base 500 mg PO qid × 7 days • Erythromycin ethylsuccinate 800 mg PO qid × 7 days • Levofloxacin 500 mg PO daily × 7 days • Ofloxacin 300 mg PO bid × 7 days
Chlamydia infections in Pregnancy[b]	• Azithromycin 1 g PO × 1 • Amoxicillin 500 mg PO tid × 7 days	• Erythromycin base 500 mg PO qid × 7 days • Erythromycin ethylsuccinate 800 mg PO qid × 7 days
Ophthalmia neonatorum from *Chlamydia*	• Erythromycin base or ethylsuccinate 50 mg/kg/day PO qid × 14 days	
Chlamydia trachomatis pneumonia in infants	• Erythromycin base or ethylsuccinate 50 mg/kg/day PO qid × 14 days	
Chlamydia infections in children < 45 kg	• Erythromycin base or ethylsuccinate 50 mg/kg/day PO qid × 14 days	
Chlamydia infections in children ≥ 45 kg and aged < 8 years	• Azithromycin 1 g PO × 1	
Chlamydia infections in children aged ≥ 8 years	• Azithromycin 1 g PO × 1 • Doxycycline 100 mg PO bid × 7 days	
Uncomplicated gonococcal infections of the cervix, urethra, pharynx, or rectum in adults or children > 45 kg	• Ceftriaxone 250 mg IM × 1 **PLUS** • Azithromycin 1 g PO × 1 **OR** • Doxycycline 100 mg daily × 7 days	

	SEXUALLY TRANSMITTED DISEASES TREATMENT GUIDELINES (CONTINUED) ADAPTED FROM CDC GUIDELINES, *MMWR.* 2010;59(RR-12):1–116.	
Infection	**Recommended Treatment**	**Alternative Treatment**
Gonococcal conjunctivitis in adults or children > 45 kg	• Ceftriaxone 1 g IM × 1	
Gonococcal meningitis or endocarditis in adults or children > 45 kg	• Ceftriaxone 1 g IV q12h	
Disseminated gonococcal infection in adults or children > 45 kg	• Ceftriaxone 1 g IV/IM daily	• Cefotaxime 1 g IV q8h • Ceftizoxime 1 g IV q8h
Ophthalmia neonatorum caused by gonococcus	• Ceftriaxone 25–50 mg/kg, not to exceed 125 mg, IV/IM × 1	
Prophylactic treatment of infants born to mothers with gonococcal infection	• Ceftriaxone 25–50 mg/kg, not to exceed 125 mg, IV/IM × 1	
Uncomplicated gonococcal infections of the cervix, urethra, pharynx, or rectum in children ≤ 45 kg	• Ceftriaxone 125 mg IM × 1	
Gonococcal infections with bacteremia or arthritis in children or adults	• Ceftriaxone 50 mg/kg (maximum dose 1 g) IM/IV daily × 7 days	
Ophthalmia neonatorum prophylaxis	• Erythromycin (0.5%) ophthalmic ointment in each eye × 1	
Bacterial vaginosis	• Metronidazole 500 mg PO bid × 7 days[c] • Metronidazole gel 0.75%, one applicator (5 g) IVag daily × 5 days • Clindamycin cream 2%, one applicator (5 g) IVag qhs × 7 days[d]	• Tinidazole 2 g PO daily × 3 days • Clindamycin 300 mg PO bid × 7 days • Clindamycin ovules 100 mg IVag qhs × 3 days

SEXUALLY TRANSMITTED DISEASES TREATMENT GUIDELINES (CONTINUED) ADAPTED FROM CDC GUIDELINES, *MMWR.* 2010;59(RR-12):1–116.		
Infection	**Recommended Treatment**	**Alternative Treatment**
Bacterial vaginosis in pregnancy	• Metronidazole 500 mg PO bid × 7 days • Metronidazole 250 mg PO tid × 7 days • Clindamycin 300 mg PO bid × 7 days	
Trichomoniasis	• Metronidazole 2 g PO × 1[c] • Tinidazole 2 g PO × 1	• Metronidazole 500 mg PO bid × 7 days[c]
Candidal vaginitis	• Butoconazole 2% cream 5 g IVag × 3 days • Clotrimazole 1% cream 5 g IVag × 7–14 days • Clotrimazole 2% cream 5 g IVag × 3 days • Nystatin 100,000-unit vaginal tablet, one tablet IVag × 14 days • Miconazole 2% cream 5 g IVag × 7 days • Miconazole 4% cream 5 g IVag × 3 days • Miconazole 100-mg vaginal suppository, one suppository IVag × 7 days • Miconazole 200-mg vaginal suppository, one suppository IVag × 3 days • Miconazole 1200-mg vaginal suppository, one suppository IVag × 1 • Tioconazole 6.5% ointment 5 g IVag × 1 • Terconazole 0.4% cream 5 g IVag × 7 days • Terconazole 0.8% cream 5 g IVag × 3 days • Terconazole 80-mg vaginal suppository, one suppository IVag × 3 days	• Fluconazole 150-mg oral tablet, one tablet in single dose
Severe pelvic inflammatory disease	• Cefotetan 2 g IV q12h **OR** • Cefoxitin 2 g IV q6h **PLUS** • Doxycycline 100 mg PO/IV bid	• Clindamycin 900 mg IV q8h **PLUS** • Gentamicin loading dose IV or IM (2 mg/kg of body weight), followed by a maintenance dose (1.5 mg/kg) q8h. Single daily dosing (3–5 mg/kg) can be substituted.

SEXUALLY TRANSMITTED DISEASES TREATMENT GUIDELINES (CONTINUED) ADAPTED FROM CDC GUIDELINES, *MMWR.* 2010;59(RR-12):1–116.		
Infection	**Recommended Treatment**	**Alternative Treatment**
Severe pelvic inflammatory disease (continued)		**OR** • Ampicillin/sulbactam 3 g IV q6h **PLUS** • Doxycycline 100 mg PO/IV bid
Mild-moderate pelvic inflammatory disease	• Ceftriaxone 250 mg IM × 1 **OR** • Cefoxitin 2 g IM × 1 **and** probenecid 1 g PO × 1 **PLUS** • Doxycycline 100 mg PO bid × 14 days +/– metronidazole 500 mg PO bid × 14 daysᶜ	
Epididymitis	• Ceftriaxone 250 mg IM × 1 **PLUS** • Doxycycline 100 mg PO bid × 10 days	• Levofloxacin 500 mg PO daily × 10 days • Ofloxacin 300 mg PO bid × 10 days
External genital warts	**Provider-Administered:** • Cryotherapy every 1–2 weeks • Podophyllin resin 10%–25% in a compound tincture of benzoin • TCA or BCA 80%–90% • Surgical removal either by tangential scissor excision, tangential shave excision, curettage, or electrosurgery	**Patient-Applied:** • Podofilox 0.5% solution or gel • Imiquimod 5% cream • Sinecatechins 15% ointment
Cervical warts	• Biopsy to exclude high-grade SIL must be performed before treatment is initiated	
Vaginal warts	• TCA or BCA 80%–90% applied only to warts, repeated weekly	
Urethral meatal warts	• Cryotherapy every 1–2 weeks • TCA or BCA 80%–90% applied only to warts, repeated weekly	
Anal warts	• Cryotherapy every 1–2 weeks • TCA or BCA 80%–90% applied only to warts, repeated weekly	• Surgical removal either by tangential scissor excision, tangential shave excision, curettage, or electrosurgery
Proctitis	• Ceftriaxone 250 mg IM × 1 **PLUS** • Doxycycline 100 mg PO bid × 7 days	

SEXUALLY TRANSMITTED DISEASES TREATMENT GUIDELINES (CONTINUED) ADAPTED FROM CDC GUIDELINES, *MMWR.* 2010;59(RR-12):1–116.		
Infection	**Recommended Treatment**	**Alternative Treatment**
Pediculosis pubis	• Permethrin 1% cream rinse applied to affected areas and washed off after 10 minutes • Pyrethrins with piperonyl butoxide applied to the affected area and washed off after 10 minutes	• Malathion 0.5% lotion applied for 8–12 hours and then washed off • Ivermectin 250 mcg/kg PO, repeated in 2 weeks
Scabies	• Permethrin cream (5%) applied to all areas of the body from the neck down and washed off after 8–14 hours • Ivermectin 200 mcg/kg PO, repeat in 2 weeks	• Lindane (1%) 1 oz or lotion (or 30 g of cream) applied in a thin layer to all areas of the body from the neck down and thoroughly washed off after 8 hours

HSV, herpes simplex virus; PO, by mouth; IM, intramuscular; IVag, intravaginally; bid, twice a day; tid, three times a day; HIV, human immunodeficiency virus; qid, four times a day; TMP-SMX, trimethoprim-sulfamethoxazole; IV, intravenous; q, every; h, hour(s); qhs, at bedtime; TCA, trichloroacetic acid; BCA, bichloroacetic acid; SIL, squamous intraepithelial lesion

[a]Treatment can be extended if healing is incomplete after 10 days of therapy.

[b]Consider concomitant treatment of gonorrhea.

[c]Avoid alcohol during treatment and for 24 hours after treatment is completed.

[d]Clindamycin cream may weaken latex condoms and diaphragms during treatment and for 5 days thereafter.

SYPHILIS

Disease Management	Organization	Date	Population	Recommendations	Comments	Source

Syphilis	IDSA	2011	Adults	• Penicillin G 2.4 million units is drug of choice for early syphilis
				  ○ CSF analysis is indicated if:
				    ○ Early syphilis infection and neurologic symptoms
				    ○ Late latent syphilis
				    • HIV-infected patients with RPR titer ≥ 1:32 or CD4 < 350 cells/mm^3
				• Patients with early syphilis do not achieve a ≥ 4-fold decline in RPR titers within 12 months
				• Doxycycline is second-line therapy for early syphilis in penicillin-allergic patients
				• Ceftriaxone is second-line therapy for neurosyphilis in penicillin-allergic patients
					• Avoid doxycycline in pregnancy	http://cid.oxfordjournals.org/content/53/suppl_3/S110.abstract

MANAGEMENT OF THYROID NODULES
Sources: AACE, JUNE 2010 AND ATA, NOVEMBER 2009

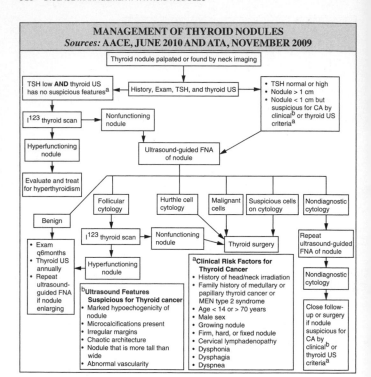

THYROID DISEASE						

Disease Management	Organization	Date	Population	Recommendations	Comments	Source

Thyroid Disease, Hyperthyroidism	AACE	2011	Adults	• Radioactive iodine uptake scan should be performed when the etiology of thyrooxicosis is unclear
				• Beta-blockade should be prescribed to elderly patients and considered for all patients with symptomatic thyrotoxicosis
				• Graves disease
				  ○ Options for Graves disease treatment:
				    - I^{131} therapy
				    - Antithyroid medications
				    - Thyroidectomy
				• Patients with Graves disease and increased risk of complications should be pretreated with methimazole and beta-blockers pror or to I^{131} therapy
				  ○ Advise smoking cessation
				  ○ Graves' ophthalmopathy should have steroids and I^{131} therapy
				• I^{131} therapy
				  ○ A pregnancy test should be checked within 48 hours of administering I^{131} therapy
				  ○ Assess patients 1–2 months after I^{131} therapy with a free T$_4$ and total T level
				  ○ Consider retreatment with I^{131} therapy if hyperthyroidism persists 6 months after I^{131} treatment
						https://www.aace.com/files/hyper-guidelines-2011.pdf

THYROID DISEASE						
Disease Management	Organization	Date	Population	Recommendations	Comments	Source
Thyroid Disease, Hyperthyroidism (continued)				• Antithyroid drug therapy 　○ Methimazole is the preferred antithyroid drug except during the first trimester of pregnancy 　○ A CBC with differential should be obtained whenever a patient taking antithyroid drugs develops a febrile illness or pharyngitis 　○ Recommend measurement of TSH receptor antibody level prior to stopping antithyroid drug therapy • Thyroidectomy 　○ Indicated for toxic multinodular goiter or toxic adenoma 　○ Wean beta-blockers post-op 　○ Follow serial calcium or intact PTH levels post-op 　○ Start levothyroxine 1. mcg/kg/day immediately post-op 　○ Check a serum TSH level 6–8 weeks post-op • Thyroid storm should be treated with beta-blockers, antithyroid drugs, inorganic iodide, corticosteroid therapy, volume resuscitation and acetaminophen		

Disease Management	Organization	Date	Population	Recommendations	Comments	Source
THYROID DISEASE, PREGNANCY AND POSTPARTUM						
Thyroid Disease, Pregnancy and Postpartum	ATA	2011	Women during and immediately after pregnancy	• Hypothyroidism in pregnancy is defined as: ○ An elevated TSH (> 2.5 mIU/L) and a suppressed FT4) ○ TSH ≥10 mIU/L (irrespective of FT4) ○ Subclinical hypothyroidism is defined as a TSH 2.5–9.9 mIU/L) and a normal FT4 • Insufficient evidence to support treatment of subclinical hypothyroidism in pregnancy • Goal therapy is to normalize TSH levels • PTU is the preferred antithyroid drug in pregnancy • Monitor TSH levels every 4 weeks when treating thyroid disease in pregnancy • Measure a TSH receptor antibody level at 20–24 weeks for any history of Graves disease • All pregnant and lactating women should ingest at least 250 mcg iodine daily • All pregnant women with thyroid nodules should undergo thyroid ultrasound and TSH testing • Patients found to have thyroid cancer during pregnancy would ideally undergo surgery during second trimester	• Surgery for well-differentiated thyroid carcinoma can often be deferred until postpartum period	http://thyroidguidelines.net/sites/thyroidguidelines.net/files/file/thy.2011.0087..pdf

TOBACCO CESSATION TREATMENT ALGORITHM
Source: U.S. PUBLIC HEALTH SERVICE

Five A's

1. Ask about tobacco use.
2. Advise to quit through clear, personalized messages.
3. Assess willingness to quit.
4. Assist to quit,[a] including referral to Quit Lines (eg, 1-800-NO-BUTTS).
5. Arrange follow-up and support.

[a]Physicians can assist patients to quit by devising a quit plan, providing problem-solving counseling, providing intratreatment social support, helping patients obtain social support from their environment/friends, and recommending pharmacotherapy for appropriate patients. Use caution in recommending pharmacotherapy in patients with medical contraindications, those smoking < 10 cigarettes per day, pregnant/breast-feeding women, and adolescent smokers. As of March 2005, Medicare covers costs for smoking cessation counseling for those who (1) have a smoking-related illness; (2) have an illness complicated by smoking; or (3) take a medication that is made less effective by smoking. (http://www.cms.hhs.gov/mcd/viewdecisionmemo.asp?id=130)

Source: Fiore MC, et al. Treating Tobacco Use and Dependence. Quick Reference Guide for Clinicians. Rockville, MD: U.S. Department of Health and Human Services. Public Health Service, October 2000.

MOTIVATING TOBACCO USERS TO QUIT

Five R's

1. Relevance: personal
2. Risks: acute, long term, environmental
3. Rewards: have patient identify (eg, save money, better food taste)
4. Road blocks: help problem solve
5. Repetition: at every office visit

		TOBACCO CESSATION TREATMENT OPTIONS[a]				
Pharmacotherapy	Precautions/ Contraindications	Side Effects	Dosage	Duration	Availability	Cost/Day[b]
First-Line Pharmacotherapies (approved for use for smoking cessation by the FDA)						
Bupropion SR	History of seizure History of eating disorder	Insomnia Dry mouth	150 mg every morning for 3 days, then 150 mg bid. (Begin treatment 1–2 weeks pre-quit)	7–12 weeks maintenance up to 6 months	Zyban (prescription only)	$5.73
Nicotine gum	—	Mouth soreness Dyspepsia	1–24 cigarettes/day: 2-mg gum (up to 24 pieces/day) 25+ cigarettes/day: 4-mg gum (up to 24 pieces/day)	Up to 12 weeks	Nicorette, Nicorette Mint (OTC only)	$5.81
Nicotine inhaler	—	Local irritation of mouth and throat	6–16 cartridges/day	Up to 6 months	Nicotrol Inhaler (prescription only)	$6.07
Nicotine nasal spray	—	Nasal irritation	8–40 doses/day	3–6 months	Nicotrol NS (prescription only)	$3.67
Nicotine patch	—	Local skin reaction Insomnia	21 mg/24 hours 14 mg/24 hours 7 mg/24 hours 15 mg/16 hours	4 weeks Then 2 weeks Then 2 weeks 8 weeks	NicoDerm CQ (OTC only), generic patches (prescription and OTC) Nicotrol (OTC only)	$3.91
Varenicline	Renal impairment	Nausea Abnormal dreams	0.5 mg QD for 3 days, then 0.5 mg bid for 4 days, then 1.0 mg PO bid	12 weeks or 24 weeks	Chantix (prescription only)	$4.22

TOBACCO CESSATION TREATMENT OPTIONS[a] (CONTINUED)

Pharmacotherapy	Precautions/ Contraindications	Side Effects	Dosage	Duration	Availability	Cost/Day[b]
Second-Line Pharmacotherapies (not approved for use for smoking cessation by the FDA)						
Clonidine	Rebound hypertension	Dry mouth Drowsiness Dizziness Sedation	0.15–0.75 mg/day	3–10 weeks	Oral clonidine–generic, Catapres (prescription only), transdermal Catapres (prescription only)	Clonidine $0.24 for 0.2 mg; Catapres (transdermal) $3.50
Nortriptyline	Risk of arrhythmias	Sedation Dry mouth	75–100 mg/day	12 weeks	Nortriptyline HCL–generic (prescription only)	$0.74 for 75 mg

FDA, Food and Drug Administration; OTC, over-the-counter; QD, every day; bid, twice daily; PO, by mouth
[a]The information contained within this table is not comprehensive. Please see package inserts for additional information.
[b]Prices from Rx for Change, the Regents of the University of California, University of Southern California, and Western University of Health Sciences.
[c]Prices based on retail prices of a national chain pharmacy; 2000.
Source: U.S. Public Health Service.

TONSILLECTOMY					

Disease Management	Organization	Date	Population	Recommendations	Comments	Source

Tonsillectomy	AAO-HNS	2011	Children	• Recommend against routine perioperative antibiotics for tonsillectomy
				• Tonsillectomy indicated for:
				  ○ Tonsillar hypertrophy with sleep disordered breathing
				  ○ Recurrent throat infections for ≥ 7 episodes of recurrent throat infection in past year; ≥ 5 episodes of recurrent throat infection per year in past 2 years; or ≥ 3 episodes of recurrent throat infection per year in past 3 years
				• Recommend post-tonsillectomy pain control
						http://www.entnet.org/HealthInformation/upload/CPG-TonsillectomyInChildren.pdf

	TREMOR, ESSENTIAL				
Disease Management	Organization	Date	Population	Recommendations	Comments	Source
Tremor, Essential	AAN	2011	Adults	• Recommend treatment with propranolol or primidone • Alternative treatment options include alprazolam, atenolol, gabapentin, sotalol, or topiramate • Recommend against treatment with levetiracetam, pindolol, trazodone, acetazolamide, or 3,4-diaminopyridine	• Unilateral thalamotomy may be effective for severe refractory essential tremors	http://www.neurology.org/content/77/19/1752.full.pdf+html

TUBERCULOSIS, MULTIDRUG-RESISTANT (MDR-TB)

Disease Management	Organization	Date	Population	Recommendations	Comments	Source
Tuberculosis, Multi-Drug-Resistant (MDR-TB)	WHO	2011	Patients with suspected or proven drug-resistant tuberculosis	• Rapid drug susceptibility testing of isoniazid and rifampicin is recommended at the time of Tb diagnosis • Recommend sputum smear microscopy and culture to monitor patients with MDR-Tb • Recommend addition of a later-generation fluoroquinolone, ethionamide, pyrazinamide, and a parenteral agent +/– cycloserine for ≥ 8 months • Recommend total treatment duration of 20 months		http://whqlit.doc.who.int/publications/2011/9789241501583_eng.pdf

URINARY INCONTINENCE, STRESS

Disease Management	Organization	Date	Population	Recommendations	Comments	Source
Urinary Incontinence, Stress	AUA	2009	Adult women	1. Recommends an exam to assess the degree of urethral mobility, pelvic floor relaxation, pelvic organ prolapse, and assess whether any urethral abnormalities exist. 2. Recommends a urinalysis. 3. Assess the post-void residual volume. 4. Surgical options for refractory stress urinary incontinence include periurethral injections, laparoscopic bladder suspensions, midurethral slings, pubovaginal slings, and retropubic suspensions.		http://www.auanet.org/content/media/stress2009-chapter1.pdf

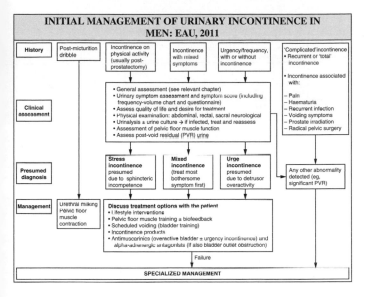

INITIAL MANAGEMENT OF URINARY INCONTINENCE IN MEN: EAU, 2011

History

- Post-micturition dribble
- Incontinence on physical activity (usually post-prostatectomy)
- Incontinence with mixed symptoms
- Urgency/frequency, with or without incontinence
- 'Complicated' incontinence
  - Recurrent or 'total' incontinence
  - Incontinence associated with:
    - Pain
    - Haematuria
    - Recurrent infection
    - Voiding symptoms
    - Prostate irradiation
    - Radical pelvic surgery

Clinical assessment

- General assessment (see relevant chapter)
- Urinary symptom assessment and symptom score (including frequency-volume chart and questionnaire)
- Assess quality of life and desire for treatment
- Physical examination: abdominal, rectal, sacral neurological
- Urinalysis ± urine culture → if infected, treat and reassess
- Assessment of pelvic floor muscle function
- Assess post-void residual (PVR) urine

Presumed diagnosis

- Stress incontinence presumed due to sphincteric incompetence
- Mixed incontinence (treat most bothersome symptom first)
- Urge incontinence presumed due to detrusor overactivity
- Any other abnormality detected (eg, significant PVR)

Management

- Urethral milking Pelvic floor muscle contraction

- Discuss treatment options with the patient
  - Lifestyle interventions
  - Pelvic floor muscle training ± biofeedback
  - Scheduled voiding (bladder training)
  - Incontinence products
  - Antimuscarinics (overactive bladder ± urgency incontinence) and alpha-adrenergic antagonists (if also bladder outlet obstruction)

Failure

SPECIALIZED MANAGEMENT

INITIAL MANAGEMENT OF URINARY INCONTINENCE IN WOMEN: EAU, 2011

| History | Incontinence on physical activity | Incontinence with mixed symptoms | Incontinence or frequency, with or without urgency incontinence | 'Complicated' incontinence • Recurrent incontinence • Incontinence associated with: - Pain - Haematuria - Recurrent infection - Significant voiding symptoms - Pelvic irradiation - Radical pelvic surgery - Suspected fistula |

Clinical assessment
- General assessment
- Urinary symptom assessment (including frequency-volume chart and questionnaire)
- Assess quality of life and desire for treatment
- Physical examination: abdominal, pelvic and perineal
- Cough test to demonstrate stress incontinence if appropriate
- Urinalysis ± urine culture → if infected, treat and reassess *if appropriate*
- Assess oestrogen status and treat as appropriate
- Assess voluntary pelvic floor muscle contraction
- Assess post-void residual urine

Presumed diagnosis

| **Stress incontinence** presumed due to sphincteric incompetence | **Mixed incontinence** (treat most bothersome symptom first) | Overactive bladder (OAB), with or without URGENCY INCONTINENCE, presumed due to detrusor overactivity | If other abnormality found eg, • Significant post void residual • Significant pelvic organ prolapse • Pelvic mass |

Management
- Life-style interventions
- Pelvic floor muscle training for SUI or OAB
- Bladder retraining for OAB
- Duloxetine* (SUI) or antimuscarinic (OAB ± urgency incontinence)

*Subject to local regulatory approval

- Other adjuncts, such as electrical stimulation
- Vaginal devices, urethral inserts

Failure

SPECIALIZED MANAGEMENT

Disease Management	Organization	Date	Population	Recommendations	Comments	Source

Urinary Tract Infections (UTIs)	ACOG EAU IDSA	2008 2010 2011	Nonpregnant women	1. Screening for and treatment of asymptomatic bacteriuria is not recommended.
				2. Recommend duration of antibiotics:
				  a. Uncomplicated cystitis: 3 days
				    i. Nitrofurantoin requires 5–7 days of therapy
				  b. Uncomplicated pyelonephritis: 7–10 days
				  c. Complicated pyelonephritis or urinary tract infection: 3–5 days after control/elimination of complicating factors and defervescence.
				3. Recommended empiric antibiotics for uncomplicated cystitis[a]:
				  a. TMP-SMX
				  b. Fluoroquinolones
				  c. Nitrofurantoin macrocrystals
				  d. Beta-lactam antibiotics are alternative agents[b]
				4. Recommended empiric antibiotics for complicated urinary tract infection or uncomplicated pyelonephritis:
				  a. Fluoroquinolones
				  b. Ceftriaxone
				  c. Aminoglycosides
					1. EAU recommends 7 days of antibiotics for men with uncomplicated cystitis.
					2. EAU suggests the following options for antimicrobial prophylaxis of recurrent uncomplicated UTIs in nonpregnant women:
					  a. Nitrofurantoin 50 mg PO daily
					  b. TMP-SMX 40/200 mg/day
					3. EAU suggests the following options for antimicrobial prophylaxis of recurrent uncomplicated UTIs in pregnant women:
					  a. Cephalexin 125 mg PO daily
						http://www.guidelines.gov/content.aspx?id=12628
						
						http://www.uroweb.org/gls/pdf/Urological%20Infections%202010.pdf
						
						http://www.guidelines.gov/content.aspx?id=2652&search=idsa+cystitis+2011

	URINARY TRACT INFECTIONS (UTIs)					
Disease Management	Organization	Date	Population	Recommendations	Comments	Source
Urinary Tract Infections (UTIs) (continued)	ACOG IDSA	2008 2011	Adult women	5. Recommended empiric antibiotics for complicated pyelonephritis: a. Fluoroquinolones b. Piperacillin-tazobactam c. Carbapenem d. Aminoglycosides • Recommend a urinalysis or dipstick testing for symptoms of a UTI: dysuria, urinary frequency, suprapubic pain, or hematuria • Empiric antibiotics for UTI ○ Trimethoprim-sulfamethoxazole × 3 days (not recommended if local resistance rate > 20%) ○ Nitrofurantoin monohydrate × 5 days ○ Fosfomycin 3 gm PO × 1 • Consider a fluoroquinolone for symptoms of pyelonephritis or for refractory UTI	4. Once urine culture and sensitivity results are known, antibiotics can be adjusted to the narrowest spectrum antibiotic.	http://guidelines.gov/content.aspx?id=12628 http://cid.oxfordjournals.org/content/52/5/e103.full.pdf+html

URINARY TRACT INFECTIONS (UTIs)						
Disease Management	Organization	Date	Population	Recommendations	Comments	Source

Urinary Tract Infections (UTIs) (continued)	AAP	2011	Febrile children 2–24 months	• Diagnosis of a UTI if:
				  ○ Pyuria ≥ 50,000 col/mL single uropathogenic organism
				  ○ Recommend a renal and bladder ultrasound in all infants 2–24 months with a febrile UTI
				• Treat febrile UTIs with 7–14 days of antibiotics
				• Antibiotic prophylaxis is not indicated for a history of febrile UTI
				• A voiding cystourethrogram (VCUG) is indicated if ultrasound reveals hydronephrosis, renal scarring, or other findings of high-grade vesicoureteral reflux, and for recurrent febrile UTIs
					• Urine obtained through catheterization has a 95% sensitivity and 99% specificity for UTI
					• Bag urine cultures have a specificity of ~63% with an unacceptably high false-positive rate. **Only useful if the cultures are negative**
						http://pediatrics.aappublications.org/content/128/3/595.full.pdf+html?sid=c1d-42b3-c89b-4fd2-9592-35908762317

aTMP-SMX only if regional *Escherichia coli* resistance is < 21%; fluoroquinolones include ciprofloxacin, ofloxacin, or levofloxacin.
bAmoxicillin-clavulanate, cefdinir, cefaclor, or cefpodoxime-proxetil. Cephalexin may be appropriate in certain settings.

LOWER URINARY TRACT SYMPTOMS (LUTS)

Disease Management	Organization	Date	Population	Recommendations	Comments	Source
Lower Urinary Tract Symptoms (LUTS)	NICE EAU	2010 2011	Adult men	1. All men with LUTS should have a thorough history and exam, including a prostate exam and review of current medications. 2. Recommends supervised bladder training exercises and consider anticholinergic medications for symptoms suggestive of an overactive bladder. 3. Recommends an alpha-blocker for men with moderate-severe LUTS. [a] 4. Consider a 5-alpha reductase inhibitor for men with LUTS with prostate size larger than 30 g. 5. For men with refractory obstructive urinary symptoms despite medical therapy, offer one of three surgeries: transurethral resection, transurethral vaporization, or laser enucleation of the prostate.		http://www.nice.org.uk/nicemedia/live/12984/48557/48557.pdf http://www.uroweb.org/gls/pdf/12_Male_LUTS.pdf

[a] Alfuzosin, doxazosin, tamsulosin, or terazosin.

DIAGNOSIS AND TREATMENT OF VENOUS THROMBOEMBOLISM (VTE) WELLS CRITERIA

Source: Deep Vein thrombosis (DVT) and Pulmonary Embolism (PE)
(Lancet. 2012; 379:1835)

Pretest probability (PTP) of VTE guides clinical evaluation
– Wells criteria for PTP of DVT and PE

DVT		PE	
VARIABLE	SCORE	VARIABLE	SCORE
Active cancer	1	Clinical evidence of DVT	3.0
Paralysis/immobilization	1	Other dx less likely than PE	3.0
Bedridden for >3 days or major surgery within 4 weeks	1	Heart rate >100	1.5
Entire leg swollen	1	Immobile >3 days or major surgery within 4 weeks	1.5
Tenderness along deep vein	1	Previous DVT/PE	1.5
Calf swelling >3 cm	1	Hemoptysis	1.0
Pitting edema (unilateral)	1	Malignancy	1.0
Collateral superficial veins	1		
Alternative dx more likely than DVT	−2		

Score and Probability-DVT
High — 3 or greater (75% risk of DVT)
Moderate — 1 or 2 (20% risk of DVT)
Low — 0 (3% risk of DVT)

Score and Probability - PE
High — 6 or greater (> 70% risk of PE)
Moderate — 2 to 6 (20–30% risk of PE)
Low — less than 2 (2–3% risk of PE)

				VENOUS THROMBOEMBOLISM (VTE)	
Disease Management	Organization/ Date	Population	Recommendations	Comments	Source
Deep Vein Thrombosis (DVT)	ACCP 2012 ACP 2011	Patients with DVT (lower and upper extremity)	• Initial heparin based regimen with unfractionated heparin (UFH) 80u/kg bolus, then 18u/kg/hour titrated to PTT, enoxaparin 1 mg/kg SQ q12h or 1.5 mg/kg SQ daily, Fondaparinux 5 mg (<50 kg), 7.5 mg (50–100 kg) or 10 mg (>100 kg) SQ daily. • Start warfarin (≤10 mg) on day 1 and overlap with heparin for at least 5 days with therapeutic INR for last 2 days. Warfarin recommended over dabigatran (oral direct thrombin inhibitor [DTI]) or rivaroxaban (direct factor Xa inhibitor). New oral anticoagulants not FDA approved as yet for treatment of DVT and PE **(see Table I).** (*NEJM* 2012; 366:1287). Knee high GCS (graduated compression stockings) (30–40 mmHg pressure at ankles) for 2 years will reduce post-thrombotic syndrome by 50%).	1. Clinical findings alone are poor predictors of DVT. 2. Early ambulation on heparin is safe. 3. With ilio-femoral thrombosis and significant swelling thrombolysis or surgical thrombectomy not recommended unless significant symptoms. 4. IVC filter indicated if pulmonary embolus while on therapeutic anticoagulation or significant uncontrolled bleeding precluding anticoagulation 5. Provoked clot-anticoagulate for 3 months if precipitating problem solved. 6. Continue anticoagulation indefinitely if provoking problem continues. 7. In cancer related clots continue LMWH, do not transition to warfarin 8. In unprovoked clot anticoagulate for 3 months then weigh risk of bleeding to benefit of prolonged anticoagulation to prevent clot – consider thrombophilia evaluation including hereditary factors and antiphospholipid antibody syndrome.	http://chestjournal. chestpubs.org/ content/ suppl/2012

VENOUS THROMBOEMBOLISM (VTE)				
Disease Management	Organization/ Date	Population	Recommendations	Comments	Source

Disease Management	Organization/ Date	Population	Recommendations	Comments	Source
Deep Vein Thrombosis (DVT) (continued)				9. Risk factors for warfarin bleeding – age >65years history of stroke, history of GI bleed and recent co-morbidity (MI, Hct<30, creatinine >1.5, diabetes). If all 4 factors present 40% risk of significant bleed in 12 months 0.4% of patients on warfarin die of bleeding yearly. (Chest. 2006; 130:1296) (AJMed. 2011; 124:111). 10. Patients with mild symptoms and good support system can be treated as outpatient. 11 Calf and ilio-femoral (IF) thrombosis with increased false negative compression ultrasound — recommend CT or MR venogram or venography for suspected IF thrombosis — for calf thrombosis follow-up CUS in 5–7 days is acceptable.	

	VENOUS THROMBOEMBOLISM (VTE)				
Disease management	Organization/ Date	Population	Recommendations	Comments	Source
Deep Vein Thrombosis (DVT) (continued)				12. If d-dimer normal with abnormal CUS in leg with previous DVT makes new clot unlikely. (JThrom Haemost. 2007; 5:1076) 13. Consider thrombophilia in patients with recurrent VTE or patients with 1st unprovoked VTE who: • are < 50 years old • family history of VTE • unusual site of thrombosis • massive venous thrombosis 14. In unprovoked VTE 3% found to have associated malignancy with another 10% diagnosed with cancer over next 2 years. (*NEJM.* 1998; 338:1169) (*Ann Int Med.* 2008; 149:323)	

[a]Surgery, cancer, hormones, pregnancy, travel, inflammatory bowel disease, nephritic syndrome, hemolytic anemia, immobilization, trauma, CHF, myeloproliferative disorders, stroke, central venous catheter, rheumatologic disorders.

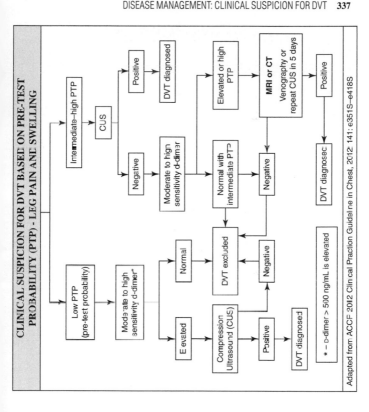

CLINICAL SUSPICION FOR DVT BASED ON PRE-TEST PROBABILITY (PTP) - LEG PAIN AND SWELLING

Low PTP (pre-test probability)

Moderate to high sensitivity d-dimer*

Elevated

Compression Ultrasound (CUS)

Positive → DVT diagnosed

Negative → DVT excluded

Normal → DVT excluded

Intermediate-high PTP

CUS

Positive → DVT diagnosed

Negative

Moderate to high sensitivity d-dimer*

Normal with intermediate PTP → DVT excluded

Elevated or high PTP

MRI or CT
Venography or repeat CUS in 5 days

Negative → DVT excluded

Positive → DVT diagnosed

* d-dimer > 500 ng/mL is elevated

Adapted from ACCF 2012 Clinical Practice Guideline in Chest, 2012; 141: e351S–e418S

	VENOUS THROMBOEMBOLISM				
Disease Management	Organization/Date	Population	Recommendations	Comments	Source
Pulmonary Embolus (PE)	ACCP 2012 ACP 2011	Diagnosed Pulmonary embolism	• Approach to initial anticoagulation is same as DVT • If patient hypotensive without high bleeding risk, systemically administered thrombolytic therapy is recommended • In a patient with acute PE associated with hypotension with contraindications to or failed thrombolysis or in shock that is likely to lead to rapid death, catheter assisted thrombus removal is indicated if appropriate expertise and resources are available • In patients whose first episode of VTE is an unprovoked PE, extended anticoagulation beyond 3 months is preferred unless high risk of bleeding	• Patients whose 1st VTE is a PE, will have a 3 fold increase risk of a 2nd clot being a PE compared to patients with DVT only (*NEJM.* 2010; 363:266) • In patients with unprovoked PE or DVT elevated d-dimer at the time of discontinuation of warfarin or 2–3 weeks after stopping anticoagulants predicts for a 3–5 fold increase in risk of clot over the next 12 months (Blood. 2010; 115:481) • The presence of a permanent IVC filter does not mandate continuous anticoagulation unless documented recurrent clot problems • Unprovoked clot has risk of recurrent clot in 1st 12 months of 8–12% vs. 3% for patients with provoked clot (*JAMA.* 2011; 305:1336). • Patients with intermediate or high PTP of PE should be treated with heparin before diagnostic work-up is complete • Asymptomatic PE (found incidentally on chest CT) should be treated with same protocol as symptomatic PE • Emerging data suggests the use of aspirin (100 mg p.o. daily) may reduce the risk of recurrent clot in patients with unprovoked VTE after 6-12 months of warfarin therapy (*NEJM.* 2012; 366:1959)	http://chestjournal.chestdubs.org/content/suppl/2012

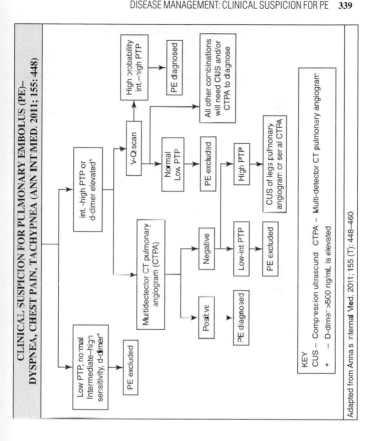

CLINICAL SUSPICION FOR PULMONARY EMBOLUS (PE)—DYSPNEA, CHEST PAIN, TACHYPNEA (ANN INT MED. 2011; 155: 448)

int.–high PTP or d-dimer elevated*

- **V-Q scan**
  - High probability int.–high PTP → **PE diagnosed**
  - Normal Low PTP → **PE excluded**
  - High PTP → CUS of legs pulmonary angiogram or serial CTPA
  - All other combinations will need CUS and/or CTPA to diagnose

- **Multidetector CT pulmonary angiogram (CTPA)**
  - Positive → **PE diagnosed**
  - Negative
    - Low-int PTP → **PE excluded**
    - High PTP → CUS of legs pulmonary angiogram or serial CTPA

Low PTP, normal Intermediate-high sensitivity, d-dimer* → **PE excluded**

KEY
CUS – Compression ultrasound   CTPA – Multi-detector CT pulmonary angiogram
* – D-dimer >500 ng/mL is elevated

Adapted from Annals Internal Med. 2011; 155 (T): 448–460

NEW ORAL ANTICOAGULANTS [a] AND WARFARIN					
Agent	Target	Dosing	Monitoring	Half-life	Time to Peak Plasma Creat
Warfarin[b]	Vitamin K Epoxide	Once daily	INR - adjusted	40 hours	72–96 hours
Dabigatran[c]	Thrombin	Fixed – once or twice daily	NONE	14–17 hours	2 hours
Rivaroxaban[c]	Factor Xa	Fixed – once or twice daily	NONE	5–9 hours (50 years old) 9–13 hours (elderly)	2.5 – 4 hours
Apixaban[c]	Factor Xa	Fixed twice daily	NONE	8–15 hours	3 hours

[a] Approved for use in atrial fibrillation and prophylaxis for orthopedic surgery but likely will be approved for treating VTE soon.
[b] If significant bleed on warfarin – give vitamin K, fresh frozen plasma, and consider prothrombin complex concentrate (PCC) or recombinant FVIIa if not controlled.
[c] If significant bleed – no standard of care. Aggressively treat source of bleed – consider PCC or recombinant FVIIa.

VERTIGO, BENIGN PAROXYSMAL POSITIONAL (BPPV)						
Disease Management	**Organization**	**Date**	**Population**	**Recommendations**	**Comments**	**Source**
Vertigo, Benign Paroxysmal Positional (BPPV)	AAO-HNS	2008	Adults	1. Recommends the Dix-Hallpike maneuver to diagnose posterior semicircular canal BPPV. 2. Recommends treatment of posterior semicircular canal BPPV with a particle repositioning maneuver. 3. If the Dix-Hallpike test result is negative, recommends a supine roll test to diagnose lateral semicircular canal BPPV. 4. Recommends offering vestibular rehabilitation exercises for the initial treatment of BPPV. 5. Recommends evaluating patients for an underlying peripheral vestibular or central nervous system disorder if they have an initial treatment failure of presumed BPPV. 6. Recommends against routine radiologic imaging for patients with BPPV. 7. Recommends against routine vestibular testing for patients with BPPV. 8. Recommends against routine use of antihistamines or benzodiazepines for patients with BPPV.	BPPV is the most common vestibular disorder in adults afflicting 2.4% of adults at some point during their lives.	http://www.entlink.net/Practice/upload/BPPV_guideline-final-journal.pdf

4
Appendices

SCREENING INSTRUMENTS: ALCOHOL ABUSE

SENSITIVITY AND SPECIFICITY OF SCREENING TESTS FOR PROBLEM DRINKING

Instrument Name	Screening Questions/Scoring	Threshold Score	Sensitivity/Specificity (%)	Source
CAGE[a]	See page 345	> 1 > 2 > 3	77/58 53/81 29/92	*Am J Psychiatr.* 1974;131:1121 *J Gen Intern Med.* 1998;13:379
AUDIT	See pages 345–346	> 4 > 5 > 6	87/70 77/84 66/90	*BMJ.* 1997;314:420 *J Gen Intern Med.* 1998;13:379

[a]The CAGE may be less applicable to binge drinkers (eg, college students), the elderly, and minority populations.

SCREENING INSTRUMENTS: ALCOHOL ABUSE

SCREENING PROCEDURES FOR PROBLEM DRINKING

1. CAGE screening test[a]

Have you ever felt the need to   Cut down on drinking?

Have you ever felt   Annoyed by criticism of your drinking?

Have you ever felt   Guilty about your drinking?

Have you ever taken a morning   Eye opener?

INTERPRETATION: Two "yes" answers are considered a positive screen. One "yes" answer should arouse a suspicion of alcohol abuse.

2. The Alcohol Use Disorder Identification Test (AUDIT)[b] (Scores for response categories are given in parentheses. Scores range from 0 to 40, with a cut-off score of ≥ 5 indicating hazardous drinking, harmful drinking, or alcohol dependence.)

1) How often do you have a drink containing alcohol?

| (0) Never | (1) Monthly or less | (2) Two to four times a month | (3) Two or three times a week | (4) Four or more times a week |

2) How many drinks containing alcohol do you have on a typical day when you are drinking?

| (0) 1 or 2 | (1) 3 or 4 | (2) 5 or 6 | (3) 7 to 9 | (4) 10 or more |

3) How often do you have six or more drinks on one occasion?

| (0) Never | (1) Less than monthly | (2) Monthly | (3) Weekly | (4) Daily or almost daily |

4) How often during the past year have you found that you were not able to stop drinking once you had started?

| (0) Never | (1) Less than monthly | (2) Monthly | (3) Weekly | (4) Daily or almost daily |

5) How often during the past year have you failed to do what was normally expected of you because of drinking?

| (0) Never | (1) Less than monthly | (2) Monthly | (3) Weekly | (4) Daily or almost daily |

SCREENING INSTRUMENTS: ALCOHOL ABUSE

SCREENING PROCEDURES FOR PROBLEM DRINKING (CONTINUED)

6) How often during the past year have you needed a first drink in the morning to get yourself going after a heavy drinking session?

(0) Never   (1) Less than monthly   (2) Monthly   (3) Weekly   (4) Daily or almost daily

7) How often during the past year have you had a feeling of guilt or remorse after drinking?

(0) Never   (1) Less than monthly   (2) Monthly   (3) Weekly   (4) Daily or almost daily

8) How often during the past year have you been unable to remember what happened the night before because you had been drinking?

(0) Never   (1) Less than monthly   (2) Monthly   (3) Weekly   (4) Daily or almost daily

9) Have you or has someone else been injured as a result of your drinking?

(0) No   (2) Yes, but not in the past year   (4) Yes, during the past year

10) Has a relative or friend or a doctor or other health worker been concerned about your drinking or suggested you cut down?

(0) No   (2) Yes, but not in the past year   (4) Yes, during the past year

[a]Modified from Mayfield D, McLeod G, Hall P. The CAGE questionnaire: validation of a new alcoholism screening instrument. *Am J Psychiatr.* 1974;131:1121.
[b]From Piccinelli M, et al. Efficacy of the alcohol use disorders identification test as a screening tool for hazardous alcohol intake and related disorders in primary care: a validity study. *BMJ.* 1997;314:420.

SCREENING INSTRUMENTS: DEPRESSION

SCREENING TESTS FOR DEPRESSION

Instrument Name	Screening Questions/Scoring	Threshold Score	Source
Beck Depression Inventory (short form)	See page 350	0–4: None or minimal depression 5–7: Mild depression 8–15: Moderate depression >15: Severe depression	*Postgrad Med.* 1972 Dec:81
Geriatric Depression Scale	See page 351	≥15: Depression	*J Psychiatr Res.* 1983;17:37
PRIME-MD® (mood questions)	1. During the past month, have you often been bothered by feeling down, depressed, or hopeless? 2. During the past month, have you often been bothered by little interest or pleasure in doing things?	"Yes" to either question[a]	*JAMA.* 1994;272:1749 *J Gen Intern Med.* 1997;12:439
Patient Health Questionnaire (PHQ-9)®	http://www.pfizer.com/phq-9/ See page 348	*Major depressive syndrome:* if answers to #1a or b and ≥ 5 of #1a–i are at least "More than half the days" (count #1i if present at all) *Other depressive syndrome:* if #1a or b and 2–4 of #1a–i are at least "More than half the days" (count #1i if present at all) 5–9: mild depression 10–14: moderate depression 15–19: moderately severe depression 20–27: severe depression	*JAMA.* 1999;282:1737 *J Gen Intern Med.* 2001;16:606

[a]Sensitivity 86%–96%; specificity 57%–75%.
®Pfizer Inc.

SCREENING INSTRUMENTS: DEPRESSION

PHQ-9 DEPRESSION SCREEN, ENGLISH

Over the last 2 weeks, how often have you been bothered by any of the following problems?

		Not at all	Several days	> Half the days	Nearly every day
a.	Little interest or pleasure in doing things	0	1	2	3
b.	Feeling down, depressed, or hopeless	0	1	2	3
c.	Trouble falling or staying asleep, or sleeping too much	0	1	2	3
d.	Feeling tired or having little energy	0	1	2	3
e.	Poor appetite or overeating	0	1	2	3
f.	Feeling bad about yourself—or that you are a failure or that you have let yourself or your family down	0	1	2	3
g.	Trouble concentrating on things, such as reading the newspaper or watching television	0	1	2	3
h.	Moving or speaking so slowly that other people could have noticed? Or the opposite—being so fidgety or restless that you have been moving around a lot more than usual?	0	1	2	3
i.	Thoughts that you would be better off dead or of hurting yourself in some way	0	1	2	3
	(For office coding: Total Score	—— =	—— +	—— +	——)

Major depressive syndrome: if ≥ 5 items present scored ≥ 2 and one of the items is depressed mood (b) or anhedonia (a). If item "i" is present, then this counts, even if score = 1.
Depressive screen positive: if at least one item ≥ 2 (or item "i" is ≥ 1).

Source: From the Primary Care Evaluation of Mental Disorders Patient Health Questionnaire (PRIME-MD PHQ). The PHQ was developed by Drs. Robert L. et al. For research information, contact Dr. Spitzer at rls8@columbia.edu. PRIME-MD® is a trademark of Pfizer Inc. Copyright © 1999 Pfizer Inc. All rights reserved. Reproduced with permission. FOR OFFICE CODING: Maj Dep Syn if answer to #2a or b and ≥ 5 of #2a–i are at least "More than half the days" (count #2i if present at all). Other Dep Syn if #2a or b and 2, 3, or 4 of #2a–i are at least "More than half the days" (count #2i if present at all).

SCREENING INSTRUMENTS: DEPRESSION

PHQ-9 DEPRESSION SCREEN, SPANISH

Durante las últimas 2 semanas, ¿con qué frecuencia le han molestado los siguientes problemas?

	Nunca	Varios días	> La mitad de los días	Casi todos los días
a. Tener poco interés o placer en hacer las cosas	0	1	2	3
b. Sentirse desanimada, deprimida, o sin esperanza	0	1	2	3
c. Con problemas en dormirse o en mantenerse dormida, o en dormir demasiado	0	1	2	3
d. Sentirse cansada o tener poca energía	0	1	2	3
e. Tener poco apetito o comer en exceso	0	1	2	3
f. Sentir falta de amor propio—o qe sea un fracaso o que decepcionara a si misma o a su familia	0	1	2	3
g. Tener dificultad para concentrarse en cosas tales como leer el periódico o mirar la televisión	0	1	2	3
h. Se mueve o habla tan lentamente que otra gente se podría dar cuenta—o de lo contrario, está tan agitada o inquieta que se mueve mucho más de lo acostumbrado	0	1	2	3
i. Se le han ocurrido pensamientos de que se haría daño de alguna manera	0	1	2	3
(For office coding: Total Score	—— =	—— +	—— +	——)

Source: From the Primary Care Evaluation of Mental Disorders Patient Health Questionnaire (PRIME-MD PHQ). The PHQ was developed by Drs Robert L. et al. For research information, contact Dr Spitzer at rls8@columbia.edu. PRIME-MD® is a trademark of Pfizer Inc. Copyright © 1999 Pfizer Inc. All rights reserved. Reproduced with permission. FOR OFFICE CODING: Maj Dep Syn if answer to #2a or b and ≥ 5 of #2a–i are at least "More than half the days" (count #2i if present at all). Other Dep Syn if #2a or b and 2, 3, or 4 of #2a–i are at least "More than half the days" (count #2i if present at all).

SCREENING INSTRUMENTS: DEPRESSION

BECK DEPRESSION INVENTORY, SHORT FORM

Instructions: This is a questionnaire. On the questionnaire are groups of statements. Please read the entire group of statements in each category. Then pick out the one statement in that group that best describes the way you feel today, that is, right now! Circle the number beside the statement you have chosen. If several statements in the group seem to apply equally well, circle each one. Sum all numbers to calculate a score.

Be sure to read all the statements in each group before making your choice.

A. Sadness
3 I am so sad or unhappy that I can't stand it.
2 I am blue or sad all the time and I can't snap out of it.
1 I feel sad or blue.
0 I do not feel sad.

B. Pessimism
3 I feel that the future is hopeless and that things cannot improve.
2 I feel I have nothing to look forward to.
1 I feel discouraged about the future.
0 I am not particularly pessimistic or discouraged about the future.

C. Sense of failure
3 I feel I am a complete failure as a person (parent, husband, wife).
2 As I look back on my life, all I can see is a lot of failures.
1 I feel I have failed more than the average person.
0 I do not feel like a failure.

D. Dissatisfaction
3 I am dissatisfied with everything.
2 I don't get satisfaction out of anything anymore.
1 I don't enjoy things the way I used to.
0 I am not particularly dissatisfied.

E. Guilt
3 I feel as though I am very bad or worthless.
2 I feel quite guilty.
1 I feel bad or unworthy a good part of the time.
0 I don't feel particularly guilty.

F. Self-dislike
3 I hate myself.
2 I am disgusted with myself.
1 I am disappointed in myself.
0 I don't feel disappointed in myself.

G. Self-harm
3 I would kill myself if I had the chance.
2 I have definite plans about committing suicide.
1 I feel I would be better off dead.
0 I don't have any thoughts of harming myself.

H. Social withdrawal
3 I have lost all of my interest in other people and don't care about them at all.
2 I have lost most of my interest in other people and have little feeling for them.
1 I am less interested in other people than I used to be.
0 I have not lost interest in other people.

I. Indecisiveness
3 I can't make any decisions at all anymore.
2 I have great difficulty in making decisions.
1 I try to put off making decisions.
0 I make decisions about as well as ever.

J. Self-image change
3 I feel that I am ugly or repulsive-looking.
2 I feel that there are permanent changes in my appearance and they make me look unattractive.
1 I am worried that I am looking old or unattractive.
0 I don't feel that I look worse than I used to.

K. Work difficulty
3 I can't do any work at all.
2 I have to push myself very hard to do anything.
1 It takes extra effort to get started at doing something.
0 I can work about as well as before.

L. Fatigability
3 I get too tired to do anything.
2 I get tired from doing anything.
1 I get tired more easily than I used to.
0 I don't get any more tired than usual.

M. Anorexia
3 I have no appetite at all anymore.
2 My appetite is much worse now.
1 My appetite is not as good as it used to be.
0 My appetite is no worse than usual.

Source: Reproduced with permission from Beck AT, Beck RW. Screening depressed patients in family practice: a rapid technic. *Postgrad Med.* 1972;52:81.

GERIATRIC DEPRESSION SCALE

Choose the best answer for how you felt over the past week

1. Are you basically satisfied with your life?	yes / no
2. Have you dropped many of your activities and interests?	yes / no
3. Do you feel that your life is empty?	yes / no
4. Do you often get bored?	yes / no
5. Are you hopeful about the future?	yes / no
6. Are you bothered by thoughts you can't get out of your head?	yes / no
7. Are you in good spirits most of the time?	yes / no
8. Are you afraid that something bad is going to happen to you?	yes / no
9. Do you feel happy most of the time?	yes / no
10. Do you often feel helpless?	yes / no
11. Do you often get restless and fidgety?	yes / no
12. Do you prefer to stay at home, rather than going out and doing new things?	yes / no
13. Do you frequently worry about the future?	yes / no
14. Do you feel you have more problems with memory than most?	yes / no
15. Do you think it is wonderful to be alive now?	yes / no
16. Do you often feel downhearted and blue?	yes / no
17. Do you feel pretty worthless the way you are now?	yes / no
18. Do you worry a lot about the past?	yes / no
19. Do you find life very exciting?	yes / no
20. Is it hard for you to get started on new projects?	yes / no
21. Do you feel full of energy?	yes / no
22. Do you feel that your situation is hopeless?	yes / no
23. Do you think that most people are better off than you are?	yes / no
24. Do you frequently get upset over little things?	yes / no
25. Do you frequently feel like crying?	yes / no
26. Do you have trouble concentrating?	yes / no
27. Do you enjoy getting up in the morning?	yes / no
28. Do you prefer to avoid social gatherings?	yes / no
29. Is it easy for you to make decisions?	yes / no
30. Is your mind as clear as it used to be?	yes / no

One point for each response suggestive of depression. (Specifically "no" responses to questions 1, 5, 7, 9, 15, 19, 21, 27, 29, and 30, and "yes" responses to the remaining questions are suggestive of depression.)

A score of ≥ 15 yields a sensitivity of 80% and a specificity of 100%, as a screening test for geriatric depression. *Clin Gerontol*. 1982;1:37.

Source: Reproduced with permission from Yesavage JA, et al. Development and validation of a geriatric depression screening scale: a preliminary report. *J Psychiatr Res*. 1982–83;17:37.

FUNCTIONAL ASSESSMENT SCREENING IN THE ELDERLY			
Target Area	**Assessment Procedure**	**Abnormal Result**	**Suggested Intervention**
Vision	Inquire about vision changes, Snellen chart testing.	Presence of vision changes; inability to read greater than 20/40	Refer to ophthalmologist.
Hearing	Whisper a short, easily answered question such as "What is your name?" in each ear while the examiner's face is out of direct view. Use audioscope set at 40 dB; test using 1000 and 2000 Hz. Brief hearing loss screener	Inability to answer question Inability to hear 1000 or 2000 Hz in both ears or inability to hear frequencies in either ear Brief hearing loss screen score ≥ 3	Examine auditory canals for cerumen and clean if necessary. Repeat test; if still abnormal in either ear, refer for audiometry and possible prosthesis.
Balance and gait	Observe the patient after instructing as follows: "Rise from your chair, walk 10 ft, return, and sit down." Check orthostatic blood pressure and heart rate.	Inability to complete task in 15 seconds	Performance-Oriented Mobility Assessment (POMA). Consider referral for physical therapy.
Continence of urine	Ask, "Do you ever lose your urine and get wet?" If yes, then ask, "Have you lost urine on at least 6 separate days?"	"Yes" to both questions	Ascertain frequency and amount. Search for remediable causes, including local irritations, polyuric states, and medications. Consider urologic referral.
Nutrition	Ask, "Without trying, have you lost 10 lb or more in the last 6 months?" Weigh the patient. Measure height.	"Yes" or weight is below acceptable range for height	Do appropriate medical evaluation.
Mental status	Instruct as follows: "I am going to name three objects (pencil, truck, and book). I will ask you to repeat their names now and then again a few minutes from now."	Inability to recall all three objects after 1 minute	Administer Folstein Mini-Mental State Examination. If score is less than 24, search for causes of cognitive impairment. Ascertain onset, duration, and fluctuation of overt symptoms. Review medications. Assess consciousness and affect. Do appropriate laboratory tests.

FUNCTIONAL ASSESSMENT SCREENING IN THE ELDERLY (CONTINUED)

Target Area	Assessment Procedure	Abnormal Result	Suggested Intervention
Depression	Ask, "Do you often feel sad or depressed?" or "How are your spirits?"	"Yes" or "Not very good, I guess"	Administer Geriatric Depression Scale or PHQ-9. If positive, check for antihypertensive, psychotropic, or other pertinent medications Consider appropriate pharmacologic or psychiatric treatment.
ADL-IADL[a]	Ask, "Can you get out of bed yourself?" "Can you dress yourself?" "Can you make your own meals?" "Can you do your own shopping?"	"No" to any question	Corroborate responses with patient's appearance; question family members if accuracy is uncertain. Determine reasons for the inability (motivation compared with physical limitation). Institute appropriate medical, social, or environmental interventions.
Home environment	Ask, "Do you have trouble with stairs inside or outside of your home?" Ask about potential hazards inside the home with bathtubs, rugs, or lighting.	"Yes"	Evaluate home safety and institute appropriate countermeasures.
Social support	Ask, "Who would be able to help you in case of illness or emergency?"	—	List identified persons in the medical record. Become familiar with available resources for the elderly in the community.
Pain	Inquire about pain.	Presence of pain	Pain inventory.
Dentition	Oral examination.	Poor dentition	Dentistry referral.
Falls	Inquire about falls in past year and difficulty with walking or balance.	Presence of falls or gait/ balance problems	Falls evaluation (see page 59).

[a]Activities of Daily Living–Instrumental Activities of Daily Living.
Source: Modified from Lachs MS, et al. A simple procedure for screening for functional disability in elderly patients. *Ann Intern Med*. 1990;112:699.
Geriatrics At Your Fingertips online edition 2008–2009. (http://www.geriatricsatyourfingertips.org, accessed 10/13/11)

SCREENING AND PREVENTION GUIDELINES IN PERSPECTIVE: PGPC 2012

The following tables highlight areas where differences exist between various organizations' guideline recommendations and areas where a new direction appears to be developing as a result of new or updated guidelines.

1. Areas of significant difference in guideline recommendations

Guidelines	Organization	Recommendations
Adolescent Alcohol Abuse	USPSTF/AAFP	Evidence insufficient
	Bright Futures/NIAAA	Screen annually
Breast CA Screening, Women aged 40–49 years	UK-NHS	Routine screening not recommended
	ACP	Mammogram and CBE yearly starting at age 40—high-risk patients (> 20% lifetime risk of breast CA) add annual MRI
	USPSTF/AAFP	Mammography ± breast examination every 1–2 years beginning at age 50. In women aged 40–50, counsel regarding risks and benefits; it should no longer be done routinely
Breast CA Screening, Women aged 50–70 years	UK-NHS	Mammography screening every 3 years
	USPSTF/AAFP	Mammography screening every 1–2 years
	ACS	Annual mammography screening
Cervical CA Screening, Women aged < 50 years	UK-NHS	Begin screening every 3 years after age 25 years
	ACS	Screen 3 years after first sexual intercourse or at age 21, screen annually (or every 2 years if liquid-based Pap smear) until age 30, then every 3 years if consecutive negative Pap smear results
Prostate CA Screening, Men aged > 50 years	USPSTF/AAFP	Do not use PSA-based screening for prostate cancer at any age—evidence suggests harms outweigh benefits
	UK-NHS	Informed decision making
	ACS	Offer annual PSA and digital rectal examination, particularly for men who defer to physician's judgment—discuss risks and benefits including treatment options and side effects of treatment
Testicular CA Screening	USPSTF/AAFP	Recommend against screening
	ACS	Perform testicular examination as part of routine CA-related checkup
Depression, Children and Adolescents	USPSTF/AAFP/ CTF/NICE	Insufficient evidence to recommend for or against screening
	Bright Futures	Annual screening for behaviors/emotions that indicate depression or risk of suicide
Family Violence and Abuse, Children and Adolescents	USPSTF/AAFP	Insufficient evidence to recommend for or against screening
	Family Violence Prevention Fund	Assess caregivers/parents and adolescent patients at least annually

SCREENING AND PREVENTION GUIDELINES IN PERSPECTIVE: PGPC 2012 (CONTINUED)

Hearing Loss, Newborns	USPSTF/AAFP	Insufficient evidence to recommend for or against screening during the postpartum hospitalization
	Joint Committee on Infant Hearing	All infants should be screened for neonatal or congenital hearing loss
Thyroid Screening, Adults	USPSTF/AAFP	Evidence insufficient to recommend for or against screening
	ATA	Screen all women aged > 35 years at 5-year intervals
Glaucoma, Adults	USPSTF/AAFP	Evidence insufficient to recommend for or against screening
	AOA	Comprehensive eye examination every 2 years ages 18–60, then every year age > 60
Diabetes Mellitus, Gestational	USPSTF/AAFP	Evidence insufficient to recommend for or against screening asymptomatic pregnant women
	ADA	Risk-assess all women at first prenatal visit

2. New directions resulting from new or updated guidelines

HIV screening: Opt-out screening for practically everyone, actively recommended against written informed consent.

Endocarditis prophylaxis: Now targets those at increased risk of complications from endocarditis, rather than risk of endocarditis.

Perioperative guidelines: New data have emerged on beta blockade that is not reflected in current guidelines. Two randomized trials of perioperative metoprolol found that perioperative metoprolol does not appear to be effective in reducing postoperative death rates among unselected patients.

Osteoporosis:
- WHO Fracture Risk Algorithm (FRAX) developed to calculate the 1-year probability of fracture to guide treatment decisions.
- Screening recommendations for men.
- Recommendation to measure and supplement serum 25-OH vitamin D levels.

Diabetes type 2 prevention: New recommendation to consider metformin for those at very high risk of developing diabetes.

CBE, clinical breast exam; CA, cancer; MRI, magnetic resonance imaging; PSA, prostate-specific antigen; HIV, human immunodeficiency syndrome.

95TH PERCENTILE OF BLOOD PRESSURE FOR BOYS

Age (years)	Systolic blood pressure (mm Hg) by percentile of height							Diastolic blood pressure (mm Hg) by percentile of height						
	5%	10%	25%	50%	75%	90%	95%	5%	10%	25%	50%	75%	90%	95%
3	104	105	107	109	110	112	113	63	63	64	65	66	67	67
4	106	107	109	111	112	114	115	66	67	68	69	70	71	71
5	108	109	110	112	114	115	116	69	70	71	72	73	74	74
6	109	110	112	114	115	117	117	72	72	73	74	75	76	76
7	110	111	113	115	117	118	119	74	74	75	76	77	78	78
8	111	112	114	116	118	119	120	75	76	77	78	79	79	80
9	113	114	116	118	119	121	121	76	77	78	79	80	81	81
10	115	116	117	119	121	122	123	77	78	79	80	81	81	82
11	117	118	119	121	123	124	125	78	78	79	80	81	82	82
12	119	120	122	123	125	127	127	78	79	80	81	82	82	83
13	121	122	124	126	128	129	130	79	79	80	81	82	83	83
14	124	125	127	128	130	132	132	80	80	81	82	83	84	84
15	126	127	129	131	133	134	135	81	81	82	83	84	85	85
16	129	130	132	134	135	137	137	82	83	83	84	85	86	87
17	131	132	134	136	138	139	140	84	85	86	87	87	88	89

95TH PERCENTILE OF BLOOD PRESSURE FOR GIRLS

Age (years)	Systolic blood pressure (mm Hg) by percentile of height							Diastolic blood pressure (mm Hg) by percentile of height						
	5%	10%	25%	50%	75%	90%	95%	5%	10%	25%	50%	75%	90%	95%
3	104	104	105	107	108	109	110	65	66	66	67	68	68	69
4	105	106	107	108	110	111	112	68	68	69	70	71	71	72
5	107	107	108	110	111	112	113	70	71	71	72	73	73	74
6	108	109	110	111	113	114	115	72	72	73	74	74	75	76
7	110	111	112	113	115	116	116	73	74	74	75	76	76	77
8	112	112	114	115	116	118	118	75	75	75	76	77	78	78
9	114	114	115	117	118	119	120	76	76	76	77	78	79	79
10	116	116	117	119	120	121	122	77	77	77	78	79	80	80
11	118	118	119	121	122	123	124	78	78	78	79	80	81	81
12	119	120	121	123	124	125	126	79	79	79	80	81	82	82
13	121	122	123	124	126	127	128	80	80	80	81	82	83	83
14	123	123	125	126	127	129	129	81	81	81	82	83	84	84
15	124	125	126	127	129	130	131	82	82	82	83	84	85	85
16	125	126	127	128	130	131	132	82	82	83	84	85	85	86
17	125	126	127	129	130	131	132	82	83	83	84	85	85	86

Source: http://www.nhlbi.nih.gov/guidelines/hypertension/child_tbl.htm, accessed 6/3/08.

BODY MASS INDEX (BMI) CONVERSION TABLE

Height in inches (cm)	BMI 25 kg/m²	BMI 27 kg/m²	BMI 30 kg/m²
	Body weight in pounds (kg)		
58 (147.32)	119 (53.98)	129 (58.51)	143 (64.86)
59 (149.86)	124 (56.25)	133 (60.33)	148 (67.13)
60 (152.40)	128 (58.06)	138 (62.60)	153 (69.40)
61 (154.94)	132 (59.87)	143 (64.86)	158 (71.67)
62 (157.48)	136 (61.69)	147 (66.68)	164 (74.39)
63 (160.02)	141 (63.96)	152 (68.95)	169 (76.66)
64 (162.56)	145 (65.77)	157 (71.22)	174 (78.93)
65 (165.10)	150 (68.04)	162 (73.48)	180 (81.65)
66 (167.64)	155 (70.31)	167 (75.75)	186 (84.37)
67 (170.18)	159 (72.12)	172 (78.02)	191 (86.64)
68 (172.72)	164 (74.39)	177 (80.29)	197 (89.36)
69 (175.26)	169 (76.66)	182 (82.56)	203 (92.08)
70 (177.80)	174 (78.93)	188 (85.28)	207 (93.90)
71 (180.34)	179 (81.19)	193 (87.54)	215 (97.52)
72 (182.88)	184 (83.46)	199 (90.27)	221 (100.25)
73 (185.42)	189 (85.73)	204 (92.53)	227 (102.97)
74 (187.96)	194 (88.00)	210 (95.26)	233 (105.69)
75 (190.50)	200 (90.72)	216 (97.98)	240 (108.86)
76 (193.04)	205 (92.99)	221 (100.25)	246 (111.59)

Metric conversion formula = weight (kg)/ height (m²)

Example of BMI calculation:
A person who weighs 78.93 kg and is 177 cm tall has a BMI of 25:
weight (78.93 kg)/height (1.77 m²) = 25

Nonmetric conversion formula = [weight (pounds)/height (inches²)] × 704.5

Example of BMI calculation:
A person who weighs 164 lb and is 68 in (or 5′ 8″) tall has a BMI of 25:
[weight (164 lb)/height (68 in²)] × 704.5 = 25

BMI categories:
Underweight = < 18.5
Normal weight = 18.5–24.9
Overweight = 25–29.9
Obesity = ≥ 30

Source: Adapted from NHLBI Obesity Guidelines in Adults: http://www.nhlbi.nih.gov/guidelines/obesity/bmi_tbl.htm, accessed 10/13/11.
BMI online calculator: http://www.nhlbisupport.com/bmi/bmicalc.htm, accessed 10/13/11.

ESTIMATE OF 10-YEAR CARDIAC RISK FOR MEN[a]

Age (years)	Points
20–34	–9
35–39	–4
40–44	0
45–49	3
50–54	6
55–59	8
60–64	10
65–69	11
70–74	12
75–79	13

Total Cholesterol	Points				
	Age 20–39	Age 40–49	Age 50–59	Age 60–69	Age 70–79
< 160	0	0	0	0	0
160–199	4	3	2	1	0
200–239	7	5	3	1	0
240–279	9	6	4	2	1
> 280	11	8	5	3	1

	Points				
	Age 20–39	Age 40–49	Age 50–59	Age 60–69	Age 70–79
Nonsmoker	0	0	0	0	0
Smoker	8	5	3	1	1

High-Density Lipoprotein (mg/dL)	Points
≥ 60	–1
50–59	0
40–49	1
< 40	2

Systolic Blood Pressure (mm Hg)	If Untreated	If Treated
< 120	0	0
120–129	0	1
130–139	1	2
140–159	1	2
≥ 160	2	3

ESTIMATE OF 10-YEAR CARDIAC RISK FOR MEN[a] (CONTINUED)

Point Total	10-Year Risk %	Point Total	10-Year Risk %		
< 0	< 1	9	5		
0	1	10	6		
1	1	11	8		
2	1	12	10		
3	1	13	12		
4	1	14	16		
5	2	15	20		
6	2	16	25		
7	3	≥ 17	≥ 30	**10-Year Risk _____ %**	
8	4				

[a]Framingham point scores.

Source: U.S. Department of Health and Human Services, Public Health Service, National Institutes of Health, National Heart, Lung, and Blood Institute. NIH Publication No. 01-3305, May 2001.
Online risk calculator: http://hp2010.nhlbihin.net/atpiii/calculator.asp

ESTIMATE OF 10-YEAR CARDIAC RISK FOR WOMEN[a]				
Age (years)	**Points**			
20–34	−7			
35–39	−3			
40–44	0			
45–49	3			
50–54	6			
55–59	8			
60–64	10			
65–69	12			
70–74	14			
75–79	16			

Total Cholesterol	**Points**				
	Age 20–39	**Age 40–49**	**Age 50–59**	**Age 60–69**	**Age 70–79**
< 160	0	0	0	0	0
160–199	4	3	2	1	1
200–239	8	6	4	2	1
240–279	11	8	5	3	2
≥ 280	13	10	7	4	2

	Points				
	Age 20–39	**Age 40–49**	**Age 50–59**	**Age 60–69**	**Age 70–79**
Nonsmoker	0	0	0	0	0
Smoker	9	7	4	2	1

High-Density Lipoprotein (mg/dL)	**Points**
≥ 60	−1
50–59	0
40–49	1
< 40	2

Systolic Blood Pressure (mm Hg)	**If Untreated**	**If Treated**
< 120	0	0
120–129	1	3
130–139	2	4
140–159	3	5
≥ 160	4	6

ESTIMATE OF 10-YEAR CARDIAC RISK FOR WOMEN[a] (CONTINUED)

Point Total	10-Year Risk %	Point Total	10-Year Risk %	
< 9	< 1	17	5	
9	1	18	6	
10	1	19	8	
11	1	20	11	
12	1	21	14	
13	2	22	17	
14	2	23	22	
15	3	24	27	**10-Year Risk _____ %**
16	4	≥ 25	≥ 30	

[a]Framingham point scores.

Source: U.S. Department of Health and Human Services, Public Health Service, National Institutes of Health, National Heart, Lung, and Blood Institute. NIH Publication No. 01-3305, May 2001.
Online risk calculator: http://hp2010.nhlbihin.net/atpiii/calculator.asp

ESTIMATE OF 10-YEAR STROKE RISK FOR MEN			
Age (years)	Points	Untreated Systolic Blood Pressure (mm Hg)	Points
54–56	0	97–105	0
57–59	1	106–115	1
60–62	2	116–125	2
63–65	3	126–135	3
66–68	4	136–145	4
69–72	5	146–155	5
73–75	6	156–165	6
76–78	7	166–175	7
79–81	8	176–185	8
82–84	9	186–195	9
85	10	196–205	10

Treated Systolic Blood Pressure (mm Hg)	Points	History of Diabetes	Points
97–105	0	No	0
106–112	1	Yes	2
113–117	2		
118–123	3		
124–129	4		
130–135	5		
136–142	6		
143–150	7		
151–161	8		
162–176	9		
177–205	10		

Cigarette Smoking	Points	Cardiovascular Disease	Points
No	0	No	0
Yes	3	Yes	4

Atrial Fibrillation	Points	Left Ventricular Hypertrophy on Electrocardiogram	Points
No	0	No	0
Yes	4	Yes	5

ESTIMATE OF 10-YEAR STROKE RISK FOR MEN (CONTINUED)

Point Total	10-Year Risk %	Point Total	10-Year Risk %	
1	3	16	22	
2	3	17	26	
3	4	18	29	
4	4	19	33	
5	5	20	37	
6	5	21	42	
7	6	22	47	
8	7	23	52	
9	8	24	57	
10	10	25	63	
11	11	26	68	
12	13	27	74	
13	15	28	79	
14	17	29	84	10-Year Risk _____ %
15	20	30	88	

Source: Modified Framingham Stroke Risk Profile. *Circulation.* 2006;113:e873–923.

ESTIMATE OF 10-YEAR STROKE RISK FOR WOMEN

Age (years)	Points	Untreated Systolic Blood Pressure (mm Hg)	Points
54–56	0	95–106	1
57–59	1	107–118	2
60–62	2	119–130	3
63–64	3	131–143	4
65–67	4	144–155	5
68–70	5	156–167	6
71–73	6	168–180	7
74–76	7	181–192	8
77–78	8	193–204	9
79–81	9	205–216	10
82–84	10		

ESTIMATE OF 10-YEAR STROKE RISK FOR WOMEN (CONTINUED)

Treated Systolic Blood Pressure (mm Hg)	Points	History of Diabetes	Points
95–106	1	No	0
107–113	2	Yes	3
114–119	3		
120–125	4		
126–131	5		
132–139	6		
140–148	7		
149–160	8		
161–204	9		
205–216	10		

Cigarette Smoking	Points	Cardiovascular Disease	Points
No	0	No	0
Yes	3	Yes	2

Atrial Fibrillation	Points	Left Ventricular Hypertrophy on Electrocardiogram	Points
No	0	No	0
Yes	6	Yes	4

Point Total	10-Year Risk %	Point Total	10-Year Risk %	
1	1	16	19	
2	1	17	23	
3	2	18	27	
4	2	19	32	
5	2	20	37	
6	3	21	43	
7	4	22	50	
8	4	23	57	
9	5	24	64	
10	6	25	71	
11	8	26	78	
12	9	27	84	
13	11	28		
14	13	29		10-Year Risk _____ %
15	16	30		

Source: Modified Framingham Stroke Risk Profile. *Circulation.* 2006;113:e873–923.

Recommended immunization schedule for persons aged 0 through 6 years—United States, 2012 (for those who fall behind or start late, see the catch-up schedule [Figure 3])

Vaccine ▼ / Age ▶	Birth	1 month	2 months	4 months	6 months	9 months	12 months	15 months	18 months	19–23 months	2–3 years	4–6 years
Hepatitis B[1]	Hep B	Hep B			HepB							
Rotavirus[2]			RV	RV	RV[a]							
Diphtheria, tetanus, pertussis[3]			DTaP	DTaP	DTaP		see footnote[a]	DTaP				DTaP
Haemophilus influenzae type b[4]			Hib	Hib	Hib[a]		Hib					
Pneumococcal[5]			PCV	PCV	PCV		PCV				PPSV	
Inactivated poliovirus[6]			IPV	IPV		IPV						IPV
Influenza[7]							Influenza (Yearly)					
Measles, mumps, rubella[8]							MMR		see footnote[a]			MMR
Varicella[9]							Varicella		see footnote[a]			Varicella
Hepatitis A[10]							Dose 1[10]				HepA Series	
Meningococcal[11]									MCV4 — see footnote[11]			

Range of recommended ages for all children

Range of recommended ages for certain high-risk groups

Range of recommended ages for all children and certain high-risk groups

This schedule includes recommendations in effect as of December 23, 2011. Any dose not administered at the recommended age should be administered at a subsequent visit, when indicated and feasible. The use of a combination vaccine generally is preferred over separate injections of its equivalent component vaccines. Vaccination providers should consult the relevant Advisory Committee on Immunization Practices (ACIP) statement for detailed recommendations, available online at http://www.cdc.gov/vaccines/pubs/acip-list.htm. Clinically significant adverse events that follow vaccination should be reported to the Vaccine Adverse Event Reporting System (VAERS) online (http://www.vaers.hhs.gov) or by telephone (800-822-7967).

1. Hepatitis B (HepB) vaccine. (Minimum age: birth)

At birth:

- Administer monovalent HepB vaccine to all newborns before hospital discharge.
- For infants born to hepatitis B surface antigen (HBsAg)-positive mothers, administer HepB vaccine and 0.5 mL of hepatitis B immune globulin (HBIG) within 12 hours of birth. These infants should be tested for HBsAg and antibody to HBsAg (anti-HBs) 1 to 2 months after completion of at least 3 doses of the HepB series, at age 9 through 18 months (generally at the next well-child visit).
- If mother's HBsAg status is unknown, within 12 hours of birth administer HepB vaccine for infants weighing ≥2,000 grams, and HepB vaccine plus HBIG for infants weighing <2,000 grams. Determine mother's HBsAg status as soon as possible and, if she is HBsAg-positive, administer HBIG for infants weighing ≥2,000 grams (no later than age 1 week).

Doses after the birth dose:

- The second dose should be administered at age 1 to 2 months. Monovalent HepB vaccine should be used for doses administered before age 6 weeks.

7. Influenza vaccines. (Minimum age: 6 months for trivalent inactivated influenza vaccine [TIV]; 2 years for live, attenuated influenza vaccine [LAIV])

- For most healthy children aged 2 years and older, either LAIV or TIV may be used. However, LAIV should not be administered to some children, including 1) children with asthma, 2) children 2 through 4 years who had wheezing in the past 12 months, or 3) children who have any other underlying medical conditions that predispose them to influenza complications. For all other contraindications to use of LAIV, see MMWR 2010;59(No. RR-8), available at http://www.cdc.gov/mmwr/pdf/rr/rr5908.pdf.
- For children aged 6 months through 8 years:
  — For the 2011–12 season, administer 2 doses (separated by at least 4 weeks) to those who did not receive at least 1 dose of the 2010–11 vaccine. Those who received at least 1 dose of the 2010–11 vaccine require 1 dose for the 2011–12 season.
  — For the 2012–13 season, follow dosing guidelines in the 2012 ACIP influenza vaccine recommendations.

- Administration of a total of 4 doses of HepB vaccine is permissible when a combination vaccine containing HepB is administered after the birth dose.
- Infants who did not receive a birth dose should receive 3 doses of a HepB-containing vaccine starting as soon as feasible (Figure 3).
- The minimum interval between dose 1 and dose 2 is 4 weeks, and between dose 2 and 3 is 8 weeks. The final (third or fourth) dose in the HepB vaccine series should be administered no earlier than age 24 weeks and at least 16 weeks after the first dose.

2. **Rotavirus (RV) vaccines.** (Minimum age: 6 weeks for both RV-1 [Rotarix] and RV-5 [RotaTeq])
- The maximum age for the first dose in the series is 14 weeks, 6 days; and 8 months, 0 days for the final dose in the series. Vaccination should not be initiated for infants aged 15 weeks, 0 days or older.
- If RV-1 (Rotarix) is administered at ages 2 and 4 months, a dose at 6 months is not indicated.

3. **Diphtheria and tetanus toxoids and acellular pertussis (DTaP) vaccine.** (Minimum age: 6 weeks)
- The fourth dose may be administered as early as age 12 months, provided at least 6 months have elapsed since the third dose.

4. **Haemophilus influenzae type b (Hib) conjugate vaccine.** (Minimum age: 6 weeks)
- If PRP-OMP (PedvaxHIB or Comvax [Hep B-Hib]) is administered at ages 2 and 4 months, a dose at age 6 months is not indicated.
- Hiberix should only be used for the booster (final) dose in children aged 12 months through 4 years.

5. **Pneumococcal vaccines.** (Minimum age: 6 weeks for pneumococcal conjugate vaccine [PCV]; 2 years for pneumococcal polysaccharide vaccine [PPSV])
- Administer 1 dose of PCV to all healthy children aged 24 through 59 months who are not completely vaccinated for their age.
- For children who have received an age-appropriate series of 7-valent PCV (PCV7), a single supplemental dose of 13-valent PCV (PCV13) is recommended for:
    — All children aged 14 through 59 months
    — Children aged 60 through 71 months with underlying medical conditions.
- Administer PPSV at least 8 weeks after last dose of PCV to children aged 2 years or older with certain underlying medical conditions, including a cochlear implant. See MMWR 2010:59(No. RR-11), available at http://www.cdc.gov/mmwr/pdf/rr/rr5911.pdf.

6. **Inactivated poliovirus vaccine (IPV).** (Minimum age: 6 weeks)
- If 4 or more doses are administered before age 4 years, an additional dose should be administered at age 4 through 6 years.
- The final dose in the series should be administered on or after the fourth birthday and at least 6 months after the previous dose.

8. **Measles, mumps, and rubella (MMR) vaccine.** (Minimum age: 12 months)
- The second dose may be administered before age 4 years, provided at least 4 weeks have elapsed since the first dose.
- Administer MMR vaccine to infants aged 6 through 11 months who are traveling internationally. These children should be revaccinated with 2 doses of MMR vaccine, the first at ages 12 through 15 months and at least 4 weeks after the previous dose, and the second at ages 4 through 6 years.

9. **Varicella (VAR) vaccine.** (Minimum age: 12 months)
- The second dose may be administered before age 4 years, provided at least 3 months have elapsed since the first dose.
- For children aged 12 months through 12 years, the recommended minimum interval between doses is 3 months. However, if the second dose was administered at least 4 weeks after the first dose, it can be accepted as valid.

10. **Hepatitis A (HepA) vaccine.** (Minimum age: 12 months)
- Administer the second (final) dose 6 to18 months after the first.
- Unvaccinated children 24 months and older at high risk should be vaccinated. See MMWR 2006;55(No. RR-7), available at http://www.cdc.gov/mmwr/pdf/rr/rr5507.pdf.
- A 2-dose HepA vaccine series is recommended for anyone aged 24 months and older, previously unvaccinated, for whom immunity against hepatitis A virus infection is desired.

11. **Meningococcal conjugate vaccines, quadrivalent (MCV4).** (Minimum age: 9 months for Menactra [MCV4-D], 2 years for Menveo [MCV4-CRM])
- For children aged 9 through 23 months 1) who persistent complement component deficiency; 2) who are residents of or travelers to countries with hyperendemic or epidemic disease; or 3) who are present during outbreaks caused by a vaccine serogroup, administer 2 primary doses of MCV4-D, ideally at ages: 9 months and 12 months or at least 8 weeks apart.
- For children aged 24 months and older with 1) persistent complement component deficiency (who have not been previously vaccinated); or 2) anatomic/functional asplenia, administer 2 primary doses of either MCV4 at least 8 weeks apart.
- For children with anatomic/functional asplenia, if MCV4-D (Menactra) is used, administer at a minimum age of 2 years and at least 4 weeks after completion of all PCV doses.
- See MMWR 2011;60:72–3, available at http://www.cdc.gov/mmwr/pdf/wk/mm6003.pdf and Vaccines for Children Program resolution No. 6/11-1, available at http://www.cdc.gov/vaccines/programs/vfc/downloads/resolutions/03-11mening-mcv.pdf, and MMWR 2011;60:1391–2, available at http://www.cdc.gov/mmwr/pdf/wk/mm6040.pdf, for further guidance including revaccination guidelines.

This schedule is approved by the Advisory Committee on Immunization Practices (http://www.cdc.gov/vaccines/recs/acip),
the American Academy of Pediatrics (http://www.aap.org), and the American Academy of Family Physicians (http://www.aafp.org).
Department of Health and Human Services • Centers for Disease Control and Prevention

Recommended immunization schedule for persons aged 7 through 18 years—United States, 2012 (for those who fall behind or start late, see the schedule below and the catch-up schedule [Figure 3])

Vaccine ▼ Age ▶	7–10 years	11–12 years	13–18 years
Tetanus, diphtheria, pertussis[1]	1 dose (if indicated)	1 dose	1 dose (if indicated)
Human papillomavirus[2]	see footnote[2]	3 doses	Complete 3-dose series
Meningococcal[3]	See footnote[3]	Dose 1	Booster at 16 years old
Influenza[4]	Influenza (yearly)		
Pneumococcal[5]	See footnote[5]		
Hepatitis A[6]	Complete 2-dose series		
Hepatitis B[7]	Complete 3-dose series		
Inactivated poliovirus[8]	Complete 3-dose series		
Measles, mumps, rubella[9]	Complete 2-dose series		
Varicella[10]	Complete 2-dose series		

Legend:
- Range of recommended ages for all children
- Range of recommended ages for catch-up immunization
- Range of recommended ages for certain high-risk groups

This schedule includes recommendations in effect as of December 23, 2011. Any dose not administered at the recommended age should be administered at a subsequent visit, when indicated and feasible. The use of a combination vaccine generally is preferred over separate injections of its equivalent component vaccines. Vaccination providers should consult the relevant Advisory Committee on Immunization Practices (ACIP) statement for detailed recommendations, available online at http://www.cdc.gov/vaccines/pubs/acip-list.htm. Clinically significant adverse events that follow vaccination should be reported to the Vaccine Adverse Event Reporting System (VAERS) online (http://www.vaers.hhs.gov) or by telephone (800-822-7967).

1. **Tetanus and diphtheria toxoids and acellular pertussis (Tdap) vaccine.**
   (Minimum age: 10 years for Boostrix and 11 years for Adacel)
   - Persons aged 11 through 18 years who have not received Tdap vaccine should receive a dose followed by tetanus and diphtheria toxoids (Td) booster doses every 10 years thereafter.
   - Tdap vaccine should be substituted for a single dose of Td in the catch-up series for children aged 7 through 10 years. Refer to the catch-up schedule if additional doses of tetanus and diphtheria toxoid-containing vaccine are needed.
   - Tdap vaccine can be administered regardless of the interval since the last tetanus and diphtheria toxoid-containing vaccine.

2. **Human papillomavirus (HPV) vaccines (HPV4 [Gardasil] and HPV2 [Cervarix]).** (Minimum age: 9 years)
   - Either HPV4 or HPV2 is recommended in a 3-dose series for females aged 11 or 12 years. HPV4 is recommended in a 3-dose series for males aged 11 or 12 years.

- For children aged 6 months through 8 years:
  — For the 2011–12 season, administer 2 doses (separated by at least 4 weeks) to those who did not receive at least 1 dose of the 2010–11 influenza vaccine. Those who received at least 1 dose of the 2010–11 vaccine require 1 dose for the 2011–12 season.
  — For the 2012–13 season, follow dosing guidelines in the 2012 ACIP influenza vaccine statement.

5. **Pneumococcal vaccines (pneumococcal conjugate vaccine [PCV] and pneumococcal polysaccharide vaccine [PPSV]).**
   - A single dose of PCV may be administered to children aged 6 through 18 years who have anatomic/functional asplenia, HIV infection or other immunocompromising condition, cochlear implant, or cerebral spinal fluid leak. See *MMWR* 2010:59(No. RR-11), available at http://www.cdc.gov/mmwr/pdf/rr/rr5911.pdf.
   - Administer PPSV at least 8 weeks after the last dose of PCV to children aged 2 years or older with certain underlying medical conditions,

- The vaccine series can be started beginning at age 9 years.
- Administer the second dose 1 to 2 months after the first dose and the third dose 6 months after the first dose (at least 24 weeks after the first dose).
- See *MMWR* 2010;59:626–32, available at http://www.cdc.gov/mmwr/pdf/wk/mm5920.pdf.

3. **Meningococcal conjugate vaccines, quadrivalent (MCV4).**
- Administer MCV4 at age 11 through 12 years with a booster dose at age 16 years.
- Administer MCV4 at age 13 through 18 years if patient is not previously vaccinated.
- If the first dose is administered at age 13 through 15 years, a booster dose should be administered at age 16 through 18 years with a minimum interval of at least 8 weeks after the preceding dose.
- If the first dose is administered at age 16 years or older, a booster dose is not needed.
- Administer 2 primary doses at least 8 weeks apart to previously unvaccinated persons with persistent complement component deficiency or anatomic/functional asplenia, and 1 dose every 5 years thereafter.
- Adolescents aged 11 through 18 years with human immunodeficiency virus (HIV) infection should receive a 2-dose primary series of MCV4, at least 8 weeks apart.
- See *MMWR* 2011;60:72–76, available at http://www.cdc.gov/mmwr/pdf/wk/mm6003.pdf, and Vaccines for Children Program resolution No. 6/11-1, available at http://www.cdc.gov/vaccines/programs/vfc/downloads/resolutions/06-11mening-mcv.pdf, for further guidelines.

4. **Influenza vaccines (trivalent inactivated influenza vaccine [TIV] and live, attenuated influenza vaccine [LAIV]).**
- For most healthy, nonpregnant persons, either LAIV or TIV may be used, except LAIV should not be used for some persons, including those with asthma or any other underlying medical conditions that predispose them to influenza complications. For all other contraindications to use of LAIV, see *MMWR* 2010;59(No.RR-8), available at http://www.cdc.gov/mmwr/pdf/rr/rr5908.pdf.
- Administer 1 dose to persons aged 9 years and older.

including a cochlear implant. A single revaccination should be administered after 5 years to children with anatomic/functional asplenia or an immunocompromising condition.

6. **Hepatitis A (HepA) vaccine.**
- HepA vaccine is recommended for children older than 23 months who live in areas where vaccination programs target older children, who are at increased risk for infection, or for whom immunity against hepatitis A virus infection is desired. See *MMWR* 2006;55(No. RR-7), available at http://www.cdc.gov/mmwr/pdf/rr/rr5507.pdf.
- Administer 2 doses at least 6 months apart to unvaccinated persons.

7. **Hepatitis B (HepB) vaccine.**
- Administer the 3-dose series to those not previously vaccinated.
- For those with incomplete vaccination, follow the catch-up recommendations (Figure 3).
- A 2-dose series (doses separated by at least 4 months) of adult formulation Recombivax HB is licensed for use in children aged 11 through 15 years.

8. **Inactivated poliovirus vaccine (IPV).**
- The final dose in the series should be administered at least 6 months after the previous dose.
- If both OPV and IPV were administered as part of a series, a total of 4 doses should be administered, regardless of the child's current age.
- IPV is not routinely recommended for U.S. residents aged 18 years or older.

9. **Measles, mumps, and rubella (MMR) vaccine.**
- The minimum interval between the 2 doses of MMR vaccine is 4 weeks.

10. **Varicella (VAR) vaccine.**
- For persons without evidence of immunity see *MMWR* 2007;56[No. RR-4], available at http://www.cdc.gov/mmwr/pdf/rr/rr5604.pdf), administer 2 doses if not previously vaccinated or the second dose if only 1 dose has been administered.
- For persons aged 7 through 12 years, the recommended minimum interval between doses is 3 months. However, if the second dose was administered at least 4 weeks after the first dose, it can be accepted as valid.
- For persons aged 13 years and older, the minimum interval between doses is 4 weeks.

This schedule is approved by the Advisory Committee on Immunization Practices (http://www.cdc.gov/vaccines/recs/acip), the American Academy of Pediatrics (http://www.aap.org), and the American Academy of Family Physicians (http://www.aap.org). Department of Health and Human Services • Centers for Disease Control and Prevention

Catch-up immunization schedule for persons aged 4 months through 18 years who start late or who are more than 1 month behind —United States • 2012

The figure below provides catch-up schedules and minimum intervals between doses for children whose vaccinations have been delayed. A vaccine series does not need to be restarted, regardless of the time that has elapsed between doses. Use the section appropriate for the child's age. Always use this table in conjunction with the accompanying childhood and adolescent immunization schedules (Figures 1 and 2) and their respective footnotes.

Vaccine	Minimum Age for Dose 1	Minimum Interval Between Doses			
		Dose 1 to dose 2	Dose 2 to dose 3	Dose 3 to dose 4	Dose 4 to dose 5
Persons aged 4 months through 6 years					
Hepatitis B	Birth	4 weeks	8 weeks and at least 16 weeks after first dose; minimum age for the final dose is 24 weeks		
Rotavirus¹	6 weeks	4 weeks	4 weeks¹		
Diphtheria, tetanus, pertussis²	6 weeks	4 weeks	4 weeks	6 months	6 months²
Haemophilus influenzae type b³	6 weeks	4 weeks if first dose administered at younger than age 12 months / 8 weeks (as final dose) if first dose administered at age 12–14 months / No further doses needed if first dose administered at age 15 months or older	4 weeks³ if current age is younger than 12 months / 8 weeks (as final dose)³ if current age is 12 months or older and first dose administered at younger than age 15 months / No further doses needed if previous dose administered at age 15 months or older	8 weeks (as final dose) This dose only necessary for children aged 12 months through 59 months who received 3 doses before age 12 months	
Pneumococcal⁴	6 weeks	4 weeks if first dose administered at younger than age 12 months / 8 weeks (as final dose) if first dose administered at age 12 months or older or current age 24 through 59 months / No further doses needed for healthy children if first dose administered at age 24 months or older	4 weeks if current age is younger than 12 months / 8 weeks (as final dose for healthy children) if current age is 12 months or older / No further doses needed for healthy children if previous dose administered at age 24 months or older	8 weeks (as final dose) This dose only necessary for children aged 12 months through 59 months who received 3 doses before age 12 months or for children at high risk who received 3 doses at any age	
Inactivated poliovirus⁵	6 weeks	4 weeks	4 weeks⁵	6 months⁵ minimum age 4 years for final dose	
Meningococcal⁶	9 months	8 weeks⁶			
Measles, mumps, rubella⁷	12 months	4 weeks			
Varicella⁸	12 months	3 months			
Hepatitis A	12 months	6 months			
Persons aged 7 through 18 years					
Tetanus, diphtheria; tetanus, diphtheria, pertussis⁹	7 years⁹	4 weeks	4 weeks if first dose administered at younger than age 12 months / 6 months if first dose administered at 12 months or older	6 months if first dose administered at younger than age 12 months	
Human papillomavirus¹⁰	9 years	Routine dosing intervals are recommended¹⁰			
Hepatitis A	12 months	6 months			
Hepatitis B	Birth	4 weeks	8 weeks (and at least 16 weeks after first dose)		
Inactivated poliovirus⁵	6 weeks	4 weeks	4 weeks⁵	6 months⁵	
Meningococcal⁶	9 months	8 weeks⁶			
Measles, mumps, rubella⁷	12 months	4 weeks			
Varicella⁸	12 months	3 months if person is younger than age 13 years / 4 weeks if person is aged 13 years or older			

1. **Rotavirus (RV) vaccines (RV-1 [Rotarix] and RV-5 [Rota Teq]).**
   - The maximum age for the first dose in the series is 14 weeks, 6 days; and 8 months, 0 days for the final dose in the series. Vaccination should not be initiated for infants aged 15 weeks, 0 days or older
   - If RV-1 was administered for the first and second doses, a third dose is not indicated.

2. **Diphtheria and tetanus toxoids and acellular pertussis (DTaP) vaccine.**
   - The fifth dose is not necessary if the fourth dose was administered at age 4 years or older.

3. **Haemophilus influenzae type b (Hib) conjugate vaccine.**
   - Hib vaccine should be considered for unvaccinated persons aged 5 years or older who have sickle cell disease, leukemia, human immunodeficiency virus (HIV) infection, or anatomic/functional asplenia.
   - If the first 2 doses were PRP-OMP (PedvaxHIB or Comvax) and were administered at age 11 months or younger; the third (and final) dose should be administered at age 12 through 15 months and at least 8 weeks after the second dose.
   - If the first dose was administered at age 7 through 11 months, administer the second dose at least 4 weeks later and a final dose at age 12 through 15 months.

4. **Pneumococcal vaccines.** (Minimum age: 6 weeks for pneumococcal conjugate vaccine [PCV]; 2 years for pneumococcal polysaccharide vaccine [PPSV])
   - For children aged 24 through 71 months with underlying medical conditions, administer 1 dose of PCV if 3 doses of PCV were received previously, or administer 2 doses of PCV at least 8 weeks apart if fewer than 3 doses of PCV were received previously.
   - A single dose of PCV may be administered to certain children aged 6 through 18 years with underlying medical conditions. See age-specific schedules for details.
   - Administer PPSV to children aged 2 years or older with certain underlying medical conditions. See *MMWR* 2010;59(No. RR-11), available at http://www.cdc.gov/mmwr/pdf/rr/rr5911.pdf.

5. **Inactivated poliovirus vaccine (IPV).**
   - A fourth dose is not necessary if the third dose was administered at age 4 years or older and at least 6 months after the previous dose.
   - In the first 6 months of life, minimum age and minimum intervals are only recommended if the person is at risk for imminent exposure to circulating poliovirus (i.e., travel to a polio-endemic region or during an outbreak).
   - IPV is not routinely recommended for U.S. residents aged 18 years or older.

6. **Meningococcal conjugate vaccines, quadrivalent (MCV4).** (Minimum age: 9 months for Menactra [MCV4-D]; 2 years for Menveo [MCV4-CRM])
   - See Figure 1 ("Recommended immunization schedule for persons aged 0 through 6 years") and Figure 2 ("Recommended immunization schedule for persons aged 7 through 18 years") for further guidance.

7. **Measles, mumps, and rubella (MMR) vaccine.**
   - Administer the second dose routinely at age 4 through 6 years.

8. **Varicella (VAR) vaccine.**
   - Administer the second dose routinely at age 4 through 6 years. If the second dose was administered at least 4 weeks after the first dose, it can be accepted as valid.

9. **Tetanus and diphtheria toxoids (Td) and tetanus and diphtheria toxoids and acellular pertussis (Tdap) vaccines.**
   - For children aged 7 through 10 years who are not fully immunized with the childhood DTaP vaccine series, Tdap vaccine should be substituted for a single dose of Td vaccine in the catch-up series; if additional doses are needed, use Td vaccine. For these children, an adolescent Tdap vaccine dose should not be given.
   - An inadvertent dose of DTaP vaccine administered to children aged 7 through 10 years can count as part of the catch-up series. This dose can count as the adolescent Tdap dose, or the child can later receive a Tdap booster dose at age 11–12 years.

10. **Human papillomavirus (HPV) vaccines (HPV4 [Gardasil] and HPV2 [Cervarix]).**
    - Administer the vaccine series to females (either HPV2 or HPV4) and males (HPV4) at age 13 through 18 years if patient is not previously vaccinated.
    - Use recommended routine dosing intervals for vaccine series catch-up; see Figure 2 ("Recommended immunization schedule for persons aged 7 through 18 years").

Recommended Adult Immunization Schedule—United States - 2012

Note: These recommendations must be read with the footnotes that follow containing number of doses, intervals between doses, and other important information.

Recommended adult immunization schedule, by vaccine and age group[1]

VACCINE ▼ AGE GROUP ►	19-21 years	22-26 years	27-49 years	50-59 years	60-64 years	≥ 65 years
Influenza [2]	1 dose annually					
Tetanus, diphtheria, pertussis (Td/Tdap) [3,*]	Substitute 1-time dose of Tdap for Td booster; then boost with Td every 10 yrs					Td/Tdap [3]
Varicella [4,*]	2 Doses					
Human papillomavirus (HPV) Female [5,*]	3 doses					
Human papillomavirus (HPV) Male [5,*]	3 doses					
Zoster [6]					1 dose	
Measles, mumps, rubella (MMR) [7,*]	1 or 2 doses					
Pneumococcal (polysaccharide) [8,9]			1 or 2 doses		1 dose	
Meningococcal [10,*]	1 or more doses					
Hepatitis A [11,*]	2 doses					
Hepatitis B [12,*]	3 doses					

*Covered by the Vaccine Injury Compensation Program

| | For all persons in this category who meet the age requirements and who lack documentation of vaccination or have no evidence of previous infection | | Recommended if some other risk factor is present (e.g., on the basis of medical, occupational, lifestyle, or other indications) | | Tdap recommended for ≥65 if contact with <12 month old child. Either Td or Tdap can be used if no infant contact | | No recommendation |

Report all clinically significant postvaccination reactions to the Vaccine Adverse Event Reporting System (VAERS). Reporting forms and instructions on filing a VAERS report are available at www.vaers.hhs.gov or by telephone, 800-822-7967.

Information on how to file a Vaccine Injury Compensation Program claim is available at www.hrsa.gov/vaccinecompensation or by telephone, 800-338-2382. To file a claim for vaccine injury, contact the U.S. Court of Federal Claims, 717 Madison Place, N.W., Washington, D.C. 20005; telephone, 202-357-6400.

Additional information about the vaccines in this schedule, extent of available data, and contraindications for vaccination is also available at www.cdc.gov/vaccines or from the CDC-INFO Contact Center at 800-CDC-INFO (800-232-4636) in English and Spanish, 8:00 a.m. - 8:00 p.m. Eastern Time, Monday - Friday, excluding holidays.

Use of trade names and commercial sources is for identification only and does not imply endorsement by the U.S. Department of Health and Human Services.

Vaccines that might be indicated for adults based on medical and other indications[1]

VACCINE ▼ INDICATION ▶	Pregnancy	Immunocompromising conditions (excluding human immunodeficiency virus [HIV])[3,4,6,7,14]	HIV infection[3,12,13,14] CD4+ T lymphocyte count < 200 cells/μL	HIV infection[3,12,13,14] CD4+ T lymphocyte count ≥ 200 cells/μL	Men who have sex with men (MSM)	Heart disease, chronic lung disease, chronic alcoholism	Asplenia[13] (including elective splenectomy and persistent complement component deficiencies)	Chronic liver disease	Diabetes, kidney failure, end-stage renal disease, except of hemodialysis	Health-care personnel
Influenza [2]	1 dose TIV annually	1 dose TIV annually	1 dose TIV or LAIV annually	1 dose TIV or LAIV annually	1 dose TIV annually	1 dose TIV annually	1 dose TIV annually	1 dose TIV annually	1 dose TIV or LAIV annually
Tetanus, diphtheria, pertussis (Td/Tdap) [3,*]	Substitute 1-time dose of Tdap for Td booster; then boost with Td every 10 yrs									
Varicella [4,*]	Contraindicated	Contraindicated		2 doses						
Human papillomavirus (HPV) Female [5,*]	3 doses through age 26 yrs	3 doses through age 26 yrs			3 doses through age 26 yrs					
Human papillomavirus (HPV) Male [5,*]	3 doses through age 26 yrs	3 doses through age 26 yrs			3 doses through age 21 yrs					
Zoster [6]	Contraindicated	Contraindicated			1 dose	1 dose	1 dose	1 dose	1 dose	
Measles, mumps, rubella (MMR) [7,*]	Contraindicated	Contraindicated			1 or 2 doses	1 or 2 doses	1 or 2 doses	1 or 2 doses	1 or 2 doses	
Pneumococcal (polysaccharide) [8,9]						1 or 2 doses	1 or 2 doses	1 or 2 doses	1 or 2 doses	
Meningococcal [10,*]			1 or more doses		1 or more doses		1 or more doses			
Hepatitis A [11,*]					2 doses	2 doses	2 doses	2 doses	2 doses	
Hepatitis B [12,*]					3 doses	3 doses	3 doses	3 doses	3 doses	

*Covered by the Vaccine Injury Compensation Program

For all persons in this category who meet the age requirements and who lack documentation of vaccination or have no evidence of previous infection

Recommended if some other risk factor is present (e.g., on the basis of medical, occupational, lifestyle, or other indications)

Contraindicated

No recommendation

The recommendations in this schedule were approved by the Centers for Disease Control and Prevention's (CDC) Advisory Committee on Immunization Practices (ACIP), the American Academy of Family Physicians (AFP), the American College of Physicians (ACP), American College of Obstetricians and Gynecologists (ACOG) and American College of Nurse-Midwives (ACNM).

These schedules indicate the recommended age groups and medical indications for which administration of currently licensed vaccines is commonly indicated for adults ages 19 years and older, as of January 1, 2011. For all vaccines being recommended on the Adult Immunization Schedule, a vaccine series does not need to be restarted, regardless of the time that has elapsed between doses. Licensed combination vaccines may be used whenever any component of the combination are indicated and when the vaccine's other components are not contraindicated. For detailed recommendations on all vaccines, including those used primarily for travelers or that are issued during the year, consult the manufacturers' package inserts and the complete statements from the Advisory Committee on Immunization Practices (www.cdc.gov/vaccines/pubs/acip-list.htm). Use of trade names and commercial sources is for identification only and does not imply endorsement by the U.S. Department of Health and Human Services.

U.S. Department of Health and Human Services
Centers for Disease Control and Prevention

Footnotes — Recommended Adult Immunization Schedule—United States - 2012

1. **Additional information**
   - Advisory Committee on Immunization Practices (ACIP) vaccine recommendations and additional information are available at http://www.cdc.gov/vaccines/pubs/acip-list.htm.
   - Information on travel vaccine requirements and recommendations (e.g., for hepatitis A and B, meningococcal, and other vaccines) available at http://www.cdc.gov/travel/page/vaccinations.htm.

2. **Influenza vaccination**
   - Annual vaccination against influenza is recommended for all persons 6 months of age and older.
   - Persons 6 months of age and older, including pregnant women, can receive the trivalent inactivated vaccine (TIV).
   - Healthy, nonpregnant persons aged 2 to 49 years without high-risk medical conditions can receive either intranasally administered live, attenuated influenza vaccine (LAIV) (FluMist), or TIV. Health-care personnel who care for severely immunocompromised persons (i.e., those who require care in a protected environment) should receive TIV rather than LAIV. Other persons should receive TIV.
   - The intramuscular or intradermal TIV are options for adults aged 18–64 years.
   - Adults aged 65 years and older can receive the standard dose TIV or the high-dose TIV (Fluzone High-Dose).

3. **Tetanus, diphtheria, and acellular pertussis (Td/Tdap) vaccination**
   - Administer a one-time dose of Tdap to adults younger than age 65 years who have not received Tdap previously or for whom vaccine status is unknown to replace one of the 10-year Td boosters.
   - Tdap is specifically recommended for the following persons:
     - pregnant women more than 20 weeks' gestation;
     - adults, regardless of age, who are close contacts of infants younger than age 12 months (e.g., parents, grandparents, or child care providers), and
     - health-care personnel.
   - Tdap can be administered regardless of interval since the most recent tetanus or diphtheria-toxoid containing vaccine.
   - Pregnant women not vaccinated during pregnancy should receive Tdap immediately postpartum.
   - Adults 65 years and older may receive Tdap.
   - Adults with an unknown or incomplete history of completing a 3-dose primary vaccination series with Td-containing vaccines should begin or complete a primary vaccination series. Tdap should be substituted for a single dose of Td in the vaccination series with Tdap preferred as the first dose.
   - For unvaccinated adults, administer the first 2 doses at least 4 weeks apart and the third dose 6–12 months after the second.
   - If incompletely vaccinated (i.e., less than 3 doses), administer remaining doses.
   - Refer to the ACIP statement for recommendations for administering Td/Tdap as prophylaxis in wound management (See footnote 1).

4. **Varicella vaccination**
   - All adults without evidence of immunity to varicella (as defined below) should receive 2 doses of single-antigen varicella vaccine or a second dose if they have received only 1 dose.
   - Special consideration for vaccination should be given to those who
     - have close contact with persons at high risk for severe disease (e.g., health-care personnel and family members of persons with immunocompromising conditions) or
     - are at high risk for exposure or transmission (e.g., teachers; child care employees; residents and staff members of institutional settings, including correctional institutions; college students; military recruits; adolescents and adults living in households with children; nonpregnant women of childbearing age; and international travelers).
   - Pregnant women should be assessed for evidence of varicella immunity. Women who do not have evidence of immunity should receive the first dose of varicella vaccine upon completion or termination of pregnancy and before discharge from the health-care facility. The second dose should be administered 4–8 weeks after the first dose.
   - Evidence of immunity to varicella in adults includes any of the following:
     - documentation of 2 doses of varicella vaccine at least 4 weeks apart;
     - U.S.-born before 1980 (although for health-care personnel and pregnant women, birth before 1980 should not be considered evidence of immunity);
     - history of varicella based on diagnosis or verification of varicella by a health-care provider (for a patient reporting a history of or having an atypical case, a mild case, or both, health-care providers should seek either an epidemiologic link to a typical varicella case or a

7. **Measles, mumps, rubella (MMR) vaccination (cont'd)**
   Rubella component:
   - For women of childbearing age, regardless of birth year, rubella immunity should be determined. If there is no evidence of immunity, women who are not pregnant should be vaccinated. Pregnant women who do not have evidence of immunity should receive MMR vaccine upon completion or termination of pregnancy and before discharge from the health-care facility.

   Health-care personnel born before 1957:
   - For unvaccinated health-care personnel born before 1957 who lack laboratory evidence of measles, mumps, and/or rubella immunity or laboratory confirmation of disease, health-care facilities should consider vaccinating personnel with 2 doses of MMR vaccine at the appropriate interval for measles and mumps or 1 dose of MMR vaccine for rubella.

8. **Pneumococcal polysaccharide (PPSV) vaccination**
   - Vaccinate all persons with the following indications:
     - age 65 years and older without a history of PPSV vaccination;
     - adults younger than 65 years with chronic lung disease (including chronic obstructive pulmonary disease, emphysema, and asthma); chronic cardiovascular diseases; diabetes mellitus; chronic renal failure or nephrotic syndrome; chronic liver disease (including cirrhosis); alcoholism; cochlear implants; cerebrospinal fluid leaks; immunocompromising conditions; and functional or anatomic asplenia (e.g., sickle cell disease and other hemoglobinopathies, congenital or acquired asplenia, splenic dysfunction, or splenectomy [if elective splenectomy is planned, vaccinate at least 2 weeks before surgery]);
     - residents of nursing homes or long-term care facilities; and
     - adults who smoke cigarettes.
   - Persons with asymptomatic or symptomatic HIV infection should be vaccinated as soon as possible after their diagnosis.
   - When cancer chemotherapy or other immunosuppressive therapy is being considered, the interval between vaccination and initiation of immunosuppressive therapy should be at least 2 weeks. Vaccination during chemotherapy or radiation therapy should be avoided.
   - Routine use of PPSV is not recommended for American Indians/Alaska Natives or other persons younger than 65 years of age unless they have underlying medical conditions that are PPSV indications. However, public health authorities may consider recommending PPSV for American Indians/Alaska Natives who are living in areas where the risk for invasive pneumococcal disease is increased.

9. **Revaccination with PPSV**
   - One-time revaccination 5 years after the first dose is recommended for persons 19 through 64 years of age with chronic renal failure or nephrotic syndrome; functional or anatomic asplenia (e.g., sickle cell disease or splenectomy); and for persons with immunocompromising conditions.
   - Persons who received PPSV before age 65 years for any indication should receive another dose of the vaccine at age 65 years or later if at least 5 years have passed since their previous dose.
   - No further doses are needed for persons vaccinated with PPSV at or after age 65 years.

10. **Meningococcal vaccination**
    - Administer 2 doses of meningococcal conjugate vaccine quadrivalent (MCV4) at least 2 months apart to adults with functional asplenia or persistent complement component deficiencies.
    - HIV-infected persons who are vaccinated should also receive 2 doses.
    - Administer a single dose of meningococcal vaccine to microbiologists routinely exposed to isolates of Neisseria meningitidis, military recruits, and persons who travel to or live in countries in which meningococcal disease is hyperendemic or epidemic.
    - First-year college students up through age 21 years who are living in residence halls should be vaccinated if they have not received a dose on or after their 16th birthday.
    - MCV4 is preferred for adults with any of the preceding indications who are 55 years and younger; meningococcal polysaccharide vaccine (MPSV4) is preferred for adults 56 years and older.
    - Revaccination with MCV4 every 5 years is recommended for adults previously vaccinated with MCV4 or MPSV4 who remain at increased risk for infection (e.g., adults with anatomic or functional asplenia or persistent complement component deficiencies).

11. **Hepatitis A vaccination**
    - Vaccinate any person seeking protection from hepatitis A virus (HAV) infection and persons with any of the following indications:
      - men who have sex with men and persons who use injection drugs;

laboratory-confirmed case or evidence of laboratory confirmation, if it was performed at the time of acute disease); or

- history of herpes zoster based on diagnosis or verification of herpes zoster by a health-care provider; or

 - laboratory evidence of immunity or laboratory confirmation of disease.

5. Human papillomavirus (HPV) vaccination

- Two vaccines are licensed for use in females, bivalent HPV vaccine (HPV2) and quadrivalent HPV vaccine (HPV4), and one HPV vaccine for use in males (HPV4).

- For females, either HPV4 or HPV2 is recommended in a 3-dose series for routine vaccination at 11 or 12 years of age, and for those 13 through 26 years of age, if not previously vaccinated. For males, either HPV4 is recommended in a 3-dose series for routine vaccination at 11 or 12 years of age, and for those 13 through 21 years of age, if not previously vaccinated. Males 22 through 26 years of age may be vaccinated.

- HPV vaccines are not live vaccines and can be administered to persons who are immunocompromised as a result of infection (including HIV infection), disease, or medications. Vaccine is recommended for immunocompromised persons through age 26 years who did not get any or all doses when they were younger. The immune response and vaccine efficacy might be less than that in immunocompetent persons.

- Men who have sex with men (MSM) might especially benefit from vaccination to prevent condyloma and anal cancer. HPV4 is recommended for MSM through age 26 years who did not get any or all doses when they were younger.

- Ideally, vaccine should be administered before potential exposure to HPV through sexual activity; however, persons who are sexually active should still be vaccinated consistent with age-based recommendations. HPV vaccine can be administered to persons with a history of genital warts, abnormal Papanicolaou test, or positive HPV DNA test.

- A complete series for either HPV4 or HPV2 consists of 3 doses. The second dose should be administered 1–2 months after the first dose; the third dose should be administered 6 months after the first dose (at least 24 weeks after the first dose).

- Although HPV vaccination is not specifically recommended for health-care personnel (HCP) based on their occupation, HCP should receive the HPV vaccine if they are in the recommended age group.

6. Zoster vaccination

- A single dose of zoster vaccine is recommended for adults 60 years of age and older regardless of whether they report a prior episode of herpes zoster. Although the vaccine is licensed by the Food and Drug Administration (FDA) for use among and can be administered to persons 50 years of age and older, ACIP recommends that vaccination begins at 60 years of age.

- Persons with chronic medical conditions may be vaccinated unless their condition constitutes a contraindication, such as pregnancy or severe immunodeficiency.

- Although zoster vaccination is not specifically recommended for health-care personnel (HCP), HCP should receive the vaccine if they are in the recommended age group.

7. Measles, mumps, rubella (MMR) vaccination

Measles component:

- A routine second dose of MMR vaccine, administered a minimum of 28 days after the first dose, is recommended for adults who
 - are students in postsecondary educational institutions;
 - work in a health-care facility; or
 - plan to travel internationally.

- Adults born before 1957 generally are considered immune to measles and mumps. All adults born in 1957 or later should have documentation of 1 or more doses of MMR vaccine unless they have a medical contraindication to the vaccine, laboratory evidence of immunity to each of the three diseases, or documentation of provider-diagnosed measles or mumps disease. For unvaccinated health-care personnel born before 1957 who lack laboratory evidence of measles immunity or laboratory confirmation of disease, health-care facilities should consider vaccinating personnel with 2 doses of MMR vaccine.

Mumps component:

- A routine second dose of MMR vaccine, administered a minimum of 28 days after the first dose, is recommended for adults who
 - are students in postsecondary educational institutions;
 - work in a health-care facility; or
 - plan to travel internationally.

- Persons who received inactivated (killed) mumps vaccine or mumps vaccine of unknown type before 1979 with either killed mumps vaccine or mumps vaccine of unknown type who are at high risk for mumps infection (e.g., persons who are working in a health-care facility) should be considered for revaccination with 2 doses of MMR vaccine.

- persons working with HAV-infected primates or with HAV in a research laboratory setting;

- persons with chronic liver disease and persons who receive clotting factor concentrates;

- persons traveling to or working in countries that have high or intermediate endemicity of hepatitis A; and

- unvaccinated persons who anticipate close personal contact (e.g., household or regular babysitting) with an international adoptee during the first 60 days after arrival in the United States from a country with high or intermediate endemicity. (See footnote 1 for more information on travel recommendations). The first dose of the 2-dose hepatitis A vaccine series should be administered as soon as adoption is planned, ideally 2 or more weeks before the arrival of the adoptee.

Single-antigen vaccine formulations should be administered in a 2-dose schedule at either 0 and 6–12 months (Havrix), or 0 and 6–18 months (Vaqta). If the combined hepatitis A and hepatitis B vaccine (Twinrix) is used, administer 3 doses at 0, 1, and 6 months; alternatively, a 4-dose schedule may be used, administered on days 0, 7, and 21–30 followed by a booster dose at month 12.

12. Hepatitis B vaccination

- Vaccinate persons with any of the following indications and any person seeking protection from hepatitis B virus (HBV) infection:

 - sexually active persons who are not in a long-term, mutually monogamous relationship (e.g., persons with more than one sex partner during the previous 6 months); persons seeking evaluation or treatment for a sexually transmitted disease (STD); current or recent injection-drug users; and men who have sex with men;

 - health-care personnel and public-safety workers who are exposed to blood or other potentially infectious body fluids;

 - persons with diabetes younger than 60 years as soon as feasible after diagnosis; persons with diabetes who are 60 years or older at the discretion of the treating clinician based on increased need for assisted blood glucose monitoring in long-term care facilities, likelihood of acquiring hepatitis B infection, its complications or chronic sequelae, and likelihood of immune response to vaccination;

 - persons with end-stage renal disease, including patients receiving hemodialysis, persons with HIV infection, and persons with chronic liver disease;

 - household contacts and sex partners of persons with chronic HBV infection; clients and staff members of institutions for persons with developmental disabilities; and international travelers to countries with high or intermediate prevalence of chronic HBV infection; and

 - all adults in the following settings: STD treatment facilities; HIV testing and treatment facilities; facilities providing drug-abuse treatment and prevention services; health-care settings targeting services to injection-drug users or men who have sex with men; correctional facilities; end-stage renal disease programs and facilities for chronic hemodialysis patients; and institutions and nonresidential daycare facilities for persons with developmental disabilities.

- Administer missing doses to complete a 3-dose series of hepatitis B vaccine to those persons not vaccinated or not completely vaccinated. The second dose should be administered 1 month after the first dose; the third dose should be given at least 2 months after the second dose (and at least 4 months after the first dose). If the combined hepatitis A and hepatitis B vaccine (Twinrix) is used, give 3 doses at 0, 1, and 6 months; alternatively, a 4-dose Twinrix schedule, administered on days 0, 7, and 21–30 followed by a booster dose at month 12 may be used.

- Adult patients receiving hemodialysis or with other immunocompromising conditions should receive 1 dose of 40 µg/mL (Recombivax HB) administered on a 3-dose schedule at 0, 1, and 6 months or 2 doses of 20 µg/mL (Engerix-B) administered simultaneously on a 4-dose schedule at 0, 1, 2, and 6 months.

13. Selected conditions for which Haemophilus influenzae type b (Hib) vaccine may be used

- 1 dose of Hib vaccine should be considered for persons who have sickle cell disease, leukemia, or HIV infection, or who have anatomic or functional asplenia if they have not previously received Hib vaccine.

14. Immunocompromising conditions

- Inactivated vaccines generally are acceptable (e.g., pneumococcal, meningococcal, and inactivated influenza [inactivated influenza vaccine]) and live vaccines generally are avoided in persons with immune deficiencies or immunocompromising conditions. Information on specific conditions is available at http://www.cdc.gov/vaccines/pubs/acip-list.htm.

PROFESSIONAL SOCIETIES AND GOVERNMENTAL AGENCIES

Abbreviation	Full Name	Internet Address
AACE	American Association of Clinical Endocrinologists	http://www.aace.com
AAD	American Academy of Dermatology	http://www.aad.org
AAFP	American Academy of Family Physicians	http://www.aafp.org
AAHPM	American Academy of Hospice and Palliative Medicine	http://www.aahpm.org
AAN	American Academy of Neurology	http://www.aan.com/professionals
AAO	American Academy of Ophthalmology	http://www.aao.org
AAO-HNS	American Academy of Otolaryngology—Head and Neck Surgery	http://www.entnet.org
AAOS	American Academy of Orthopaedic Surgeons and American Association of Orthopaedic Surgeons	http://www.aaos.org
AAP	American Academy of Pediatrics	http://www.aap.org
ACC	American College of Cardiology	http://www.acc.org
ACCP	American College of Chest Physicians	http://www.chestnet.org
ACIP	Advisory Committee on Immunization Practices	http://www.cdc.gov/vaccines/recs/acip
ACOG	American Congress of Obstetricians and Gynecologists	http://www.acog.com
ACP	American College of Physicians	http://www.acponline.org
ACR	American College of Radiology	http://www.acr.org
ACR	American College of Rheumatology	http://www.rheumatology.org
ACS	American Cancer Society	http://www.cancer.org
ACSM	American College of Sports Medicine	http://www.acsm.org
ADA	American Diabetes Association	http://www.diabetes.org
AGA	American Gastroenterological Association	http://www.gastro.org
AGS	The American Geriatrics Society	http://www.americangeriatrics.org
AHA	American Heart Association	http://www.americanheart.org
ANA	American Nurses Association	http://www.nursingworld.org
AOA	American Optometric Association	http://www.aoa.org
ASA	American Stroke Association	http://www.strokeassociation.org
ASAM	American Society of Addiction Medicine	http://www.asam.org

PROFESSIONAL SOCIETIES AND GOVERNMENTAL AGENCIES (CONTINUED)		
Abbreviation	**Full Name**	**Internet Address**
ASCCP	American Society for Colposcopy and Cervical Pathology	http://www.asccp.org
ASCO	American Society of Clinical Oncology	http://www.asco.org
ASCRS	American Society of Colon and Rectal Surgeons	http://www.fascrs.org
ASGE	American Society for Gastrointestinal Endoscopy	http://asge.org
ASHA	American Speech-Language-Hearing Association	http://www.asha.org
ASN	American Society of Neuroimaging	http://www.asnweb.org
ATA	American Thyroid Association	http://www.thyroid.org
ATS	American Thoracic Society	http://www.thoracic.org
AUA	American Urological Association	http://auanet.org
BASHH	British Association for Sexual Health and HIV	http://www.bashh.org
	Bright Futures	http://brightfutures.org
BGS	British Geriatrics Society	http://www.bgs.org.uk/
BSAC	British Society for Antimicrobial Chemotherapy	http://www.bsac.org.uk
CDC	Centers for Disease Control and Prevention	http://www.cdc.gov
COG	Children's Oncology Group	http://www.childrensoncologygroup.org
CSVS	Canadian Society for Vascular Surgery	http://csvs.vascularweb.org
CTF	Canadian Task Force on Preventive Health Care	http://www.ctfphc.org
EASD	European Association for the Study of Diabetes	http://www.easd.org
EAU	European Association of Urology	http://www.uroweb.org
ERS	European Respiratory Society	http://ersnet.org
ESC	European Society of Cardiology	http://www.escardio.org
ESCDPCP	European and Other Societies on Cardiovascular Disease Prevention in Clinical Practice	http://www.escardio.org
ESH	European Society of Hypertension	http://www.eshonline.org

PROFESSIONAL SOCIETIES AND GOVERNMENTAL AGENCIES (CONTINUED)		
Abbreviation	**Full Name**	**Internet Address**
IARC	International Agency for Research on Cancer	http://screening.iarc.fr
ICSI	Institute for Clinical Systems Improvement	http://www.icsi.org
IDF	International Diabetes Federation	http://www.idf.org
NAPNAP	National Association of Pediatric Nurse Practitioners	http://www.napnap.org
NCCN	National Comprehensive Cancer Network	http://www.nccn.org/cancer-guidelines.html
NCI	National Cancer Institute	http://www.cancer.gov/cancerinformation
NEI	National Eye Institute	http://www.nei.nih.gov
NGC	National Guideline Clearinghouse	http://www.guidelines.gov
NHLBI	National Heart, Lung, and Blood Institute	http://www.nhlbi.nih.gov
NIAAA	National Institute on Alcohol Abuse and Alcoholism	http://www.niaaa.nih.gov
NICE	National Institute for Health and Clinical Excellence	http://www.nice.org.uk
NIDCR	National Institute of Dental and Craniofacial Research	http://www.nidr.nih.gov
NIHCDC	National Institutes of Health Consensus Development Program	http://www.consensus.nih.gov
NIP	National Immunization Program	http://www.cdc.gov/nip
NKF	National Kidney Foundation	http://www.kidney.org
NOF	National Osteoporosis Foundation	http://www.nof.org
NTSB	National Transportation Safety Board	http://www.ntsb.gov
SCF	Skin Cancer Foundation	http://www.skincancer.org
SGIM	Society of General Internal Medicine	http://www.sgim.org
SKI	Sloan-Kettering Institute	http://www.mskcc.org/mskcc/html/5804.cfm
SVU	Society for Vascular Ultrasound	http://www.svunet.org
UK-NHS	United Kingdom National Health Service	http://www.nhs.uk
USPSTF	United States Preventive Services Task Force	http://www.ahrq.gov/clinic/uspstfix.htm
WHO	World Health Organization	http://www.who.int/en

Index